Nanotechnology in Drug Delivery: Design and Applications

Nanotechnology in Drug Delivery: Design and Applications

Editor: Miranda Cowan

AMERICAN
MEDICAL PUBLISHERS
www.americanmedicalpublishers.com

AMERICAN MEDICAL PUBLISHERS
www.americanmedicalpublishers.com

Cataloging-in-Publication Data

Nanotechnology in drug delivery : design and applications / edited by Miranda Cowan.
p. cm.
Includes bibliographical references and index.
ISBN 979-8-88740-292-5
1. Drug delivery systems. 2. Nanotechnology. 3. Nanoparticles. 4. Drugs--Design.
5. Pharmaceutical technology. 6. Pharmaceutical biotechnology. I. Cowan, Miranda.
RS199.5 .N363 2023
615.6--dc23

American Medical Publishers,
41 Flatbush Avenue,
1st Floor, New York,
NY 11217, USA

ISBN 979-8-88740-292-5 (Hardback)

Contents

Preface

Nanotechnology is a science and engineering discipline that deals with designing, producing, and using structures, devices and systems by manipulating atoms and molecules at the nanoscale. There are several applications of nanotechnology in various sectors, including information technology, security, medicine, transportation, energy, food safety and environmental science. The major objective of the application of nanotechnology in drug delivery is to improve treatments with targeted delivery and fewer side effects. It is generally performed through the usage of designed nanomaterials, as well as forming delivery systems from nanoscale molecules like liposomes. There are various advantages of applying nanotechnology in drug delivery systems, such as providing site-specific targeting in order to reduce the accumulation of drug within healthy tissue. Furthermore, it facilitates effective treatment by retaining the drug for a sufficient time in the body. This book explores the design and applications of nanotechnology in drug delivery systems. The various studies that are constantly contributing towards advancing technologies and evolution of this field are examined in detail. This book will help new researchers by foregrounding their knowledge in this branch of science.

Various studies have approached the subject by analyzing it with a single perspective, but the present book provides diverse methodologies and techniques to address this field. This book contains theories and applications needed for understanding the subject from different perspectives. The aim is to keep the readers informed about the progresses in the field; therefore, the contributions were carefully examined to compile novel researches by specialists from across the globe.

Indeed, the job of the editor is the most crucial and challenging in compiling all chapters into a single book. In the end, I would extend my sincere thanks to the chapter authors for their profound work. I am also thankful for the support provided by my family and colleagues during the compilation of this book.

Editor

1

Nano Carrier Drug Delivery Systems for the Treatment of Neuropsychiatric Disorders: Advantages and Limitations

Yana Zorkina [1,2,*], Olga Abramova [1], Valeriya Ushakova [1,3], Anna Morozova [1,2], Eugene Zubkov [1], Marat Valikhov [1], Pavel Melnikov [1], Alexander Majouga [4] and Vladimir Chekhonin [1,5]

1. Department Basic and Applied Neurobiology, V.P. Serbsky Federal Medical Research Centre of Psychiatry and Narcology, 119034 Moscow, Russia; abramova1128@gmail.com (O.A.); ushakovavm@yandex.ru (V.U.); hakurate77@gmail.com (A.M.); zubkov@ngs.ru (E.Z.); marat.valikhov@gmail.com (M.V.); proximopm@gmail.com (P.M.); chekhoninnew@yandex.ru (V.C.)
2. Healthcare Department, Mental-Health Clinic No. 1 Named after N.A. Alexeev of Moscow, 117152 Moscow, Russia
3. Department of Biology, Lomonosov Moscow State University, 119992 Moscow, Russia
4. D. Mendeleev University of Chemical Technology of Russia, 125047 Moscow, Russia; rector@muctr.ru
5. Department of Medical Nanobiotechnology, Pirogov Russian National Research Medical University, 117997 Moscow, Russia

* Correspondence: zorkina.ya@serbsky.ru;

Abstract: Neuropsychiatric diseases are one of the main causes of disability, affecting millions of people. Various drugs are used for its treatment, although no effective therapy has been found yet. The blood brain barrier (BBB) significantly complicates drugs delivery to the target cells in the brain tissues. One of the problem-solving methods is the usage of nanocontainer systems. In this review we summarized the data about nanoparticles drug delivery systems and their application for the treatment of neuropsychiatric disorders. Firstly, we described and characterized types of nanocarriers: inorganic nanoparticles, polymeric and lipid nanocarriers, their advantages and disadvantages. We discussed ways to interact with nerve tissue and methods of BBB penetration. We provided a summary of nanotechnology-based pharmacotherapy of schizophrenia, bipolar disorder, depression, anxiety disorder and Alzheimer's disease, where development of nanocontainer drugs derives the most active. We described various experimental drugs for the treatment of Alzheimer's disease that include vector nanocontainers targeted on β-amyloid or tau-protein. Integrally, nanoparticles can substantially improve the drug delivery as its implication can increase BBB permeability, the pharmacodynamics and bioavailability of applied drugs. Thus, nanotechnology is anticipated to overcome the limitations of existing pharmacotherapy of psychiatric disorders and to effectively combine various treatment modalities in that direction.

Keywords: nanocarriers; schizophrenia; bipolar disorder; depression; anxiety; Alzheimer's disease; BBB

---

1. Introduction

According to statistics, one in four people in the world afflicts with various mental or neurological illnesses at some point of their lives. Around 450 million people currently suffer from such conditions, placing mental disorders among the leading causes of ill and disability worldwide [1].

There is a great clinical need for development a new-generation of psychoactive drugs, because the global burden of mental illness continues to increase. Despite the wide range of existing drugs with psychotropic and neurotropic activity, there has been no significant success in treating mental illness. This may be because it takes time to achieve an effective concentration of drugs, with which side effects are associated. This, in turn, forces clinicians to change their treatment methods frequently.

Preparations in their usual form (pills or injections) have many obstacles in their way to achieve the desired effect. These include poor bioavailability, low absorption (food effect), first-pass metabolism, drug toxicity and dose-dependent side effects.

The concept of nanotherapy includes systems with sizes of 10–100 nm and unique physiological and chemical properties. Nanopreparations are distinguished by their plasticity and modified surface properties, flexibility and controlled release of the active drug substance. Nanotherapeutics provide targeted delivery of central nervous system (CNS) active drugs to the brain [2], which is essential for drugs aimed at treating mental illness. An example of such preparations is biodegradable, biocompatible polymers, which are non-immunogenic and non-toxic to cells. Their increased solubility and targeted delivery result in an increased concentration of drugs in cells and tissues, thereby increasing the bioavailability of drug molecules. Therefore, nanoparticles (NPs) application demonstrates a variety of advantages in comparison with other methods of drug administration as intranasal, transdermal, oral and intravenous administration (Table 1).

Table 1. Advantages of nanoparticles (NPs) administration (adm.) compared to other methods of drug delivery for CNS treatment.

Property	NPs	Intranasal Adm.	Transdermal Adm.	Oral Adm.	Intravenous Adm.
Controlled release	Available	Not available	Available	Not available	Not available
BBB penetration	• Does not depend on the properties of drug • Target ligands • Transcytosis, endocytosis and exocytosis and others.	• Does not depend on the properties of drug • Direct transport	Depends on the properties of drug	Depends on the properties of drug	Depends on the properties of drug
Ability to targeted delivery	High	Not available	Not available	Not available	Not available
Bioavailability	High	High	Poor	Poor	Poor
Hepatic first-pass metabolism	Prevent	Prevent	Prevent	Not prevent	Not prevent
Toxicity	Less pronounced side effects because of lower concentrations of therapeutic drugs and more stable release characteristics.	Less pronounced side effects because of lower concentrations of therapeutic drugs and direct transport through BBB.	Less pronounced side effects because of lower concentrations of therapeutic drugs and more stable release characteristic	High chance and dose-depended side effects	High chance and dose-depended side effects

Currently, various types of nanotherapy for mental disorders, including polymeric nanoparticles, solid lipid nanoparticles (SLN), nanostructured lipid carriers (NLC), nanoemulsions, nanogels, carbon nanotubes and liquid crystalline nanoparticles with neuroprotective properties [3] are being investigated.

In our review we will present current data on promising areas of nanotherapy in the field of mental and neurodegenerative illnesses, such as schizophrenia, bipolar disorder, depression, anxiety and Alzheimer's disease.

2. Drug Transport through the Blood Brain Barrier

Despite significant progress in understanding the molecular and cellular mechanisms of brain disorders and the development of strategies for their treatment, efficient drug delivery to the central nervous system is an important problem today [4]. One of the most significant barriers in the central nervous system that interferes with drug delivery compounds is the blood brain barrier (BBB). Its functions include not only transporting nutrients and oxygen to the brain from the bloodstream, but also protection of the CNS from neurotoxic substances [5]. The BBB consists of several types of cells such as: endothelial cells, astrocytes, perivascular macrophages and pericytes [6]. The impermeability of the BBB for many molecules is due to the tight contacts between endothelial cells, which in turn form the proteins occludins, claudins and adhesion molecules [7]. Together with tight junctions of endothelial cells, a specialized extracellular matrix and a basement membrane from collagen IV type, laminin, fibronectin, tenascin and proteoglycans provide controlled BBB permeability [8]. The most studied pathways of substances through the BBB are the so-called passive or transcellular diffusion, facilitated diffusion and active transport. Transcellular transport of substances occurs through active and passive diffusion. In the case of active transport in the transfer of molecules, there are three types of transport systems in the BBB: receptor-mediated transport, which carries out the transfer of macromolecules; carrier proteins that transport sugars, amino acids, organic anions and cations, neurotransmitters and metabolites; active transport by proteins of the adenosine triphosphate binding cassette family [9]. Proteins of the adenosine triphosphate binding cassette family, such as P-glycoprotein, make the BBB impermeable to drugs [10].

One of the key problems today is the development of drugs for the treatment of CNS diseases, which will pass through the BBB. For effective therapeutic response the necessary concentration of the drug should accumulate in the right body region and remain maintained enough time to achieve that response. In other organs and tissues, the drug concentration has to stay minimal for side effects reduction. In that case, the presence of BBB significantly complicates the delivery of drugs into brain tissue.

To solve that problem, many methods have been developed to date, such as: violation of the integrity of tight contacts using hypertonic solutions (arabinose and mannitol) [11]; vasoactive drugs (leukotriene C4, IL-2, TNF-α, IFN-γ and bradykinin) [12] and directed ultrasound [13].

Other methods of overcoming the BBB are direct injection of drugs into the brain tissue. In these techniques, it is possible to distinguish intrathecal or intraventricular administration of drugs for direct delivery into the cerebrospinal fluid, intranasal administration and administration of biodegradable substances [14].

High concentrations of drugs in the brain can be achieved by intrathecal administration. Compared to systemic administration, this method allows the use of low doses of drugs and does not require changes in the integrity of BBB. However, this is an invasive strategy and can lead to increased intracranial pressure and neurotoxicity [15].

Intranasal delivery is another method of direct transport of a therapeutic agent for treating various diseases and CNS disorders. This method is based on the connection between the olfactory nasal lining mucosa and the circulation of cerebrospinal fluid next to the olfactory bulbs [16]. Intranasal delivery of pharmaceuticals is a non-invasive, safe and promising method of treatment.

One of the promising methods to overcome BBB is the loading of drugs into nanocontainers that are characterized by relatively small size and ability to cross the BBB. Using this method of drug delivery significantly increases substances bioavailability and reduces the side effects.

The mechanisms of NPs transportation through BBB can be classified into tree main types [17]:

- Transient opening of BBB is induced by a stimulus derived from bioactive components on the surface of nanoparticles, or by a stimulus derived from the "nanoeffects" or "nanotoxicity" of nanoparticles. This opening promotes the diffusion of drug conjugates into brain tissue;
- The adsorption of nanocarrier conjugates on the surface of capillary endothelium cells facilitates the release of the drug from carriers on the cell surface. This process increases the concentration gradient of the drug and promotes the diffusion of substances into the brain;
- Transcytosis, endocytosis and exocytosis of nanocarriers by capillary endothelial cells of the brain provides direct penetration of the substances into brain tissue.

Figure 1 describes the main pathways of nanoparticles entering the brain: mechanisms for BBB penetration and transport across the cell membrane.

Basically, there are three main mechanisms of NPs cellular uptake [18]. The first one is pinocytosis, which is divided into macro- and micropinocytosis, depending on the nanocarrier size and the type of targeted cell. Another method of nanotherapeutics uptake is clathrin-mediated endocytosis or receptor-mediated endocytosis [18]. This process is based on the formation of clathrin-coated endocytic vesicles. The third way to load NPs into cells is caveolae-dependent endocytosis with calveolar vesicles generation. This type of endocytosis is commonly found in endothelial and muscle cells [18].

In the brain different types of neural cells, including neurons, astrocytes, oligodendrocytes and microglia can represent a target for drug delivery. Targeting ability of nanotherapeutic agents depends on NPs functionality and sometimes requires the presence of specific molecules. Neuron-specific delivery is rather difficult because neurons have a non-phagocytic nature in comparison to glial cells. In some studies, neuron-specific targeting was achieved by the properties of connecting ability of loaded substances. To enhance the neuronal targeting, active strategies such as utilizing ligands with dopamine [19], and rabies virus glycoprotein peptide (RVG and RDP peptide) [20] have being used. Receptor-mediated endocytosis strategies are commonly used to induce neuron uptake of NPs. For example, nanocarriers coated with apolipoprotein E can be uptaken by neurons through the agency of the lipoprotein-binding receptors on neurons surface [21].

Astrocytes are also very promising targets for nanomedicine. Commonly NPs can be transported into astrocytes via phagocytosis. Their targeting can affect the neurotransmitters release (e.g., glutamate, γ-aminobutyric acid, glycine and histamine), which is crucial for the maintenance of neuronal excitability [22].

Oligodendrocytes are specialized neural cells, where their role is to myelinate the axons in CNS. Properties of their surface can simplify drug delivery via nanopreparations. In particular, NG-2 chondroitin sulphate proteoglycans are expressed on oligodendrocyte precursor cells, which represent useful targets for specific NPs like poly(lactic-co-glycolic acid (PLGA). Such nanocarriers loaded with leukemia inhibitory factor can increase myelin repair [23].

Targeting of microglia or macrophages is also a promising direction for nanomedicine. It is known, that clathrin-mediated endocytosis serves as the major pathway for microglia to uptake NPs. NPs with a larger surface area demonstrate higher uptake efficiency, because clathrin-mediated endocytosis is carried out by the binding of clathrin receptor with the surface of nanocarriers. This property was manifested by the experiments demonstrated that gold NPs with "urchin-mimicking" geometry were absorbed more effectively by microglial cells compared to spherical and rod-like gold NPs [24]. In addition to clathrin-mediated endocytosis, mannose receptors and macrophage scavenger receptors have also been implicated in playing a role in nanocarriers uptake in non-activated microglia [25,26]. There are two main ways to affect microglia or macrophages with nanotherapy. The first one allows controlling microglia/macrophages population by inhibition of infiltrating monocytes/macrophages. For these reason cytotoxic drugs, such as clodronate, glucocorticoids, doxorubicin and methotrexate are usually applied. For example, it was demonstrated that locally delivered methylprednisolone encapsulated into PLGA nanoparticles dramatically reduced the number of macrophages/reactive microglia [27]. The second way to modulate glial cells functions is the use of control release of cytokines via NPs.

Therefore, various research groups are developing nanocontainer systems for drug delivery. There are several types of using nanoparticles with different advantages and disadvantages. In the following we will consider the types of nanoparticles and their way of penetration through BBB, which is necessary for the treatment of neuropsychiatric disorders.

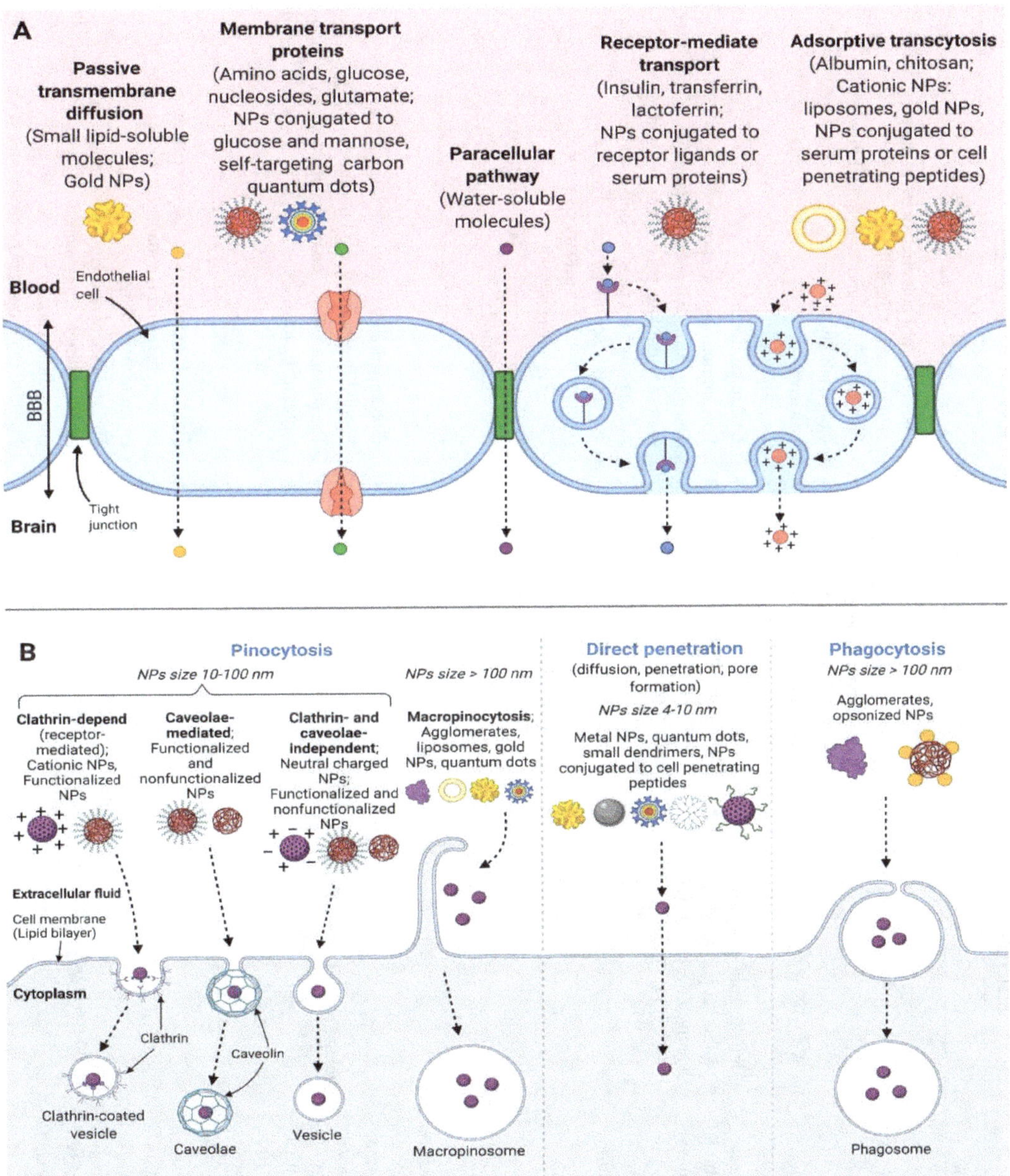

Figure 1. The main pathways of nanoparticles entering the brain. (**A**) The main mechanisms for blood brain barrier (BBB) penetration. (**B**) The mechanisms of nanoparticle transport across the cell membrane. BBB—blood-brain barrier; NPs—nanoparticles.

3. Categories of Nanocarriers

Currently the spectrum of nanoparticles used for targeted drug delivery is quite wide. Such nanocontainers can be divided into three main groups: polymeric nanoparticles (NPs), lipid-based NPs and inorganic NPs (Table 2).

Table 2. Various categories of nanocarriers.

Nanocarrier	Description	Materials	BBB Penetration	Advantages	Disadvantages	References
Polymer-Based Nanocarrier Systems						
Polymeric NPs	The colloidal carriers are obtained from biodegradable and biocompatible natural or synthetic polymers into which drugs are loaded in either solid-state or solution.	Alginate, chitosan, gelatin, cellulose, polyacrylate, polyanhydride, PLGA, PACA, PCL, PEI, PLA, PEG.	• The NPs are permeated the BBB through the tight junctions. The NPs are retained in the brain blood capillaries and are adsorbed of the NPs to the capillary walls. • Endocytosis by the endothelial cells. • Transcytosis. • The inhibition of the efflux system by using polysorbate 80 as the coating agent. • The surface functionalization with targeting ligands.	• The significant potential for brain drug delivery across the BBB. • Biocompatibility and biodegradability • Good stability. • Low cost. • Less toxicity. • Ease in production. • Low immunogenic response. • The mucoadhesive polymers (alginate, chitosan, cellulose, gelatin) can be used intranasally to bypass the BBB. Can be used as gelling/viscosity building agents to conquer nasal mucociliary clearance. • Controlled drug release. • The surface groups can be conjugated with targeting ligands.	• Uncertain potential toxicity. • Slow degradability.	[28–33]
Polymeric micelles	The core–shell structure from amphiphilic blocks copolymers that aggregate in aqueous solutions to form spheroidal NPs with a hydrophobic core and hydrophilic surface.	PEG, PLGA, cholesterol conjugated polyoxyethylene sorbitol oleate.	The surface functionalization with targeting ligands.	• Biocompatibility. • Possibility of solubilizing lipophilic drugs. • The surface groups can be conjugated with targeting ligands.	The efficiency delivering across the intact BBB still needs further investigation.	[17]
Dendrimers	The monodisperse symmetric molecules that comprise a series of branching units around an inner core, which have a spheroidal shape and radially crowded layers.	Poly(amido amide) (PAMAM)	The internalization by brain capillary endothelial cells through a clathrin- and caveolane-mediated energy-depending endocytosis, also partly through macropinocytosis.	• The core is loosely packed in comparison to the periphery and is suitable for the entrapment of drugs. • The presence of numerous surface groups allows for high drug payload and multifunctionality. • The surface groups can be conjugated with targeting ligands.	Potential toxicity.	[17,30–32]

Table 2. *Cont.*

Nanocarrier	Description	Materials	BBB Penetration	Advantages	Disadvantages	References
			Lipid-Based Nanocarrier System			
				Less or no toxicity, biodegradability, and ability to successfully deliver biomolecules, DNA, RNA, genes, antibodies, etc.		
Liposomes	The spherical vesicles with different sizes (20 nm to 100 μm), with an aqueous inner core enclosed by unilamellar or multilamellar phospholipid bilayers. Liposomes may have different surface charges and uni-, bi- or multi-lamellar structures.	Sphingomyelin, phosphatidyl choline, glycerophospholipids, cholesterol, phosphatidylcholine, cardiolipin.	• Receptor-mediated and adsorption-mediated endocytosis (for small liposomes with a diameter not larger than 100 nm) • The surface functionalization with targeting ligands • Cationization of the conjugated ligands is another method to improve BBB transport rate of liposomes. • Interactions of liposomes with cells can be realized by: adsorption, fusion, endocytosis, and lipid transfer.	• Good biocompatibility. • Non-toxic. • Widely investigated. • Encapsulate both hydrophilic and lipophilic drugs. • Increase the solubility of drugs. • Improve pharmacokinetic properties and protect the drugs from enzymatic degradation. • Reduction of harmful side effects of drugs. • Improving therapeutic effectiveness of drugs.	• Opsonization and rapid clearance by macrophages of the mononuclear phagocytic system organs. This can be fixed by using surface coatings, such as PEG. • Low drug transport rate. • Poor stability. • Difficulty of binding ligands to the surface as a result of the small number of available surface groups and steric hindrance.	[28–30,32,33]
Solid lipid NPs	Nano-sized dispersions of biocompatible lipids	The lipid core consists of triglycerides, diglycerides, monoglycerides, fatty acids, steroids, stearic acid or waxes stabilized by various surfactants	• The surface functionalization with targeting ligands • Can be used intranasally to bypass the BBB. The use of cationic lipids can improve mucoadhesion in the nasal cavity by promoting electrostatic interactions with mucus. • Endocytosis by the endothelial cells. • Adsorptive-mediated transcytosis of cationic NPs.	• Good physical stability • The capability to deliver lipophilic drugs dispersed in the hydrophobic core into cells. • Improves bioavailability of drugs. • Increases drug loading ability. • Controlled drug release. • Reduced cytotoxicity of drugs. • Reduces the RES uptake, increases the retention and circulation time and protect drugs from degradation. • The surface groups can be conjugated with targeting ligands.	• Easy clearance by the reticuloendothelial system • Low loading capacity • Drug expulsion after crystallization Relatively high water content of the dispersions.	[29,30,33]

Table 2. *Cont.*

Nanocarrier	Description	Materials	BBB Penetration	Advantages	Disadvantages	References
Nanoemulsions	Colloidal droplet system of oil-in-water (O/W) or water-in-oil (W/O) formulations stabilized with surface-active agents Oil droplet size of nanoemulsions ranges from 10 to 100 nm, making them interesting systems to improve drug delivery	Edible oils, such as flaxseed oil, pine-nut oil, hemp oil, fish oil as well as safflower oil and wheat-germ oil, biocompatible surfactants such as egg phosphatidylcholine which is one of the components of cell membrane lipids, deoxycholic acid, stearylamine, dioleoyltrimethyl ammonium propane.	• The surface functionalization with targeting ligands • Receptor-mediated endocytosis of cells	• Biocompatibility. • The ability to solubilize hydrophobic or hydrophilic drugs. • Improves the bioavailability of the drug. • The surface groups can be conjugated with targeting ligands.	• Thermodynamic instability. • Instability upon storage. • Immediate drug release.	[17,32,33]
Inorganic Nanoparticles						
Mesoporous Silica NPs	Silica xerogels and mesoporous silica nanoparticles	*N*-Cetyltrimethylammonium bromide, Tetraethoxysilane	Transcytosis of vascular endothelial cells (PEGylated NPs)	• Good biocompatibility. • Stability. • Highly porous framework. • High drug loading efficiency. • Controlled drug release.	• Potential toxicity and adverse effect showed by recent studies • Contribute to the level increase of reactive oxygen species • Can induce the elevated production of malondialdehyde and decreased glutathione level	[30,34]
Gold NPs			• Adsorption-mediated endocytosis • Diffusion	• Can easily penetrate cells because of their small size, high efficiency in cellular uptake. • Easy conjugation to biomolecules. • Can be easy functionalized by surface modification (small size, large surface area and pore volume, high reactivity).	Drug delivery efficiency needs further investigation.	[34]

Table 2. *Cont.*

Nanocarrier	Description	Materials	BBB Penetration	Advantages	Disadvantages	References
Carbon nanotubes	Graphitic sheets rolled into single-walled or multiple walled tubes with an enormous surface area	Graphitic sheets	• The surface functionalization with targeting ligands. • PEG-modified carbon nanotubes also exhibited the capability of crossing the BBB.	• Biocompatibility. • Efficient loading of multiple molecules.	• Potential toxicity. • Drug delivery efficiency needs further investigation. • Contribute to the level increase of reactive oxygen species. • Similarity in carcinogenic potential between carbon nanotubes and asbestos. • Can cause necrosis or apoptosis of macrophage cell lines and changes in cell morphology. • Can induce proinflammatory response. • Cannot be functionally integrated into the biological systems unless surface functionalization.	[30]
Iron oxide NPs	Iron oxide nanoparticles, which are also known as super paramagnetic nanoparticles	Iron oxide	Ability to cross the blood-brain barrier. Mechanisms of internalization and overall biodistribution are closely associated with their surface chemistry and hydrodynamic sizes.	• Easy biodegradable (degraded iron can be absorbed by hemoglobin). • Non-toxicity. • Chemical stability in physiological conditions. • Can be visualized by magnetic resonance imaging and it can be used for MR-imaging. • Generate heat after exposure to an alternating magnetic field and can be used for magnetic hyperthermia and temperature-triggered drug release • The possibility of using passive and active drug delivery strategies. • Possibility of chemical modification by coating the iron oxide cores with various shells.	Tend to aggregate into larger clusters.	[17,30,31,34]

PLGA—polylactic acid-co-glycolic acid, PACA—poly (alkyl cyanoacrylate), PCL—polycaprolactone, PEI, polyethyleneimine, PLA—poly(lactic acid), PEG—poly(ethylene glycol), RES—reticular endothelial system.

3.1. Polymeric Nanoparticles

This class includes polymer-based nanoparticles and micelles and dendrimers (Table 2).

Nanoparticles based on polylactide acid (PLA) and poly (lactic-co-glycolic acid) (PLGA) developed over several decades have proved to be a promising alternative system for delivering drugs to the brain, primarily due to their high biocompatibility and low toxicity. They have uncomplicated synthesis methods (emulsification, evaporation, solvent replacement method (deposition), solvent diffusion method, etc.) and are metabolized into lactic and glycolic acids using a simple mechanism. So, they are biodegradable, with optimal sizes ranging from 100 to 200 nm. PLGA/PLA nanoparticles are U.S. Food and Drug Administration (FDA) certified and can be used in implants, biodegradable scaffolds and human medicines.

The therapeutic molecules encapsulated in polymer nanoparticles can form the following thermodynamically stable structures, depending on the loading method. Either they are nanospheres where the drug is loaded across the entire polymer matrix or only on its surface, or they are nanocapsules where the active substance is surrounded by a polymer shell.

The surface of such particles is easily modifiable, both with ligands for target delivery and molecules that promote adsorption on target cells. Thus, using the example of the anticonvulsant Clonazepam contained in the PLGA matrix, it was possible to achieve effective delivery of the drug through BBB by conjugating the poloxamer-188 to the surface of the NP [35]. Conclusion in PLGA nanocarriers curcumin solved the problem of its insolubility in water, and conjugation with Tet-1 made it possible to increase nanoparticles capture in the treatment of Alzheimer's disease (AD) [36].

Polymer nanoparticles penetrate the BBB through endocytosis. They can also avoid the phagocytosis of the reticular endothelial system, thereby increasing the concentration of drugs in the brain [37]. In vitro studies have shown that the use of polymer nanoparticles increases the delivery of drugs to the brain. For example, improved delivery of curcumin (in the treatment of AD) is more effective in reducing oxidative stress, inflammation and plaque load.

3.1.1. Dendrimers

Dendrimers are monodisperse symmetrical macromolecules consisting of a series of branched blocks around the inner nucleus. The spherical structure of dendrimers consists of the core, layers of branched, repeating blocks coming out of the core and functional end groups on the outer layer [17].

In the treatment of brain diseases, polyamidoamine dendrimers are most commonly used among dendrimers. For example, there is a study on the use of encapsulated carbamazepine (an antiepileptic drug) for the treatment of AD [38].

3.1.2. Micelles

Micelles consist of amphiphilic block copolymers. They aggregate in aqueous solutions to form stable spheroidal nanostructures that have a hydrophobic core and hydrophilic surface.

The micelles are promising agents for delivering drugs to the brain. This is made possible by the dissolution of poorly soluble substances in the hydrophobic nucleus area and the ability to conjugate with certain target ligands [17].

3.2. Lipid-Based NPs

This type of nanoparticles includes liposomes, solid lipid nanoparticles, nanoemulsions and exosomes (Table 2).

3.2.1. Liposomes

Liposomes are the family of nanostructures, the main characteristic of which is a spherical shape and lipid bilayer. Optimal sizes range from 100 to 200 nm. The first FDA approved nanodrug in 1995 was Doxil represented a preparation based on liposomes [39]. Over the next 2 decades all types of liposome forms, methods of construction and modifications have been developed [40]. For example, liposomal nanoparticles produced by microfluidics were constructed. These nanocarriers allow increasing the percentage of drug loading and obtaining a balanced size of nanocontainer [41]. Generally, liposomes are characterized by the high biocompatibility, biodegradability, improved bioavailability and stability of therapeutic agents [42]. Moreover, they are able to modify the surfaces for active targeting [43]. Nanoparticles structure allows the incorporation of auxiliary lipids such as dioleylphosphatidylethanolamine (DOPE) or cholesterol. DOPE is able to conjugate with other lipids when exposed to low pH, which promotes increased efficiency of loading into cytosol and favor endosomes construction [44]. Cholesterol provides structural stability. The linkers are sensitive to different biological stimuli and contribute to the release of the drug under certain conditions. For example, modifications of gold nanoshells liposomes mediating by chitosan can provide liver protection [45]. Opsonization and capture by macrophages of the organs of the mononuclear phagocytic system obstructs the delivery of drugs via unmodified liposomes. Modification with polyethylene glycol (PEG) increases nanoparticles circulation time and reduces cell capture [17].

The using of liposomal constructions for BBB crossing has been investigated for decades [43]. Liposomes are modified for targeting transcytosis through CNS endothelium via the liposomal surface functionalization with biologically active ligands, such as peptides, antibodies or small molecules. G-Technology® (FDA approved technology) is another method for transformation of the liposomal surface. It represents a strategy for using glutathione-PEGylated liposomes, which are able to bind with glutathione transporter [46].

Thus, liposomes are promising candidates for BBB penetration and targeting delivery of therapeutic agents.

3.2.2. Solid Lipid Nanoparticles

Unlike liposomes, this type of nanoparticles does not possess a lipid layer, but is characterized by the presence of a solid lipid core matrix that can encapsulate lipophilic molecules. Solid lipid nanoparticles (SLNs) are nanoscale suspensions of biologically compatible lipids such as triglycerides, fatty acids or waxes stabilized by bioactive substances possessing a hydrophile-lipophile balance [17].

Such nanoparticles are also subjected to surface modification, which significantly increases the efficiency of drug transporting through BBB [47]. As containers for drug delivery, they demonstrate a high level of biocompatibility, biodegradability and the ability to transform the surface with target bioactive molecules. However, their hydrophobicity promotes easier clearance by the reticuloendothelial system (RES), which alleviates nanoparticles effectiveness.

3.2.3. Nanoemulsion

Nanoemulsions are heterogeneous dispersions of the composition "oil in water" (O/W) or "water in oil" (W/O), stabilized by surfactants. The diameter of the internal phase in such nanosystems is reduced to a nanometric scale. Due to their properties, nanoemulsions demonstrate the ability to carrier both hydrophobic (O/W) or hydrophilic (W/O) drugs. The surface of these nanoparticles can also be modified with bioactive ligands. Delivery of drugs via nanoemulsions is carried out through receptor-mediated endocytosis of cells.

Compared to other nanocarriers, the preponderance of nanoemulsions for BBB penetration is the ability to use safe oils. In addition, the application of this type of nanoparticles possesses a number of useful biological properties due to the presence of essential omega-3 and omega-6 fatty acids in the oils [17].

3.3. Inorganic NPs

Inorganic nanoparticles represent solid nanosize objects consisting of inorganic materials such as silicon dioxide, carbon nanotubes, metal or metal oxide. This type of nanoparticles is widely used for visualization research, including neuroimaging.

To facilitate penetration through BBB, they are covered with several polymers such as polysaccharides, polyacrylamide, poly(vinyl alcohol), poly(*N*-vinyl-2-pyrrolidone), PEG and PEG-containing copolymers. The most commonly used covering polymer is PEG. These surface modifications enhance nanoparticles stability, improve water solubility and allow modifying of the particle surface with vector molecules [48]. In addition, such PEGylation of nanocontainers averts the capture of particles by the RES and prevents non-specific interactions with opsonin proteins [49].

Besides PEG covering inorganic nanoparticles are also modified with lactoferrin (Lf). It is interesting that this conjunction demonstrated better efficiency during BBB penetration than PEG because of Lf-receptor-mediated transcytosis of cerebral endothelial cells [50].

In addition to chemical modification, the physical properties of inorganic nanoparticles can also be changed for an increase of penetration through BBB. For example, Fe_3O_4 nanoparticles demonstrate the ability to be magnetized in the presence of a magnetic field. It has been shown that superparamagnetic iron oxide nanoparticles (SPIONs) contained magnetite (Fe_3O_4) and maghemite (c-Fe_2O_3) can cross human brain microvascular endothelial cells via an external magnet pressure. Therefore, this mechanism demonstrates the ability of BBB penetration and targeted drug delivery to the brain to be carried out by the magnetic force-mediated dragging of SPIONs through the BBB. Such property of iron oxide nanoparticles as magnetism can be applied for diagnostics and simultaneous therapy of neurodegenerative diseases [51]. Along with iron nanocarriers gold nanoparticles can also penetrate through BBB and can be administered for therapy of neuropsychiatric diseases [52].

Nevertheless, despite the advantages of these types of nanoparticles, they exhibit potential toxicity due to their nondegradability. For this reason, their application requires further research.

4. Drug Delivery for Depression

Depression is a widespread disorder, affecting almost 350 million people worldwide [53]. Depressive symptoms influence quality of life of patients and aggravate the course of comorbid diseases. Depression pathogenesis affects various neurobiological processes including HPA axis activity, monoamine systems functioning, neurogenesis, neuroinflammation, etc. [54]. Traditional medications for the treatment of depression are antidepressants with different mechanisms of action affecting monoamine neurotransmission in the brain.

Antidepressants are divided into several classes according to its mechanisms [55].

- Tricyclic antidepressants (TCAs) block the reuptake of monoamine neurotransmitters (primarily serotonin and norepinephrine) presynaptically.
- Monoamine oxidase inhibitors (MAOIs) amplify concentration of monoamines in the synaptic cleft by the blockage of monoamine oxidase enzymes.

- Selective serotonin reuptake inhibitors (SSRIs) selectively block the reuptake of serotonin. This group of drugs demonstrates decreased side-effects in comparison to other classes of antidepressants.
- Serotonin and norepinephrine reuptake inhibitors (SNRIs) produce dual inhibition of serotonin and norepinephrine reuptake.
- Norepinephrine-dopamine reuptake inhibitors block the action of norepinephrine and dopamine transporters thereby inducing reuptake suppression.
- Norepinephrine reuptake inhibitors block norepinephrine and epinephrine reuptake via norepinephrine transporter inhibition.
- Serotonin antagonists and reuptake inhibitors (SARIs) act by antagonizing serotonin receptors such as 5-HT2A and inhibiting the reuptake of serotonin, norepinephrine and/or dopamine. Most of them also act as α1-adrenergic receptor antagonists. The majority of the currently marketed SARIs belong to the phenylpiperazine class of substances.
- NMDA receptor antagonists deactivate NMDA glutamate receptors. This class of antidepressants characterizes as rapid-action drugs and includes such substances as ketamine and esketamine.

In spite of the variety of therapy methods, depression treatment is still a serious concern among psychiatrists. A major study by the National Institute of Mental Health found that less than 50% of people are completely recovered from symptoms of depression even after taking two different antidepressants. Moreover, many of those who respond to treatment soon become depressed again, even though they continue to take their medication [55].

Effectiveness of antidepressant therapy depends on the concentration of the drug in the brain. Conventional oral and parenteral therapies are limited because it requires the drug to cross the BBB.

Antidepressants in dosage forms that manageably release the drug directly into the brain reduce their systemic effects, side effects, drug interactions and ultimately bypass pharmacoresistant problems.

At present, quite a few research groups are busy studying the pharmacokinetics, pharmacodynamics and efficacy of antidepressant nanodrugs. Their research are at various stages: from nanoproducts design to preclinical and clinical stages of testing. So far, none of the antidepressants with targeted delivery to the brain have passed the FDA.

Literature analysis suggests that the intranasal administration of nanotherapy (where the drug is encapsulated in nanoparticles) is the most advantageous way to deliver a whole set of antidepressants of different classes to the brain [56,57]. Moreover, this is consistent with the assumption that a faster start of action accompanied by prolonged circulation of active molecules increases efficiency. Polymer nanoparticles are the most frequently investigated among the various nanosystems (Table 3).

Table 3. Summary of nanotechnology-based systems applied in the treatment of depression, anxiety and schizophrenia.

Drug	Nanocarrier	Components	PS, nm	ZP, mV	EE, %	LC, %	PDI	In Vivo Route of Administration	Outcomes	References
					Depression					
Agomelatine	PLGA NPs	PLGA, PM407	116,06 ± 3523	−22.7	96	-	<0.3	i.n.	Prominent antidepressant activity	[58]
Agomelatine	Polymeric NPs	Propylene glycol, Plu F68, Ethanol, Transcutol HP.	107.64	−15	81.91	-	0.209	t.d.	Penetration enhancement of drug	[59]
Baicalein	Solid lipid NPs.	*N*-Acetyl Pro-Gly-Pro (to binding to neutrophil CXCR2 receptor), GMS, PM188, 1,2-dipalmitoyl-sn-glycero-3-phospho choline.	<100	−13.5, −12.6	98.7, 99.1	-	-	i.v.	The enhanced concentration of drug in the basolateral amygdala. Antidepressant effect in vitro and in vivo.	[60]
BDNF	Polyion complex formulation of BDNF (nano-BDNF)	Human recombinant BDNF, PEG-poly(L-glutamate) diblock copolymer	95	-	-	-	0.165	i.v.	Significant reduction in cerebral tissue loss. Improved memory/cognition, reduced post-stroke depressive phenotypes, and maintained myelin basic protein and brain BDNF levels.	[61]
HU-211 and curcumin	Solid lipid dual-drug NPs	Polyoxyethylene (40) stearate, stearic acid, and lecithin.	58.77 ± 1.7	−21.7 ± 0.4	-	0.74 ± 0.02, 18.34 ± 1.06	-	i.p.	Protection of PC12 cells from corticosterone-induced apoptosis. Antidepressant-like effect and enhanced fall latency in rotarod test, improved level of dopamine in the mice blood. NPs can deliver more curcumin to the brain and thus produce a significant increase in neurotransmitters level in brain tissue, especially in the hippocampus and striatum.	[62]
Curcumin and dexanabinol	Solid lipid NPs	Stearic acid, lecithin, polyoxyethylene stearate.	-	−22.6 ± 0.9	19.12 ± 1.43, 0.81 ± 0.04	-	-	-	NPs exerted antidepressant activity by targeting the endocannabinoid/CB1 receptor system.	[63]
Curcumin	Nanocapsules	Organic phase PCL, capric caprylic triglycerides, 106 sorbitan monoestearate, acetone	291–312	From −22 to −36	Close to 100%	-	-	via gavage	Antidepressant-like and antioxidant effects in a mouse model of Alzheimer's disease. NPs were more effective than the free curcumin.	[64]
Duloxetine	Nanostructured lipid carriers	GMS, capryol 136 PGMC, Plu F-68, sodium taurocholate	80.17–127.73	-	-	-	-	i.n., i.v.	Better brain targeting efficiency than DLX solution when administered intranasally. Decreased side effects.	[65]
Folic acid	Niosomes	Different nonionic surfactants (Span 20, Span 60, Span 80, Tween 20, Tween 80, CL)	3050–5625	-	69.42	-	-	i.n.	Niosomes prepared with span 60 and CL in the ratio of 1:1 (50 mg: 50 mg) showed higher EE and better in vitro drug release of 64.2% at the end of 12 hrs and therefore considered as optimized formulation. About 48.15% of the drug was found to be absorbed through the nasal cavity at the end of 6 hrs.	[66]
Lithium carbonate	CS nanocomposites	CS, sodium tripolyphosphate anions, Tween 80.	90.68–220.81	+37.9	87 ± 1.21	28.87	-	p.o.	Reversed degenerative changes and gliosis in depression-induced animal models. Fortified targeted drug delivery and restrained adverse effects.	[67]

Table 3. *Cont.*

Drug	Nanocarrier	Components	PS, nm	ZP, mV	EE, %	LC, %	PDI	In Vivo Route of Administration	Outcomes	References
Minocycline hydrochloride (MH)	CS NPs	Tween 80, CS. Two types of NPs: MH loaded NPs, Tween 80 coated MH encapsulated NPs.	-	-	-	-	-	i.p.	NPs improved the therapeutic efficacy as well as safety of MH.	[68]
Selegiline hydrochloride	Thiolated CS NPs	CS, thioglycolic acid.	215 ± 34.71	+17.06	70 ± 2.71	-	0.214 ± 0.042	i.n.	Attenuation of the oxidative stress and restoring of the activity of the mitochondrial complex. Antidepressant-like effect in vivo	[69]
Silymarin	Nanostructured lipid carriers	Precirol solid lipid, Labrafac Lipophile oil.	519.00 ± 28.67	−12.95 ± 1.58	90.00 ± 3.20	-	0.66 ± 0.05	p.o.	Antidepressant-like effect, comparable with fluoxetine in mice. Significantly higher brain concentration by 12.46 fold superior to silymarin.	[70]
Thymoquinone (TQ)	Solid lipid NPs	Tween 80, GMS, PM188.	188.66 ± 8.94	−12.32 ± 1.04	68.60 ± 4.82	-	0.319 ± 0.04	p.o.	Higher amount of TQ reached the target region after administration. Higher levels of monoamines 5 hydroxytryptamine, dopamine and norepinephrine as compared to TQ suspension were demonstrated.	[71]
Tramadol HCl	CS NPs with mucoadhesive thermo-reversible gel.	CS, Thermo reversible mucoadhesive Plu-HPMC	152.0 ± 9.56	+31 ± 2.21	85 ± 3.23	-	0.143 ± 0.003	i.n.	Antidepressant-like effect in rat model of depression.	[72]
Trefoil factor 3 (TFF3)	cRGD-modified liposomes	Cyclic RGD (cRGD) peptide with high affinity for integrin receptors of leukocytes, soybean phosphatidylcholine, DSPE-PEG (PEG 2000), DSPG, CL	133	−21.8	27.6	-	-	i.p.	Brain targeted delivery in a murine model. Antidepressant-like effect of direct intra-basolateral amygdala administration of TFF3 solution in rats subjected to chronic mild stress.	[73]
Venlafaxine	CS NPs	CS glutamate.	167 ± 6.5	+23.83 ± 1.76	79.3 ± 2.6	32.25 ± 1.63	0.367 ± 0.045	i.n.	Enhanced uptake of venlafaxine to the brain.	[74]
Venlafaxine	PLGA NPs	PLGA, two ligands (Tf and TfRp) against transferrin receptor (TfR) to enhance access to brain across BBB.	206.3 ± 3.7	−25	48–50	10–12	0.041 ± 0.017	i.n.	Plain NPs demonstrated the highest ability to reach the brain vs. functionalized NPs.	[75]
Venlafaxine	Alginate NPs	-	-	-	-	-	-	i.n., i.v., p.o.	Improved antidepressant-like activity in comparison with the venlafaxine (i.n. and oral form). The greater brain/blood ratios for VNPs (i.n.)	[76]
$Zn^{(2+)}$	PLGA NPs conjugated with glycopeptides	Antibodies against NCAM1 and CD44, PLGA conjugated with tetramethylrhodamine and glycopeptides.	190–210	From −0.5 to −10	-	-	-	-	NPs were able to cross the BBB and to deliver Zn(2+) ions at non-toxic concentrations. Easily modified for preferential targeting of specific cell populations.	[77]
Anxiety Disorders										
Peptide antisauvagine-30 (ASV-30)	Iron oxide NPs	Fe_2O_3, 3-aminopropyltriethoxysilane	5 ± 1	-	-	-	-	i.p.	Systemically administered NPs were observed in the brain. Association with neurons and reduced amphetamine withdrawal-induced anxiety in rats without affecting locomotion were demonstrated.	[78]

Table 3. *Cont.*

Drug	Nanocarrier	Components	PS, nm	ZP, mV	EE, %	LC, %	PDI	In Vivo Route of Administration	Outcomes	References
BUH	Thiolated CS NPs	CS, thiolated CS.	226.7 ± 2.52	-	81.13 ± 2.8	49.67 ± 5.5	-	i.n.	The brain concentration achieved after intranasal administration was significantly higher than after administration of BUH (i.v. and i.n.). Excellent bioadhesion.	[79]
BUH	Nanovesicles	Two types of nanovesicular in situ gels (P407-based and carbopol 974P-based). Span 20, Span 40, Span 60, CL, stearylamine, dicetylphosphate.	-	-	56.67–70.57	-	-	i.n.	Higher level of permeability for carbopol formulation in comparison to PM formulations. A 3.26 times increase of BUH bioavailability when loaded into the carbopol nanovesicular in situ gel in comparison to control (i.n.).	[80]
Diazepam	PLGA NPs	PLGA, PVA.	250	−23.3	66	-	-	-	In vitro drug release analysis showed sustained release of drug from nanoparticles. Correspondence to Korsmeyer–Peppas model.	[81]
Gallic acid (GA)	CS NPs	CS, Tween 80 (for coating (cGANP batch)). Two types of NPs: Ligand coated NPs (cGANP) and uncoated NPs (GANP).	103.33 ± 2.28	-	93.62	-	-	i.p.	Improved anxiolytic activity in mice. The plasma nitrite level decreased in GA, GANP and cGANP (most pronounced for cGANP) treated group as compared to saline treated control group while no change in plasma corticosterone levels was observed after any treatment.	[82]
Schizophrenia and Bipolar Disorders										
Aripiprazole (ARP)	Solid lipid NPs	Tristearin, Tween 80, sodium taurocholate.	85.05–2042	From -4.25 to −17.5	57.65–81.70	9.28–31.54	0.241–0.682	p.o.	Improved bioavailability of aripiprazole (1.6-fold compared to plain drug suspension). Enhancement of absorption and minimizing of the first-pass metabolism.	[83]
Aripiprazole	PCL NPs	PCL	199.2 ± 5.65	−21.4 ± 4.6	69.2 ± 2.34	-	-	i.n., i.v.	The enhanced brain targeting efficiency	[84]
Asenapine maleate	CS coated nanostructured lipid carrier	GMS, oleic acid, Tween 80, glycol CS.	184.2 ± 5.59	+18.83 ± 1.19	83.52 ± 2.59	-	-	i.n.	2.3 and 4 fold higher systemic and brain bioavailability compared to pure asenapine solution (i.n.).	[85]
Asenapine maleate	Transfersomes	SPC and sodium deoxycholate (SDC).	126.0	−43.7	54.96	-	0.232	t.d.	Significant increase of bioavailability after transdermal application compared with oral route.	[86]
Haloperidol	Lectin-functionalized, PEG–PLGA NPs	Mixture of Maleimide-PEG–PLGA and Me-PEG–PLGA, Solanum tuberosum lectin (STL).	132 ± 20	14.4 ± 0.1	73.2 ± 0.8	0.85 ± 0.01	0.07–0.22	i.n.	Increase of the brain tissue haloperidol concentrations by 1.5-3-fold compared to non-STL-NPs and other routes of administration.	[87]
Lithium carbonate	CS NPs	CS	162–419	+ 30	-	-	-	-	CS increased cellular uptake of lithium.	[88]
Lurasidone hydrochloride (LH)	Solid lipid NPs	GMS, PM188, sodium deoxycholate.	139.8 ± 5.5	−30.8 ± 3.5	79.10 ± 2.50	-	-	p.o.	Improved bioavailability of LH via lymphatic uptake along with improved therapeutic effect in MK-801 induced schizophrenia model in rats.	[89]
Lurasidone hydrochloride	Nanolipid carrier	Capryol 90, Tween 80, and Transcutol P.	207.4 ± 1.5	-	92.12 ± 1.0	-	0.392 ± 0.15	i.n.	2-fold increase of the drug concentration in the brain when compared with pure drug solution (i.n.)	[90]

Table 3. *Cont.*

Drug	Nanocarrier	Components	PS, nm	ZP, mV	EE, %	LC, %	PDI	In Vivo Route of Administration	Outcomes	References
Lurasidone	Mixed polymeric micelles	Plu F127, Gelucire 44/14.	175	-	97.8	-	-	i.n., i.v.	Improved brain distribution as well as kinetics of lurasidone via the intranasal route. The sustained release of lurasidone hydrochloride from micelles with better permeability and bioavailability.	[91]
Olanzapine	Solid lipid NPs	Two types of NPs with GMS and tripalmitin. Stearylamine, Tween 80.	165, 110	+66.50, +35.3	96.3, 67.2	-	0.34, 0.726	i.v.	23-fold increased bioavailability of olanzapine in brain and decreased clearance.	[92]
Olanzapine	Nanostructured lipid carriers	Mucoadhesive NPs was prepared by using carbopol 974P (MNLC (C)) and the combination of PM 407 and of HPMC K4M (MNLC (P + H)).	88.95 ± 1.7	−22.62 ± 1.9	88.94 ± 3.9	-	0,31 ± 0,01	i.n.	Nose-to-brain delivery of olanzapine MNLC (P + H) was considered as an effective and safe for CNS disorders.	[93]
Olanzapine	Micellar nanocarriers	Plu® mixture of L121 and P123 in different ratios.	58.55 ± 2.47	-	75.03 ± 2.35	1.84 ± 0.06	0.27 ± 0.03	i.n., i.v.	The micelles (i.n.) demonstrated a conciliation between kinetic and thermodynamic stability, controlled drug-release characteristics and evoked minor histopathological changes in sheep nasal mucosa.	[94]
Olanzapine	Nanocapsules	Copolymer-functionalized PCL	254.9 ± 12.1	+22.2 ± 1.2	99.00 ± 0.05	-	0.03 ± 0.01	i.n.	Controlled release, improved retention of the drug on the nasal mucosa under continuous wash was demonstrated. Increased brain uptake and improved prepulse inhibition deficit induced by apomorphine in rats.	[95]
Olanzapine	CS NPs	CS. NPs were prepared with 20 or 60% loading.	208 ± 29 322 ± 18	-	86.7 ± 7.1, 87.6 ± 5.2	17.2 ± 1.4, 52.3 ± 3.1	-	i.n., i.v.	Olanzapine administered via intranasal CS NPs demonstrated the potential to improve the efficacy of systemic absorption thereby offering an efficient method of administration in noncompliant patients.	[96]
Olanzapine	PLGA NPs	PLGA, PM407, acetone, acetonitrile, tetrahydrofuran.	91.2 ± 5.2	−23.7 ± 2.1	68.91 ± 2.31	8.613 ± 0.288	0.120 ± 0.018	i.n., i.v.	6.35 and 10.86 times higher uptake than pure olanzapine solution (i.v. and i.n.) in vivo	[97]
Paliperidone	Nanolipomers	PCL as a polymeric core, Lipoid S75, and Gelucire® 50/13 as a lipid shell and PVA as a stabilizing agent.	168.2 ± 0.7	−23.1	87.27 ± 0.098	-	0.22	p.o.	Sustained release up to 24 h and better ex vivo intestinal permeation for paliperidone compared to the corresponding polymeric, solid lipid NPs and drug suspension.	[98]
Paliperidone	in situ Gels	Carbopol 934, HPMC K4M, HP-β-CD in the form of inclusion complex of PLPD as nasal absorption enhancer.	-	-	-	-	-	i.n.	In vitro and ex vivo drug permeation, exhibited mucoadhesion and sustained drug release. The formulation containing HP-β-CD complex of paliperidone demonstrated higher level of drug permeation through sheep nasal mucosa without injury of nasal mucosa architecture.	[99]

Table 3. *Cont.*

Drug	Nanocarrier	Components	PS, nm	ZP, mV	EE, %	LC, %	PDI	In Vivo Route of Administration	Outcomes	References
Paliperidone palmitate	Micelles	D-alpha-tocopheryl polyethylene glycol 1000 succinate	26.5 ± 4.8	92.61 ± 2.5	-	-	-	i.m.	Improved antipsychotic effect and decreased adverse effects after micellar formulation application.	[100]
Paliperidone	Microemulsion	Muco-adhesive polymer, oleic acid	27.31 ± 1.86	−38.65 ± 2.39	-	-	0.241 ± 0.05	i.n., i.v.	Higher brain paliperidone concentrations compared to pure drug (i.v.)	[101]
Risperidone	Proteinoid NPs	Amino acids l-glutamic acid, l-phenylalanine, l-histidine, poly (l-lactic acid), PEG	86 ± 3	−16 ± 1	-	20 ± 0.1	-	i.v.	Enhanced antipsychotic activity compared to pure risperidone in mice	[102]
Risperidone	CS NPs	CS, tween 80, PM 188.	86	+36.6	77.96 ± 1.50	13–37	0.287	i.n.	Reduced stereotypical behavior score in experimental animals and reversed amphetamine effect.	[103]
Risperidone	Solid lipid NPs	Compritol 888 ATO, Plu F-127.	0.148 ± 0.028	−25.35 ± 0.45	59.65 ± 1.18	59.65 ± 1.18	0.148 ± 0.03	i.n., i.v.	Effective brain targeting in mice in vivo	[104]
Risperidone	Nanoemulsion	CS, capmul MCM, transcutol, propylene glycol	16.7 ± 1.21	−9.15 ± 2.14	98.86 ± 1.21	-	0.191 ± 0.04	i.n., i.v.	Effective delivery of significant amount of risperidone to the brain after intranasal administration.	[105]
Risperidone	Functionalized liposomes	Conventional liposomes consisting of SPC/CL, cationic liposomes containing SPC/CL/stearylamine, PEGylated liposomes consists of SPC/CL/distearylphosphatidy lethanolamine-mPEG-2000	98.51 ± 6.82	−28.6 ± 3.62	58.86 ± 1.38	-	0.103–0.324	i.n., i.v.	Liposomal formulations provided enhanced bioavailability, less clearance rate, higher mean residential time and better response in vivo compared to conventional formulations.	[106]
Risperidone	CS lipid NPs	CS	132.7	-	-	7.6	-	i.n., i.v.	Increased nose to brain drug delivery compared to pure drug suspension of equivalent dose.	[107]
Quetiapine fumarate	Solid lipid NPs in situ gel	Heat-melting GMS, Span 80, butanol, PM407, PM188.	307.1 ± 17.7	+ 57.2 ± 0.24	97.6 ± 0.58	-	-	i.n., i.v., p.o.	Stable and effective brain delivery, amelioration of the damages induced by MK-801 in rat model of schizophrenia.	[108]
Quetiapine fumarate	Nanoemulsion system	HLBs of Emalex LWIS 10, PEG 400, Transcutol P, Capmul MCM, Tween 80.	144 ± 0.5	−8.131 ± 1.8	-	-	0.193 ± 0.04	i.n.	2-fold increase of the drug release compared to pure drug. Better direct nose-to-brain drug transport.	[109]
Quetiapine Fumarate	Liposome	Egg phosphatidylcholine, CL	139.6	−32.1	75.63 ± 3.77	-	-	i.n.	Higher level of diffusion. Better potential to deliver drugs to the brain than by the pure solution.	[110]
Quetiapine fumarate	Microemulsion with and without CS	CS, methyl-β-cyclodextrin, Capmul MCM EP, labrasol, Tween 80, Transcutol-P.	35.31 ± 1.71	20.29 ± 1.23	-	-	0.249 ± 0.03	i.n., i.v.	Enhanced brain uptake of quetiapine and improved bioavailability.	[111]
Quetiapine fumarate	CS NPs	CS, sodium tripolyphosphate	131.08 ± 7.45	+ 34.4 ± 1.87	89.93 ± 3.85	-	0.252 ± 0.064	i.n., i.v.	Significantly higher brain/blood ratio and 2 folds higher nasal bioavailability in the brain in comparison to pure drug solution (i.n.).	[112]

BBB—Blood-brain barrier; NPs—nanoparticles; PS—particle size; ZP—zeta potential; EE—drug entrapment efficiency; LC—loading capacity; PDI—polydispersity index; i.m.—Intramuscular route of administration; i.n.—intranasal route of administration; i.p.—intraperitoneal route of administration; i.v.—intravenous route of administration; p.o.—per oral route of administration; t.d.—transdermal route of administration; BDNF—brain-derived neurotrophic factor; BUH—Buspirone hydrochloride; CL—cholesterol; CS—chitosan; GMS—glyceryl monostearate; HPMC—hydroxypropyl methyl cellulose K4M; PCL—poly(ε-caprolactone); PEG—(poly(ethylene glycol); PLGA—poly(lactic-co-glycolic acid); Plu—pluronic; PM—poloxamer; PVA—polyvinyl alcohol; SPC—soya-phosphatidylcholine.

4.1. TCAs

Doxepin is one of the tricyclic antidepressants used for depression treatment. During the last few years doxepin was also investigated as a nanoform. In particular, doxepin in the form of thermoreversible biogel or chitosan and glycerophosphate or polyethylenenglycol demonstrated lower local toxicity and significant effectiveness in the forced swim test [113].

4.2. MAOIs

Antidepressants from MAOIs class have been also investigated for targeting drug delivery. For example, a selective inhibitor of MAO type B—Selegiline was loaded into nanoparticles for depression treatment. It was demonstrated that thiolated chitosan nanoparticles developed by Singh et al. (2016) enhanced the nasal delivery of selegiline and produced antidepressant-like effect in rats [69].

4.3. SSRIs

SSRIs have also being studied as potential nanopreparations. Paroxetine as nanoemulsion form [114] and fluoxetine as ion sensitive in situ nasal gel [115], showed significant responses in locomotor activity level and immobility in injected rats compared to control groups.

Citalopram is also one of the SSRIs. It belongs to the few drugs that can be used safely in childhood psychiatric disorders treatment. Along with other SSRIs Citalopram was loaded in interpenetrating polyelectrolytes nanocomplexes (composed of chitosan: pectin in a 3:1 ratio) constructed by Kamel and colleagues [116]. During experiment researchers demonstrated extended drug release pattern, higher serotonin brain level up to 24 h, more rapid onset of action and more extended behavioral effects in rats with depressive-like behavior treated with these complexes compared to pure citalopram.

Sertraline is another SSRI drug characterized by poor water-solubility and low oral bioavailability. Sertraline-loaded solid lipid nanoparticles improved the drug releasing. In particular, the maximum plasma concentration after nanoparticles injection was 10-fold higher compared to pure drug. Moreover, Sertraline-loaded SLN were found to be stable at 4 °C for 6 months of the study period [117].

4.4. SNRIs

One of the promising antidepressants for targeting delivery is venflaksin hydrochloride (SNRI). There are several ways to deliver it into the brain, for example by Lutrol F127 [118], nanoparticle-based NLC gel [56], alginate–chitosan nanoparticles (AGNPs) [119]. It was shown that nanoparticles loaded with venlafaxine hydrochloride produced a more pronounced effect after intranasal administration in vivo in comparison to oral administration of equivalent dose [118,119]. Desvenlafaxine is another preparation that belongs to that class of drugs. It represents an active metabolite of venlafaxine also investigated in PLGA-chitosan nanoparticles [120].

Duloxetine (SNRI) is another antidepressant that demonstrated better response in NLC [47]. The scintigraphy images are consistent with the biodistribution and pharmacokinetic studies, having revealed a high uptake of duloxetine into the rat brain [47].

4.5. SARIs

Serotonin antagonists and reuptake inhibitors are drugs characterized by antidepressant, anxiolytics and hypnotics effects. This class of substances includes trazodone and nefazodone. These drugs were also loaded into nanoform. In particular, Casolaro et al. (2015) constructed hydrogels bearing L-phenylalanine (Phe-Nip3) or L-valine (Ava2) residues, with citalopram and trazodone. Hydrogel form showed improved release of these drugs compared to pure substances [121].

4.6. Other Drugs

Agomelatine is atypical antidepressant that both stimulates melatonin receptors (MT1 and MT2) and blocks 5-HT2C-receptors. This drug is characterized by low side-effects because it does not counteract with other serotonin receptors, does not affect reuptake of monoamines and does not interact with adrenergic, cholinergic, dopamine, histamine and GABA receptors. Nevertheless, agomelatine has a low biological half-life coupled with extensive hepatic first-pass metabolism [59]. In that context the loading of preparation into nanoform could improve its therapeutic effect. Thus, it was demonstrated that intranasal administration of Agomelatine-loaded poly-lactic-co-glycolic acid nanoparticles shown significant antidepressant-like effect in rats [58]. Another type of nanoparticles was developed by Shinde et al. (2020) and represented polymeric nanoparticles with Agomelatine for transdermal use. These nanocarriers demonstrated good permeability across rat skin [59].

Another type of irregular antidepressant is flavonoid Baicalein. Chen and colleagues constructed solid lipid NPs loaded with Baicalein [60]. These NPs were modified with *N*-Acetyl Pro-Gly-Pro (PGP) peptide, which is characterized by high specific binding affinity to neutrophils through the CXCR2 receptor. When associated with neutrophils, these particles can penetrate through the BBB and reach targets in the brain.

Along with research of classical antidepressants in nanoforms, it is quite interesting to study various peptides and neurotrophins as antidepressant treatment. In this regard, challenging data concern the proven neuroprotective and antidepressant properties of the brain-derived neurotrophic factor (BDNF). In vitro experiments showed that BDNF delivery using the adenoviral vector produce neuroprotective effects. AAV-Syn-BDNF-EGFP virus vector maintains brain cell viability and preserves the neural network functional structure in the late posthypoxic period [122].

It was found that intranasal administration of BDNF-HA2TAT/AAV to normal mice produce an antidepressant effect in the forced swimming test, but only with chronic treatment. No statistical difference was found in the forced swim test after acute intranasal injection of the AAV to the mice. After the BDNF-HA2TAT/AAV administration to the animals with the chronic mild stress model of depression the successful therapeutic effect was demonstrated in the tail suspension test and forced swim test, but not in open field test [123]. Moreover, the female mice were more sensitive to the drug administration. One of the possible explanations is that the prevalence of depression in females is much higher than that in males [124].

Therefore, different nanocontainer forms of drugs have been developed for the treatment of depression. Such systems contain not only the most popular antidepressants, such as SNRI and SSRI, but also various original forms including vector systems for target delivery in the brain. Application of nanocarriers could help to reduce side effects and to improve drugs bioavailability.

5. Drug Delivery for Anxiety Disorders

Anxiety disorders are the largest group of mental disorders in most Western societies. Essential features of anxiety disorders are excessive and persistent fear, avoidance of perceived threats and panic attacks in certain instances. Although the pathophysiology of anxiety disorders is not fully understood, targeting systems for their treatment are of interest. Drugs for treating anxiety disorders include medications that affect serotonergic, adrenergic, glutamatergic, endocannabinoid systems and various neuropeptides [125]. First of all, tranquilizers with anxiolytic, myorelaxing, sedative and anticonvulsant activity are used for the treatment of anxiety disorders. Many anxiolytic drugs are derived from benzodiazepine and affect benzodiazepine receptors (second generation anxiolytics). However, there is also a spectrum of tranquilizers aimed at other therapeutic targets. Examples include such drugs as buspirone, meprobamate, benactin, etc. Significant progress has been made in the development of formulations and psychosocial treatment strategies for anxiety disorders. However, symptoms persist in many patients despite improvements in therapy. Randomized controlled trials of anxiety disorders pharmacotherapy report a response rate of 40–70% and a remission rate of 20–47%. Anxiety disorders are considered as resistant to treatment when there are residual symptoms or when symptoms do not improve at all after some form of therapeutic intervention. The optimal use of available medication and the development of new pharmacological strategies and agents promise to improve this situation [126].

Polymer nanocarriers are used to develop delivery forms for therapeutic drugs against anxiety disorders. Nanoparticles created from biodegradable polymers such as PLGA are widely studied as drug delivery systems because of their two important properties, such as biocompatibility and controlled drug release. For example, replicable spherical diazepam PLGA nanoparticles have been developed and characterized by Bohrey and colleagues [81]. Chitosan is another natural carbohydrate polymer with ideal for nanoparticles polymer carrier properties such as biocompatibility, biodegradability, non-toxicity and low cost. It exhibits bioadhesive properties and the ability to significantly increase permeability for hydrophilic compounds. Chitosan with thiol groups provides much higher adhesion properties.

Buspirone is a drug belonging to the group of tranquilizers using for anxiety disorders treatment. It is a complete agonist of 5-HT1A presynaptic serotonin receptors, which leads to a decrease of serotonin release and the resulting reduction of anxiety symptoms. Buspirone also acts as a partial agonist of the post-synaptic serotonin receptors, which contribute to the release of serotonin in synapses, resulting in increased serotonin concentration and reduced depression. Additionally, buspirone inhibits the dopamine receptors D2 [127]. Bari et al. (2015) loaded buspirone hydrochloride into polymeric thiolated chitosan nanoparticles for intranasal administration. Ex vivo study carried out via the porcine mucin binding efficiency test demonstrated excellent bioadhesion. Moreover, the drug concentration in the brain after the intranasal injection was significantly higher than after pure Buspirone hydrochloride administration [79]. Along with chitosan nanoparticles construction two types of nanovesicular in situ gels (based on carbopol 974P and poloxamer 407) were developed for delivery of buspirone hydrochloride. The carbopol composition showed higher permeability compared to the poloxamer. It was demonstrated that buspirone hydrochloride has low bioavailability of about 4% after oral administration due to first pass metabolism. Nevertheless, the bioavailability of buspirone hydrochloride increased by 3.26 times when used in the composition of the nanovesicular gel of carbopol compared to the nasal solution of a pure drug [80].

Gallic acid has significant anxiolytic activity, which may be due to its antioxidant properties and reduced nitrite levels in plasma. Chitosan nanoparticles coated with Tween 80 ligand were used to deliver gallic acid to the brain. Behavioral studies have shown that GA nanoparticles significantly improve anxiolytic activity in mice. Nitrite levels decrease in plasma was most pronounced in the group that received the nanoparticle with loaded with drugs. This may have been due to the reduction in plasma nitrite levels by gallic acid. This effect was improved by the increase of GA brain absorption through the nanoparticles application [82].

Inorganic nanoparticles are also used to create delivery systems for anxiety disorders. Many peptides and their analogues cannot effectively cross the BBB. For that reason, Vinzant and colleagues conjugated peptide antisauvagine-30 (ASV-30) with iron oxide nanoparticles [78]. It was shown that ASV-30 peptide affects corticotrophin releasing factor type 2 receptors when directly injected into the brain and thus reduces anxious behavior in animals. Imaging studies demonstrated that iron oxide + ASV-30 particles were present in the brain and were associated with neurons, including those that express CRF2 receptors after intraperitoneal injection. Brain distribution studies were affirmed nanoparticles anxiolytic activity in rats [78].

Currently, the range of application of anxiolytic drugs and their assortment are quite wide. These drugs include preparations of benzodiazepine-line and non-benzodiazepine anxiolytics. Nevertheless, not many nanocontainer forms have been developed for the standard medicines using for anxiety disorders treatment. The loading of other types of drugs in nanocarriers besides the usual forms of anxiolytics could help to improve the treatment of anxiety disorders and to prevent aggravation into depression or severe generalized form.

6. Drug Delivery for Schizophrenia and Bipolar Disorders

Schizophrenia is a complex endogenous mental disorder characterized by cognitive and emotional symptoms that significantly reduce the quality of life of patients [128]. The main drugs used to treat the pathology are antipsychotic drugs that reduce the increased dopaminergic transmission in the brain of patients. Atypical antipsychotics of a new generation, characterized by a narrower range of side effects compared to the first generation, are also used to treat bipolar disorder, along with lithium and antiepileptic drugs [129].

The first drug for the treatment of schizophrenia, chlorpromazine, was first used in 1952, but already in the 60s researchers tried to develop long-acting substances consisting of an antipsychotic agent and fat-soluble solution [130].

Despite the fact that new antipsychotic drugs have appeared on the market, providing greater efficiency with significantly reduced side effects, delivery systems of antipsychotic drugs are still in the stage of conventional drug forms, such as tablets, capsules and solutions, and need to be dosed 2–4 times a day. There is no doubt that new drug delivery systems, such as stable and controlled release systems, will be useful for antipsychotics. They should reduce the frequency of dosing, increase bioavailability of the drug and improve adherence of the therapy course [131].

The drug delivery system produces less pronounced side effects than the original drugs, because they provide lower inpatient concentrations of therapeutic drugs and more stable release characteristics than oral drugs. Thus, such combined drugs increase exposure to oral medications, further reducing morbidity and mortality [132]. As nanocarriers bypass the gastrointestinal tract, such a type of therapy reduces the amount of medication needed and can minimize some peripheral side effects, including hepatotoxicity and hyperprolactinemia [130].

Nanocontainer systems based on PLA were developed in 1989 for chlorpromazine—the first antipsychotic agent [131].

Since then atypical neuroleptics have appeared and become widespread in medical practice. A lot of publications about nanocontainers involve drugs with olanzapine—a second-generation or atypical antipsychotic, which selectively binds to central dopamine D2 and serotonin (5-HT(2c)) receptors. It has poor bioavailability due to hepatic first-pass metabolism and low permeability into the brain due to efflux by P-glycoproteins [133]. Due to its low oral bioavailability, researchers have created various container preparations [134]. Joseph et al. 2017 conducted research on glyceryl monostearate nanoparticles with olanzapine [133]. A longer release of the drug within 48 hours was shown, compared with 8 hours of the antipsychotic action of pure olanzapine solution. Pervaiz and colleagues described the release of olanzapine loaded in PNA (poly(*N*-isopropylacrylamide-co-acrylic acid)) microgels for 72 h [135]. In vitro bioaccessibility research of Jawahar and colleagues indicated $5\frac{1}{2}$-fold increase in oral bioavailability for nano structured lipid carriers with olanzapine [134]. Cyclodextrins containers were also used for this neuroleptic [136]. An in vitro study on kinetics of clozapine solid lipid nanoparticles showed an increase in lymphatic bioavailability of the drug and its steady release up to 48 h [137]. The study done by Shafaat and coworkers demonstrated that clozapine nanoemulsions resulted in 4.4-fold increase in bioavailability and better drug loading capacity of hydrophobic drug molecules compared with marketed drug formulation [138]. There are also studies on the intranasal introduction of nanoparticles with olanzapine [94]. Nanoparticles containing olanzapine (PLGA) have been shown to be more effectively delivered to the brain by intranasal administration of poly(lactic-co-glycolic acid) nanoparticles [97]. Olanzapine-SLNs showed a 23-fold increase in the relative bioavailability of olanzapine in the brain after nasal administration [92]. The innovative therapeutic approach represents a new form of pharmaceuticals—transdermal drug delivery systems—"patches" containing lipid nanocontainers with this neuroleptic [139]. In addition to improving bioavailability, a study [140] with biodegradable polymeric lipid-core nanocapsules and a decrease in extrapyramidal side effects were shown for polymeric nanoparticles polycaprolactone [141]. Animal model studies have demonstrated improved therapeutic efficacy compared to pure olanzapine [141].

Lurasidone (another atypical antipsychotic) was loaded into SLNs. Its improved therapeutic effect in MK-801 induced schizophrenia model in rats after oral administration was shown [89].

Aripiprazole, a second-generation (or atypical antipsychotic), is poorly soluble and undergoes extensive hepatic metabolism and P-glycoprotein efflux, which lead to reduced in vivo efficacy and increased dose-related side effects. Solid lipid nanoparticles with aripiprazole enhance bioaccessibility of this neuroleptic [83]. In another study, intranasal administration of poly-caprolactone nanoparticles showed a 2-fold increase in aripiprazole distribution in rat brain when compared to aripiprazole nanoparticles administered intravenously [84]. An interesting study was devoted to buccoadhesive chitosan films with aripiprazole. Ex vivo nanocrystal loaded buccal films FAPZ 14 have the potential to provide a faster availability of aripiprazole. The aim of the present study was to design a mucoadhesive dosage form for buccal delivery of aripiprazole, which could provide a rapid drug delivery to the systemic circulation [142].

The same mucoadhesive drug delivery systems were created for riperidone, another atypical neuroleptic used to treat schizophrenia and bipolar disorder. A mucoadhesive buccal tablet formulation of risperidone allowed 90% release of the drug over 8 h, thereby providing direct systemic delivery of risperidone [143]. Risperidone-loaded solid lipid nanoparticles drug release and transport studies illustrated the advantages of oral delivery over poorly water-soluble drugs such as risperidone [144,145]. Pharmacokinetic studies of NLCs of iloperidone 2-fold increase in the % drug targeting efficiency relative to iloperidone pure drug suspension [146]. The pharmacokinetic study revealed almost 8.30-fold increase in oral bioavailability of iloperidone NLCs as compared to the plain drug solution. The nanoemulsions of riperidone also showed improved bioavailability and brain uptake [147]. Intranasal administration of risperidone-loaded mucoadhesive nanoemulsion demonstrated higher efficacy, enhanced brain targeting and higher drug transport to the brain in Swiss albino rats, when compared with intranasal risperidone solution and risperidone nanoemulsion intravenously [105]. In another study, riperidone was enclosed in biodegradable proteinoids. These systems were synthesized by thermal step-growth polymerization from the amino acids L-glutamic acid, L-phenylalanine and L-histidine and poly (L-lactic acid). Behavioral studies on mice found enhanced antipsychotic activity compared to free risperidone.

Quetiapine fumarate, a second generation atypical antipsychotic drug has a plasma half-life of 6h, hence requires frequent administration to maintain effective therapeutic concentration. The increase in bioavailability of mucoadhesive microemulsion Quetiapine during intranasal injection is shown [111].

Azenapine appeared on market in 2009. It was a new atypical antipsychotic for the treatment of schizophrenia and bipolar disorder. However, it had the same disadvantage—low bioavailability when used orally (less than 2%). Most of this drug is metabolized in the liver. The antipsychotic activity of azenapine is thought to be due to antagonistic activity on D2 dopamine and 5-HT2A serotonin receptors. To improve its bioavailability some of the researchers developed sublingual film, intranasal and injectable formulations of azenapine [86]. Shreya et al. (2016) used transfersomes, deformable elastic liposomes loaded with azenapine and transdermal plasters, as a drug formulation. Transfersomes as a drug carrier showed increasing the transdermal permeation and bioavailability of azenapine during in vitro and in vivo experiments.

Lithium medications—psychotropic drugs from the group of normotimists—are historically the first drugs of this group, discovered in 1949. However, they remain essential in the treatment of affective disorders, primarily manic and hypomaniacal phases of bipolar disorder [148]. They are also used to prevent its exacerbation and to treat severe and resistant depression. Their important property is to get rid of suicidal thoughts, so they can prevent suicide.

Lithium ions have a variety of effects on the nervous system, particularly as an antagonist of sodium ions in nerve and muscle cells. In this way, they weaken the nerve impulse (this also explains one of the frequent side effects of lithium preparations: muscle weakness). Lithium also affects the metabolism and transport of monoamines (noradrenaline and serotonin) and increases the sensitivity of some areas of the brain to dopamine. According to some data, the main role in the mechanism of action of lithium is its ability to block the activity of enzymes involved in the synthesis of inositol, which plays a role in regulating the sensitivity of neurons.

The treatment with lithium bipolar disorders is based on its property to selectively inhibit kinase 3 glycogen synthase activity [149]. In addition, it was found that in mania, there is an irregular increase in the activity of proteinkinase C, and a recent study has shown that lithium inhibits its activity. Thus, lithium, like other PkC inhibitors, exhibits antimaniac properties.

Formulations with lithium are the standard drugs for the treatment of bipolar disorders [148]. In one work, the researchers concluded lithium carbonate in chitosan nanoparticles to improve bioavailability. It is postulated that the encapsulation of lithium carbonate within chitosan nanoparticles enables the drug to overcome the intracellular degradative blocks such as endosomes and lysosomes. The ion chelation route was used for encapsulating lithium carbonate [88].

Neuroleptics therapy frequently used for schizophrenia and bipolar disorder treatment requires constant use of drugs and thereby induces various side effects. The loading of drugs into nanocontainers for the controlled release is modern and relevant approach. In addition to targeted delivery and increased bioavailability, it reduces the doses and side effects of antipsychotics, often accompanied its application.

7. Drug Delivery for Alzheimer's Disease

Currently, the most intensive development of drugs based on nanocontainer systems is being carried out to treat AD. The progress of modern medicine has significantly increased average life expectancy. At the same time, the risks of neurodegenerative diseases rise with age. For example, the percent of people suffering from the most frequent neurodegenerative pathology, AD, in the ages from 65 to 74 is 3% and in the ages from 75 to 84 is already 17%. AD is a progressive disorder characterized by memory, cognition and behavioral impairment (dementia), which eventually leads to mood fluctuation and fatal delirium [150].

The action of the existing drug groups is directed on the pathogenesis blocks presumed as the hypotheses of AD pathogenesis.

Hypotheses of AD development can be divided into several main causes [32,151].

- Accumulation of β-amyloid (Aβ(1 $\rightarrow$ 40) and Aβ(1 $\rightarrow$ 42)), which is resulted from pathologic proteolysis of amyloid precursor protein (APP). The aggregates of this protein are toxic and induce neurodegeneration, cytotoxicity and inevitably leading to dementia manifestations.
- Tau accumulation. It is known that a normal mature neuron produces three microtubule-associated protein (MAP) taus; MAP1A, MAP1B and MAP2. These proteins are responsible for the promotion of the assembly and stability of microtubules. The biological activity of tau is regulated by its phosphorylation level. For example, in the brain of AD patients, tau hyperphosphorylates abnormally, which impairs its binding to microtubules; leading to the accumulation of neurofibrillary tangles and dementia development. Several anti-tau therapies including lithium, valproate and nicotinamide have been already investigated for the prevention of Tau protein hyperphosphorylation.
- Progressive decline of acetylcholine concentration. This is the earliest hypothesis of AD progression. It was demonstrated that AD is accompanied by substantial presynaptic cholinergic deficit, which expresses as a reduced choline uptake and acetylcholine release in the brain. That leads to memory and cognition impairment. Drugs that eliminate these symptoms include acetylcholinesterase inhibitors (AChEs) such as tacrine, donepezil, rivastigmine and galantamine.
- NMDA excitotoxicity. Some experimental and neuropathological evidence suggests that glutamatergic system is also involved in the neurodegenerative progression. NMDA receptor is essential for the control of synaptic plasticity and memory function. It is activated by glutamate and glycine, allowing Ca2+ and Na+ influx. It was demonstrated that the hyperexcitability of

NMDA receptors induces Ca2+ overload, eventually leading to apoptosis and producing cognitive impairments. The drug that affects this pathogenesis block is memantine (NMDA inhibitor).

- Abnormality of mitochondria energy metabolism. It is suggested that genetic mutations alter the regulation of the electron transport chain complex enzymes, which are capable of generating ROS. That leads to cell apoptosis and neurodegeneration.

Figure 2 describes the main pathological pathway of Alzheimer's disease and therapy methods, targeted to these mechanisms.

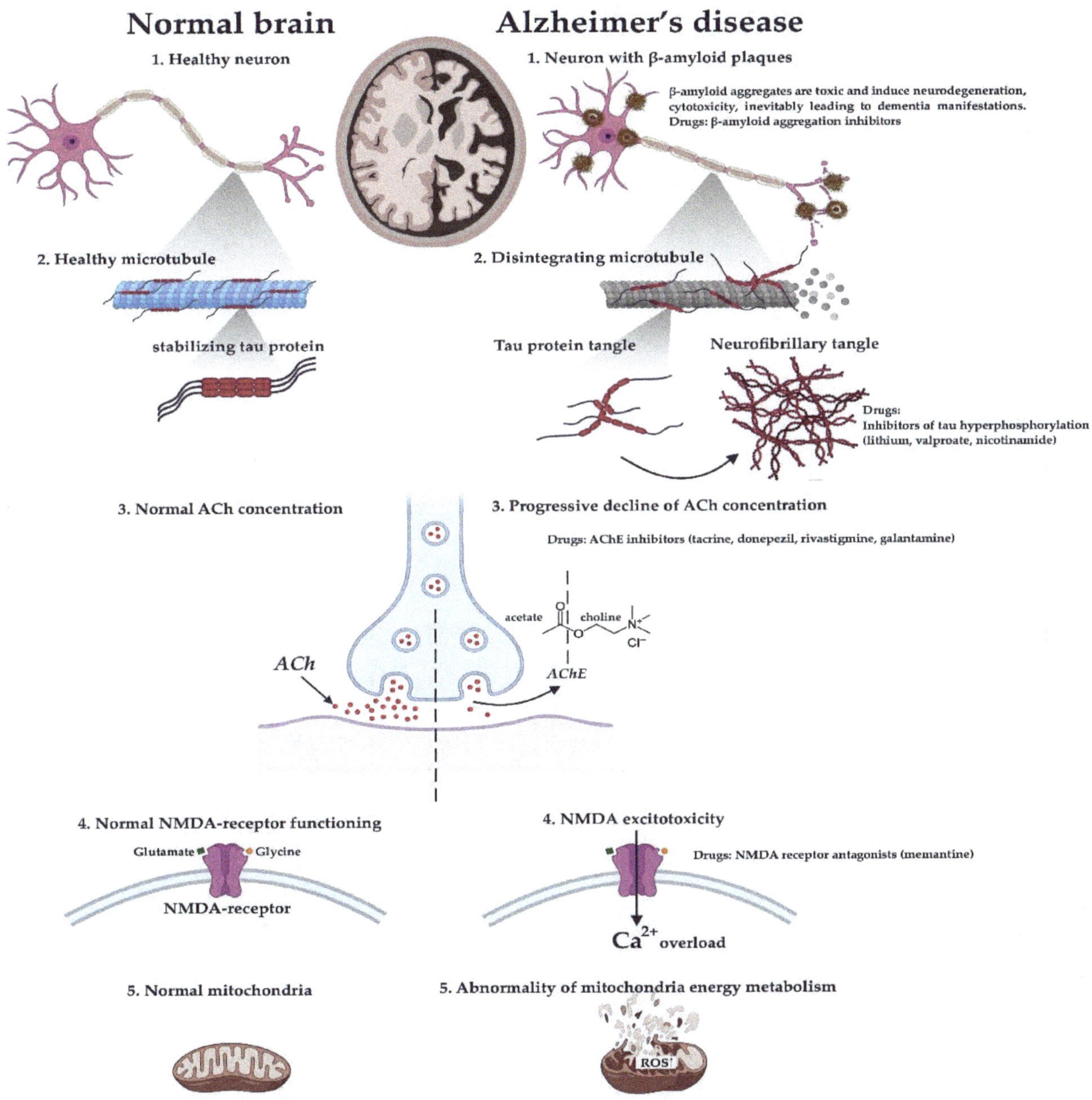

Figure 2. The main pathological pathway of Alzheimer's disease and therapy methods, targeted to these mechanisms. Ach—acetylcholine, AChE—acetylcholine esterase, ROS—reactive oxygen species, NMDA—N-methyl-D-aspartate.

Currently, nanoparticles with various therapeutic mechanism associated with AD pathogenesis have been developed (Table 4).

Table 4. Summary of nanotechnology-based systems applied in the treatment of Alzheimer's disease.

Drug	Nanocarrier	Targeting Ligand	Components	PS, nm	ZP, mV	EE, %	LC, %	PDI	In Vivo Route of Administration	Outcomes	References
Amyloid—Related Nanoparticles											
Pioglitazone	Nano lipid carriers	-	Tripalmitin, MCM, stearyl amine	211.4 ± 3.54	+14.9 ± 1.09	70.18 ± 4.5	-	0.257 ± 0.108	i.n.	The NC significantly improved the nasal permeability of pioglitazone ex-vivo.	[152]
BACE1 siRNA	Solid lipid NPs	Peptide derived from rabies virus glycoprotein (RVG-9R)	CS-coated and uncoated NPs	419.47 ± 24.36, 469.71 ± 49.07	−12.52 ± 0.99, +14.47 ± 0.19	-	-	0.26 ± 0.09, 0.30 ± 0.04	i.n.	The siRNA permeated the monolayer (Caco-2) to a greater extent when released from any of the studied formulations than from bare siRNA, and primarily from CS-coated NPs.	[153]
siRNA against BACE1	Nano complexes CT/siRNA, composed of CGN-PEG-PDMAEMA and Tet1-PEG-PDMAEMA (1:1)	CGN peptide, Tet1 peptide	PEGylated poly(2-(*N,N*-dimethylamino) ethyl methacrylate) (PEG-PDMAEMA)	70–80	+10	-	-	-	i.v.	The NC entered the cytoplasm of the neuron cells, inducing effective gene silence (about 50% decrease in BACE1 mRNA levels) and reversing synaptic injury. The NC significantly decreased BACE1 mRNA and the amyloid plaques, suppressed phosphorylated tau protein levels, and promoted hippocampal neurogenesis. NC restored the cognitive performance of the AD transgenic mice to the level of wild-type control.	[154]
Plasmid DNA encoding BACE1-AS siRNA, D-peptide	PEGylated DGL NPs	Peptide from rabies virus glycoprotein (RVG29)	Dendrigraft poly-L-lysines 10 (DGL), α-Malemidyl-ω-*N*-hydroxysuccinimidylpolyethyleneglycol.	110	+ 7.72 ± 2.80	-	-	0.3	i.v.	Successful codelivery of drugs crossed the BBB. Simultaneous delivery of the therapeutic peptide into brain led to the reduction of neurofibrillary tangles. The memory loss rescue in AD mice was also observed.	[155]
BACE1 siRNA	Dendrimer NPs	Apolipoprotein A-I (ApoA-I), NL4 peptide.	Dendrigraft poly-L-lysines, α-Maleimide-ω-*N*-hydroxysuccinimidylPEG	79.26	+3.53	97.05	-	0.216	-	The NC effectively targeted both BBB and PC12 cells and down-regulated BACE1 gene expression in PC12 cells.	[156]
Cyclophosphamide	Theranostic nanovehicles	Putrescine modified $F(ab')_2$ fragment of antiamyloid antibody, IgG4	CS, MRI contrast agent, pentasodiumtripolyphosphate,	239 ± 4.1	11.9 ± 0.5	-	21,7 ± 1,31	-	i.v.	NPs successfully targeted cerebrovascular amyloid.	[157]

Table 4. *Cont.*

Drug	Nanocarrier	Targeting Ligand	Components	PS, nm	ZP, mV	EE, %	LC, %	PDI	In Vivo Route of Administration	Outcomes	References
Peptide iA5	PLGA NPs	Anti-transferrin receptor monoclonal antibody (OX26), anti-A (DE2B4)	PLGA	166 ± 2	−13 ± 1	63 ± 9	-	0.10 ± 0.04	-	The uptake of NPs with a controlled delivery of the peptide iA5 was substantially increased compared to the NPs without monoclonal antibody functionalization.	[158]
Peptide H102	PEG-PLA NPs	TGN and QSH peptides.	PEG-PLA	125.5.10 ± 2.26	−29.33 ± 0.15	58.49 ± 0.86	0.54	0.127. ± 0.010	i.v.	This dual-functional drug delivery system effectively increased the H102 accumulation at brain Aβ42 concentrated in the hippocampal region and provided better neuroprotective effects in the AD model mice.	[159]
-	Liposomes and solid lipid NPs	Phosphatidicacid, cardiolipin	Monosialogangliosides, disialogangliosides, trisialoganglioside, sphingomyelin, CL, diphosphatidylglycerol, 1-palmitoyl-oleoyl-PC, phosphatidylethanolamine, Sephadex G75.	145, 76	−37.89, −43.30	-	-	-	-	NPs with surfacephosphatidic acid and cardiolipin demonstrated pronounced affinity to Aβ1e42 fibrils	[160]
-	Liposomes	Peptide from the apolipoprotein-E receptor- binding domain, phosphatedic acid.	Dimyristoyl-PA, sphingomyelin, CL.	121 ± 7	−18.7 ± 4	-	-	0.15	i.p.	Decrease of the total brain-insoluble amyloid peptide was demonstrated. Amelioration of mice impaired memory was observed.	[161]
-	Liposomes	MethoxyXO4	DSPE-PEG, CL, DPPC.	150	-	-	-	-	i.v.	The NPs appeared to cross the BBB and to bind with Aβ plaque deposits, marketing the parenchymal amyloid deposits and vascular amyloid.	[162]
-	Apolipoprotein E3 NPs	High density lipoprotein	Lipid free ApoE3, DMPC.	27.9 ± 8.9	−4.07 ± 0.83	-	-	0.30	i.v.	Four-week daily treatment with NPs decreased Aβ deposition, attenuated microgliosis, ameliorated neurologic changes, and rescued memory deficits in an AD animal model.	[163]
-	Monodisperse iron Oxide NPs	Monoclonal antibody against fibrillar human amyloid-β	-	8	-	-	-	-	i.v.	The targeting ability of NPs to cerebrovascular amyloid was demonstrated.	[164]
-	Gold NPs	peptide CLPFFD, peptide sequence THRPPMWSPVWP	Gold (III) chloride hydrate.	13 ± 1.7	−41 ± 2	-	-	-	i.p.	Increase of the permeability of the conjugate into the brain was shown.	[165]

Table 4. *Cont.*

Drug	Nanocarrier	Targeting Ligand	Components	PS, nm	ZP, mV	EE, %	LC, %	PDI	In Vivo Route of Administration	Outcomes	References
-	Gold NPs	-	Gold NPs, polyoxometalate with Wells–Dawson structure, Aβ1-40 peptide	21.7	−36.8	-	-	-	i.v.	NPs inhibited Aβ aggregation, dissociated Aβ fibrils and decreased Aβ -mediated peroxidase activity and Aβ -induced cytotoxicity.	[166]
-	Gold NPs	-	Gold colloid solution	10 ± 2	-	-	-	-	-	NPs disrupted insulin amyloid fibrillation resulting in construction of fibrils that are shorter and more compact.	[167]
-	PEG-coated cerium oxide NPs	Aβ antibody	PEG	-	−37	-	-	-	-	The rescue of neuronal survival was demonstrated.	[168]
Tau–Related Nanoparticles											
Nicotin-amide	Solid lipid NPs	-	Stearic acid, phospholipon® 90G, sodium taurocholate. Three types of particles functionalized by phosphatidic acid, polysorbate 80, phosphatidylserine.	124 ± 0.8	−46.1 ± 0.65	41.3 ± 0.41	-	-	i.p., i.v.	The phosphatidylserine-functionalized NPs improved the cognition, preserving the neuronal cells and reducing tau hyperphosphorylation in a rat model of AD.	[169]
Methylene blue	PLGA NPs	-	PLGA-b-PEG	136.5 ± 4.4	-	-	-	-	-	The reduction of both endogenous and over expressed tau protein levels in human neuroblastoma SHSY-5Y and HeLa cells was shown.	[170]
-	Protein-capped metal NPs	-	Two types of NPs: iron oxide (Fe_3O_4) NPsare capped with hydrolytic proteins from fungi, cadmium sulfide (CdS) NPs are capped with the mixture of four different proteins.	10–20	-	-	-	-	-	CdS NPs demonstrated dual properties of inhibition and disaggregation of Tau.	[171]
Acetylcholinesterase Inhibitors											
Gal	Solid lipid NPs	-	Plu F127, Tween 80, glyceryl behenate.	92.0 ± 3.51	−17.22 ± 1.1	83.42 ± 0.63	-	0.380 ± 0.16	p.o.	NPs restored memory in cognitive deficit rats. Increased bioavailability compared to the plain drug was demonstrated.	[172]

Table 4. *Cont.*

Drug	Nanocarrier	Targeting Ligand	Components	PS, nm	ZP, mV	EE, %	LC, %	PDI	In Vivo Route of Administration	Outcomes	References
Gal	Flexible liposomes	-	Propylene glycol, soya PC, CL	112 ± 8	−49.2 ± 0.7	83.6 ± 1.8	-	-	i.n., p.o.	The efficiency of acetylcholinesterase inhibition was greatly enhanced by i.n. administration compared with p.o. administration, especially after loading of the drug in flexible liposomes.	[173]
Gal	Nano-emulsions	-	PLGA	21.5 ± 0.25	−11.18 ± 0.89	98.47 ± 0.43	56.87 ± 3.48	-	-	Non-cytotoxic drug-loaded NPs have been obtained with high encapsulation efficiencies and sustained drug release, maintaining drug pharmacological activity.	[174]
Gal	CS complex NPs	-	CS, Tween 80, sodium tripolyphosphate	-	-	-	-	-	i.n.	NPs exhibited a significant decrease of AChE protein level and activity in rat brains.	[175]
Gal	CS NPs	-	CS, sodium tripolyphosphate.	190 ± 1.159	+ 31.6 ± 9.75	23.34	9.86	0.276 ± 0.006	i.n.	NPs were detected in the olfactory bulb, hippocampus, orbitofrontal and parietal cortices 1 h after i.n. administration.	[176]
Donepezil	Liposomes	-	CL, PEG, DSPC.	102 ± 3.3	−28.31 ± 0.85	84.91 ± 3.31	-	0.28 ± 0.03	i.n.	The bioavailability of drug in the plasma and in the brain increased significantly. The formulation was safe and free from toxicity	[177]
Donepezil	Nano suspension	-	CS, tripolyphosphate.	150–200	-	92–96	40–48	0.341	i.n.	No mortality, hematological changes, body weight variations and toxicity in animals were observed.	[178]
Donepezil	Mango gum polymeric NPs	-	CS, mango gum, Span 80. NPs were prepared by two methods.	135. 55, 95.1 2	+ 8.2 5, + 25.9 2	72 ± 3.62, 85 ± 2.14	51 ± 5.42, 76 ± 2.26	0.53, 0.26	i.v.	The brain targeting was achieved.	[179]
Donepezil	PLGA-b-PEG nanoparticles	-	PLGA, PEG, Plu F68.	174-240	From −11.32 to −20.49	52–61	-	0.20–0.36	-	NPs crossed the BBB and showed a controlled release profile in this system. NPs administration caused a significant dose-dependent decrease in both gene and protein expression levels of IL-1b, IL-6, GM-CSF and TNF-a.	[180]
Hup	Nano structured lipid carriers	-	Cetyl Palmitate, Miglyol®812, soybean PC, Solutol HS15®	120	−22.93 ± 0.91	89.180.28	1.460.05	-	-	A burst release at the initial stage and followed by a prolonged release of drug from NPs was up to 96 h.	[181]

Table 4. *Cont.*

Drug	Nanocarrier	Targeting Ligand	Components	PS, nm	ZP, mV	EE, %	LC, %	PDI	In Vivo Route of Administration	Outcomes	References
Hup	Micro emulsion, solid lipid NPs, nano-structured lipid carriers.	-	Glyceryl monostearate, glyceryl mono-dicaprylate, TranscutolP, Tween 80, triethanolamine.	119–148	From −4 to −20	60.05 ± 5.84	-	0.3–0.422	t.d.	In vitro permeation profiles in rat skin exhibited zero-order kinetics. The significant improvement in cognitive function in mice was observed.	[182]
Hup	Nanoemulsion	Lf	Isopropyl myristate, Capryol 90, Cremophor EL, Labrasol.	15.24 ± 0.67	−4.48 ± 0.97	-	-	0.128 ± 0.025	i.n.	Intranasal Lf-nanoemulsion significantly enhanced drug delivery to the brain compared to pure nanoemulsion.	[183]
Hup	Mucoadhesive and targeted PLGA NPs	Lf	N-trimethylated CS, PLGA 5050 2A.	153.2 ± 13.7	+35.6 ± 5.2	73.8 ± 5.7	-	0.229 ± 0.078	i.n.	The NPs facilitated the distribution of drug in the brain.	[184]
Tacrine	In situ gels	-	Plu F127, Plu F68, CS, PEG 8000	-	-	-	-	-	i.n.	The enhanced nasal residence time, improved bioavailability, increased brain uptake of the drug and decreased exposure of metabolites were shown.	[185]
Tacrine	Albumin NPs carrying beta cyclodextrin and two beta cyclodextrin derivatives	-	Beta cyclodextrinderivatives, hydroxypropyl beta cyclodextrin, sulphobutylether beta cyclodextrin.	177–266	From −10 to −10.9	85–91	12.5–22.0	0.228–0.327	i.n.	The presence of the different beta cyclodextrins affected drug loading and differently modulated NPs mucoadhesiveness and drug permeation.	[186]
Tacrine	CS NPs	-	CS, Polysorbate 80	41 ± 7	+34.7 ± 1.5	77–83	10,86 ± 0,30	-	i.v.	The NPs coated with 1% Polysorbate 80 altered the biodistribution pattern of NPs.	[187]
Riv	Nano structured lipid carriers	-	Glyceryl monosterate, Capmul MCM C8, lecithin, stearylamine, Tween 80	123.2 ± 2.3	32 ± 1.2	68.3 ± 3.4	-	-	i.n., i.v.	The faster regain of memory loss in amnesic mice with 5-fold decrease in escape latency with NC compared to plain rivastigmine solution was shown.	[188]
Riv	Liposomes	-	1,2-Diacyl-sn-glycero -3-phosphocholine, dihexadecyl phosphate, CL	67,51–528.7	From −6.6 to −25.1	75–97	-	0.612–0.755	Subcutaneously	NPs resulted in faster memory regain and amelioration of metabolic disturbances in AD rats.	[189]

Table 4. *Cont.*

Drug	Nanocarrier	Targeting Ligand	Components	PS, nm	ZP, mV	EE, %	LC, %	PDI	In Vivo Route of Administration	Outcomes	References
Riv	Liposomes	-	Soya lecithin, CL	10.0 ± 2.8 μm	-	80.0 ± 5.0	-	-	i.n., p.o.	Intranasal liposomes demonstrated a longer half-life in the brain than intranasally or orally administered pure drug.	[190]
Riv	Liposomes	Cell penetrating peptide	DSPE-PEG, CL, egg PC	178.9 ± 11.7	−8.6 ± 2.4	30.5 ± 8.0	-	0.333 ± 0.032	i.n., i.v.	i.n. administration demonstrated the capacity to improve rivastigmine distribution and adequate retention in CNS regions compared to i.v. administration.	[191]
Riv	Liposomes	-	CL, DPPC, methyl cellulose, dimethyl-β-CD, sodium taurocholate	3.37 ± 0.00 μm	−4.30 ± 0.66	25,2	-	-	p.o., i.p.	The highest acetylcholinesterase inhibition was observed for rivastigmine-sodium-taurocholate liposomes.	[192]
Riv	PLGA NPs, PBCA NPs	-	PLGA, PBCA	135.6 ± 4.2, 146.8 ± 2.7	−23.7 ± 1.18, −3.9 ± 0.58 m	74.46 ± 0.76, 57.32 ± 0.91	-	-	i.v.	The faster regain of memory loss in amnesic mice with both PLGA and PBCA NPs compared to rivastigmine solution was demonstrated.	[193]
Riv	CS NPs	-	CS, Polysorbate 80	45,16 ± 1,56	35.08 ± 1. 5	83.26 ± 3.1	43.48 ± 1.3 0	-	i.v.	The Polysorbate 80 Coated CS NPs of rivastigmine was formulated and evaluated for brain delivery.	[194]
Riv	CS NPs	-	CS	185.4 ± 8.4	38.4 ± 2.85	85.3 ± 3.5	43.37 ± 3.9	0.391 ± 0.065	i.n., i.v.	NPs demonstrated better brain targeting efficiency and represented a promising approach for i.n. delivery of rivastigmine for the treatment and prevention of AD.	[195]
Others											
p38 MAPK inhibitor PH797804	Nanoemulsion-based CS nanocapsules	-	Span 85, oleic acid, Tween 20, CS.	406.1	−18.5 ± 2.9	21.5 ± 2.7	3.5 ± 0.5	0.287	i.n.	The p38 MAPK inhibitor encapsulated in CS nanocapsules reduces p38 MAPK activity in brain cells in the cerebral cortex and hippocampus to a lower extent.	[196]
Erythropoie-tin	Solid lipid NPs	-	Glycerin monostearate, Span 80, Span 60, dichloromethane, Tween 80	219.9 ± 15.6	−22.4 ± 0.8	-	-	(0.187 ± 0.03	i.p.	NPs reduced the oxidative stress, and beta-amyloid plaque deposition in the hippocampus more effectively than the pure drug. The memory was significantly restored in cognitive deficit rats treated with NPs.	[197]

Table 4. *Cont.*

Drug	Nanocarrier	Targeting Ligand	Components	PS, nm	ZP, mV	EE, %	LC, %	PDI	In Vivo Route of Administration	Outcomes	References
Piperine	Monoolein cubosomes	-	Peceol®, Tween 80, poloxamer, Cremophor.	167.00 ± 10.49	−34.60 ± 0.47	86.67 ± 0.62	-	0.18 ± 0.01	p.o.	The NPs significantly enhanced drug cognitive effect and even restored cognitive function to the normal level.	[198]
NAP	High density lipoprotein nanostructure	Mono sialotetrahexosyl ganglioside (GM1)	apoE3-reconstituted high density lipoprotein (rHDL), 1,2-dimyristoyl-sn-glycero3-phosphocholine (DMPC) liposome	25.42 ± 1.18	−15.70 ± 0.93	64.39 ± 12.84	-	0.218	i.n.	Protection of neurons from cell toxicity, a reduction of Aβ deposition and a rescue of memory in AD model mice were demonstrated.	[199]
NAP	PEG-PCL NPs	Lf	PEG-PCL, coumarin-6.	88.4 ± 7.8	23.56 ± 0.96	47.61 ± 2.36	0.62 ± 0.013	0.22 ± 0.033	i.n.	The neuroprotective and memory improvement effect of Lf-NP was observed. These results were also confirmed by the evaluation of acetylcholinesterase, choline acetyltransferase activity and neuronal degeneration in the mice hippocampus.	[200]
Metal chelatorclio-quinol	Gold NP-capped mesoporous silica	-	Mesoporous silica NPs (*N*-Cetyl trimethylammonium bromide, tetraethoxysilane)	52.13	+26.7	-	-	-	i.v.	The NPs reduced the cell membrane disruption, microtubular defects and apoptosis.	[201]
Selenium, sialic acid	Sialic acid modified selenium NPs	Peptide-B6	Sodiumselenite,	95	−14.4	-	-	-	-	The high permeability across the BBB was shown. The effectively inhibition Aβ aggregation was demonstrated. Therefore, NC did not disaggregate preformed Aβ fibrils into non-toxic amorphous oligomers.	[202]
Resveratrol, grape extract	Solid lipid NPs	Antitransferrin receptor mono clonal antibody (OX26 mAb)	Cetylpalmitate, polysorbate 80.	254 ± 17	−4.0 ± 0.1	92 ± 7, 95 ± 2	-	0.23 ± 0.05	-	The cellular uptake of the OX26 NPs was substantially more efficient than that of normal NPs and NPs functionalized with an unspecific antibody.	[203]
Resveratrol (Res)	Delivery system MSe-Res/Fc-β-CD/Bor	-	Mesoporous nano-selenium (MSe), β-CD, borneolBor)	160	-	>70	-	-	i.v.	NC inhibited aggregation of Aβ, mitigated oxidative stress, suppressed tau hyperphosphorylation and improving memory impairment in AD mice.	[204]
Memantine	Polyamido amine (PAMAM) dendrimers	Lf	PAMAM	131.72 ± 4.73	+ 20.13 ± 0.94	71.1 ± 4.84	-	0.16 ± 0.025	i.v.	A significant improvement in behavioral responses was demonstrated.	[205]

Table 4. *Cont.*

Drug	Nanocarrier	Targeting Ligand	Components	PS, nm	ZP, mV	EE, %	LC, %	PDI	In Vivo Route of Administration	Outcomes	References
Lipoyl–memantine	Solid lipid NPs	-	Stearic acid	170	−33.8	88	-	0.072	Through the gastrointestinal tract	The NPs demonstrated low toxicity.	[206]
Amlodipine	Diamond NPs	-	Nanodiamond powder	31.1 ± 8.2	-	41	-	-	-	The highest percentage of loaded amlodipine onto nanodiamond particles was achieved in alkaline medium using 2 mMNaOH at a corresponding pH of 8.5.	[207]
Curcumin	Low density lipoprotein mimic nanostructured lipid carrier	Lf	Carboxylated PEG (100) monostearate, CL, glycerol trioleate	103.8 ± 0.6	−5.80 ± 0.73	96.51 ± 1.87	2.60 ± 0.17	0.15 ± 0.022	i.v.	The Lf NPs could effectively permeate BBB and preferentially accumulate in the brain. Superior efficacy of Lf NPs in controlling the damage associated with AD.	[208]
Curcumin	RBC membrane camouflaged HSANPs	T807, tri phenyl phosphine (TPP)	Amino-T807, carboxy-TPP, PEG, red blood cell (RBC) membrane, human serum albumin (HAS).	<120	-	88.43 ± 1.25	4.87 ± 1.04	-	i.v.	The NPs relieved AD symptoms by mitigating mitochondrial oxidative stress and suppressing neuronal death.	[209]
Curcumin, NGF	Liposomes	Wheat germ agglutinin (WGA), cardiolipin (CL)	CL, soybean PC, 1,2-Dipalmitoylsn-glycero-3-phosphocholine.	122–142	−5.2 to −18.3	20.5–56.7	-	-	i.v.	The NPs inhibited the expression of phosphorylated p38, prevented neurodegeneration of cells, enhanced the quantities of p-neurotrophic tyrosine kinase receptor type 1 and p-extracellular signal-regulated kinase 5.	[210]
Curcumin, selenium	PLGA nanospheres	-	PLGA, selenium NPs	160 ± 5	-	-	11.5	Low	i.v.	The NPs provided the enhanced therapeutic efficacy in AD lesions.	[211]
Curcumin or dexamethasone	Polymeric nanocore	Antiamyloid antibody IgG4.1	CS, gadolinium-diethylene triamine pentaacetic acid, hydroxypropyl-beta-cyclodextran, Magnevist®, 125I	145 ± 5,4, 157,6 ± 3,4	7,7 ± 0,4, 4,5 ± 0,5	-	-	-	i.v.	The NPs targeted cerebrovascular amyloid deposits selectively.	[212]
Andrographolide	Human albumin NPs	-	Human albumin	210.4 ± 3.2	−20.3 ± 1.5	99.1 ± 0.2	-	0.10 ± 0.01	i.v., i.p.	In the step-down inhibitory avoidance test, NPs improved mice performance. The presence of NPs both in the pE3-Aβ plaque surroundings and inside the pE3-Aβ plaque was observed. The anti-inflammatory activity was shown.	[213]

Table 4. *Cont.*

Drug	Nanocarrier	Targeting Ligand	Components	PS, nm	ZP, mV	EE, %	LC, %	PDI	In Vivo Route of Administration	Outcomes	References
Flurbiprofen	Dendrimer NPs	-	Phenylalanine	-	-	-	-	-	-	Efficiency of NC influence on the γ-secretase enzyme in target cells was shown. Eventual drug release by hydrolysis of the carrier was demonstrated.	[214]
Tarenflurbil (TFB)	Solid lipid NPs, PLGA NPs	-	Monostearate, stearic acid, soya lecithin, Tween 20, PLGA, DMAB, PF-68, PVA	169.87 ± 10.98, 133.13 ± 7.82	−23.13 ± 2.32, −30.25 ± 2.11	57.81 ± 5.32, 64.11 ± 2.21	−10	0.24 ± 0.04, 0.21 ± 0.02	i.n.	The absolute bioavailability of the NPs was higher than TFB solution suspension.	[215]
Metformin	Nano liposomes	-	Phosphatidylserine.	148.3 ± 5.6	−34.8 ± 2.8	37 ± 2.3	-	<0.3	i.p.	The learning and memory parameters significantly improved in AD-rats treated with NPs. The decreased cytokine levels of IL1-β, TNF-α and TGF-β in hippocampal tissues were shown. A reduction in inflammatory and necrotic neural cells, and an increase neurogenesis was demonstrated.	[216]
Saxagliptin	CS-L-valine based NPs	L-valin	CS, BocL-valine	385 ± 21	+ 0.554 ± 0.110	56.23 ± 13.44	-	0.574 ± 0.125	i.p.	The NPs were highly stable in the plasma releasing only a minute after administration of the drug. Pronounced accumulation of drug from the NPs was demonstrated. The pure substance showed no detectable amount of the drug after 24 h.	[217]
NGF	Liposomes	Lf	CL, DSPE-PEG, DPPC, PEPEG	About 110	From −3 to −11	-	-	-	-	Lf/NGF-liposomes comprising CL and DPPC were physically stable with high biocompatibility to HBMECs and HAs cells.	[218]
NGF	Liposomes	P-aminophenyl-a D manno-pyrano-side, apolipo protein E	Soybean PC, phosphatidic acid, DPPC, cardiolipin, DSPE-PEG, CL	<170	From −4 to −10	35.1 ± 3.2	-	-	-	NPs were capable to enhance the NGF delivery across the BBB. NPs recognized a low-density lipoprotein receptor expressed by SK-N-MC cells and yielded neuroprotective effect on the neuronal degeneration induced by fibrillar Aβ1–42.	[219]

Table 4. *Cont.*

Drug	Nanocarrier	Targeting Ligand	Components	PS, nm	ZP, mV	EE, %	LC, %	PDI	In Vivo Route of Administration	Outcomes	References
NGF	Liposomes	Cereport trans-ferrin	L-α-PC, DPPC, CL, DSPE-PEG-carboxy.	152-189	from −4.5 to −8.5	31.2 ± 2.8	-	-	-	Covering of NPs with cereport and transferrin was effective in carrying NGF across the BBB and rescued the apoptosis of SK-N-MC cells after neurotoxic treatment with Aβ1–42.	[220]
Fibroblast growth factor	PEG-PLGA NPs	Solanum tubero-sum lectin	PEG-PLGA	118.7	−31,18	69.21	0.0462	-	i.n.	Neuroprotective effect in AD rats was demonstrated.	[221]
Pituitary adenylate cyclaseactivating Polypeptide (PACAP38) coupled to a docosahexaenoic acid (DHA: an ω-3 polyunsaturated fatty acid)	Pep-lipid nanostructures and liquid crystalline nanocarriers	-	PACAP-DHA/MO (nonlamellar lipid monoolein)/DHA/ vitamin E/VPGS-PEG1000 and MO/DHA/vitamin E/VPGS-PEG1000	~100	-	-	-	-	-	Multicompartment nanocarriers with PACAP and DHA are promising therapy strategies for neurodegenerative disorders. PACAP is neuropeptide ligand of the PAC1 membrane receptor (a class B GPCR). PACAP demonstrate antiapoptotic effects in neuronal and non-neuronal cells, neuroprotive and neurotransmitter properties, can act as neurotrophic factor, attenuates Aβ amyloid toxicity. DHA plays a crucial role in the control of the phospholipid membrane organization, act as lipid trophic factor, demonstrated antiapoptotic, neuroprotective effect, take part in inflammatory cell signaling. Vitamin E reduces oxidative stress, demonstrates anti-inflammatory, cardio and neuroprotective effects, inhibit lipid peroxidation.	[222]
-	Amphiphilic yellow-emissive carbon dots (Y-CDs)	-	Citric acid, o-phenylenediamine.	3.4 ± 1.0	−15.3	-	-	-	Injected into the heart.	Y-CDs entered cells to inhibit the overexpression of human amyloid precursor protein and β-amyloid.	[223]
-	Nanosystem CB-Gd-Cy5.5	Holera toxin B subunit (CB)	Chelated gadolinium (Gd), Cyanine5.5 (Cy5.5).	110	−11.0	-	-	-	i.n.	The nanosystem was accumulated in the hippocampus and demonstrated good magnetic resonance imaging capability satisfying the monitoring of AD at the different stages.	[224]

Table 4. *Cont.*

Drug	Nanocarrier	Targeting Ligand	Components	PS, nm	ZP, mV	EE, %	LC, %	PDI	In Vivo Route of Administration	Outcomes	References
-	Fe_3O_4 NPs loaded with PEG-PLGA nano composite	Anti-transferrin mono clonal antibody (OX26) receptor	Fe_3O_4NPs, PEG, PLGA.	95	-	76.2	18.1	-	-	The significant in vitro drug release and cell viability were shown.	[225]
-	Carboxyl magnetic nano containers	-	Fluorescent Carboxyl Magnetic Particles, Yellow, 1% *w/v*	700–900	-	-	-	-	i.v.	The magnetic NPs crossed the normal BBB in mice after subjection to external electromagnetic fields of 28 mT (0.43 T/m) and 79.8 mT (1.39 T/m).	[226]
-	Gold NPs	-	Gold NPs suspension	5	−47.7 ± 10.9	-	-	-	i.p.	The NPs improved the acquisition and retention of spatial learning and memory in Aβ treated rats. Expression of BDNF, cAMP, CREB and stromal interaction molecules, e.g., STIM1 and STIM2 was increased.	[227]

AD—Alzheimer's disease; Aβ—amyloid-β peptide; BBB—Blood–brain barrier; NC—nanocarrier; NPs—nanoparticles; PS—particle size; ZP—zeta potential; EE—drug entrapment efficiency; LC—loading capacity; PDI—polydispersity index; i.m.—Intramuscular route of administration; i.n.—intranasal route of administration; i.p.—intraperitoneal route of administration; i.v.—intravenous route of administration; p.o.—per oral route of administration; t.d.—transdermal route of administration; BDNF—brain-derived neurotrophic factor; CL—cholesterol; CS—chitosan; DPPC—1,2-dipalmitoyl-sn-glycero-3- phosphocholine; DMPC—1,2-dimyristoyl-sn-glycero-3-phosphocholine; DSPC—1,2-distearyl-sn-glycero-3-phosphocholine; DSPE-PEG—1,2-distearoyl-sn-glycero-3- phosphoethanolamine-N-[carboxy(polyethylene glycol); Gal—galantamine hydrobromide; Hup—huperzine A; Lf—lactoferrin; NAP—neuroprotective peptide NAPVSIPQ; NGF—neuron growth factor; PC—phosphatidylcholine; PEG—(poly(ethylene glycol); PEG-PCL—poly(ethylene glycol)-co-poly(ε-caprolactone) copolymer; PEPEG—1,2-dipalmitoyl-sn-glycero-3-phosphoethanol- amine-N-[methoxy(polyethylene glycol)-2000]; PLA—poly(lactic acid); PLGA—poly(lactic-co-glycolic acid); PVA—polyvinyl alcohol; siRNA—small interfering RNAs; Plu—pluronic; Riv—rivastigmine;.

7.1. Nanoparticles with High Affinity to Aβ1–42 Peptide

This type of nanocarriers represents a completely new approach to treating AD. Such a method includes application of multifunctional nanoparticles modified by antitransferrin antibodies in combination with MAbs-IgG domains and transferrin ligands for delivery of the iAβ5 peptide, inhibiting the aggregates associated with AD [228]. Another strategy involves monoclonal antibodies (MAbs) targeting Aβ fibril formation [164]. For example, Kuo with coauthors investigated various modifications of gold nanoparticle systems loaded with the neuron growth factor in combination with transferrin, lactoferrin, p-aminophenyl-alpha-d-mannopyranoside and apolipoprotein E and added peptide sequence [218–220]. This sequence interacts with the transferrin receptor present in the microvascular endothelial cells of the blood–brain barrier, thus causing an increase in the permeability of the conjugate in brain, as shown by experiments in vitro and in vivo. It is highly relevant for the therapeutic applications of gold nanoparticles for molecular surgery in the treatment of neurodegenerative diseases such as AD. By irradiation with weak microwaves, Ab aggregates bound to the conjugate peptide sequence with a gold nanoparticle were destroyed by local dissipation of the absorbed energy in vitro [165]. Along with gold nanoparticles PLGA nanoparticles with surface functionalized by antitransferrin receptor monoclonal antibody (OX26) and anti-Aβ (DE2B4) have also been developed for the delivery of encapsulated iAβ5 into the brain. This system efficacy and toxicity were evaluated with porcine brain capillary endothelial cells (PBCECs) used as a BBB model [158].

Another form of nanocarriers [162] presents the construction of Aβ-targeted stealth liposomal nanoparticles using the Aβ-targeted lipid conjugate DSPE-PEG with Methoxy-XO4, which interconnect with amyloid. It was demonstrated that these nanoparticles selectively bind to amyloid plaques in the brain tissue of APP/PSEN1 transgenic mice. Ex vivo analyses of brain samples showed that injected nanoparticles efficiently bind both parenchymal plaques and cerebral amyloid angiopathy associated amyloid throughout the brain [162]. Along with other nanocarriers PEG coated and anti-Ab antibody-conjugated antioxidant (cerium oxide) nanoparticles were developed, and their effects on neuronal survival and BDNF signaling pathway were examined. For this nanoparticles protective effect against oxidative stress and Ab-mediated neurodegeneration were reported. In particular, these nanoforms specifically targets the Ab aggregates, produce an antioxidant effect and thereby perform neuroprotection [168].

β-sheet breaker peptides compose a class of compounds that are highly potent in Aβ1−42- or α-synuclein-inflicted cell toxicity neutralization. β-sheet breaker peptides are highly effective for Aβ amyloidogenesis inhibition as they are homologous to regions of the β-sheet hydrophobic carboxyl segments [229]. These peptides represent oligopeptides structurally analogous to specific epitopes of Aβ. Such substances have been also loaded in nanocarriers for Aβ-targeted delivery. It was demonstrated that the use of gold nanoparticles loaded with LPFFD peptide induces Aβ-aggregate inhibition, Aβ fibrils dissociation and Aβ-mediated peroxidase reduction [166]. TGN TGNYKALHPHNG and QSH D-enantiomeric peptide QSHYRHISPAQV were also conjugated to the surface of the nanoparticles for blood–brain barrier transport and Aβ42 targeting. Nanoparticles implication enhanced bioavailability of drug in the brain and produced neuroprotective effects in the mouse model of AD in vivo [159]. In another work [230] researchers developed a dual-functional nanoparticle drug delivery system loaded with β-sheet breaker peptide H102 (HKQLPFFEED). This peptide was encapsulated into liposomes to reduce the degradation level and was administrated nasally to increase brain penetration. It was demonstrated that the nanosystem application recovered spatial memory impairment in AD model rats both in a low dose and in a high dose [230].

Liposomes are frequently used for drug delivery during targeted AD therapy. For example, liposome nanoparticles are loaded with Aβ1–42 ligands with high affinity, phosphatidic acid and cardiolipin phospholipids [160]. Another research demonstrates the induction of amyloid degradation via administration of apolipoprotein E3-reconstituted high-density lipoprotein nanoparticles bond with Aβ oligomers [163]. Therapeutic effect was also reported for bifunctional liposomes, loaded with phosphatidic acid and peptide derived from apolipoprotein-E receptor-binding domain. In particular, peptide implication allowed penetrating through BBB and phosphatidic acid use caused Aβ aggregates degradation in APP/PS1 transgenic mice [161]. Thus, liposome administration reduced amyloid concentration and improved cognitive function in transgenic mice [161].

Nanoparticles using Congo Red/Rutin/MNP are another method of AD treatment. It was shown that the intranasal administration of Congo Red/Rutina-MNP contributed to the dissipation of amyloid plaques in MRI, increased drug delivery and reduced the production of active oxygen forms and Aβ-induced cytotoxicity in vitro. The intravenous administration of such nanosystems also increased the detection of amyloid aggregates, prevented memory deficit and neurological disorders in transgenic APPswe/PS1dE9 mice in vivo [231].

Multifunctional nanoparticles are being also used for diagnostic and therapy of other pathologies associated with Aβ accumulation. One of them is cerebral amyloid angiopathy described as a condition resulted from Aβ protein lodgment within the walls of cerebral vascular cells. The peptide accumulation leads to vascular inflammation and periodic hemorrhagic strokes. Therapeutic nano-transportable vehicles containing a polymeric core of chitosan-conjugated magnetivist (magnetic resonance imaging (MRI) contrast agent) have been developed for the treatment and early diagnosis cerebral amyloid angiopathy [157]. Cyclophosphamine, an agent that suppresses inflammation of brain vessels, was also loaded into the THB nanonucleus, and a Putreskin-modified F(ab′)2 fragment of an antiamyloid antibody, IgG4.1 (pF(ab′)24.1), was bound to the surface of the nanonucleus to target the cerebrovascular amyloid. Similar systems have already been tested in vitro with human endothelial cells (hCMEC/D3) and in vivo in laboratory mice [157]. It has been shown that other anti-inflammatory and antiamyloidogenic agents capable of reducing the inflammation of cerebrovascular vessels can also be loaded into such nanotransport systems [212].

7.2. Drugs Directed on the Inhibition of Tau Aggregation

Tau represents an intracellular protein, playing a crucial role in the microtubules stabilization. It was demonstrated that tau protein could respond to various factors via aggregates formation. The accumulation of these aggregates induces neurofibrillary tangles conglomeration in neurons and neurodegeneration. As the peptide contains two hexapeptide motifs in the repeat region, after pathological impact tau can randomly coil into the β-sheet structure and perform aggregation.

By now serious research has been done in the field of protein aggregation prevention in neurodegenerative diseases. In spite of investigation of various drugs from different classes like peptide inhibitors, natural substances, etc., little success was achieved. Some research has been performed in the area of nanoparticles, which offers a challenge in AD treatment improvement.

For example, a tau aggregation suppressor phenothiazine was loaded in polymer-based (PLGA-PEG) hydrophobic–glutathione coated nanoparticles [170]. Moreover, for some types of nanocarriers aggregation inhibitory activity were demonstrated of its own accord. The cadmium sulfide and iron oxide (Fe_3O_4) nanoparticles inhibit tau fibrillization in vitro. Despite its antiaggregation activity and excellent delivery properties, the in vivo experiments are hampered by interfering molecular species [171].

Red blood cell membrane-coated PLGA particles with T807 can also be used as a resource for tau aggregation inhibition. As T807 demonstrates high permeability for neurons and pronounced p-tau-specific tracing activity, it can be considered as a therapeutic agent of targeted delivery for AD treatment. One more virtue of that type of nanocarriers is red blood cell membranes, characterized by low immunogenicity and long half-life in the circulation, which allow performing effective drug delivery. Synergetic action of T807 with triphenylphosphine (TPP) produces an inhibitory effect on key components of AD pathogenesis associated with tau-phosphorylation and prevents neurodegeneration. Thus, the systemic administration red blood cell PLGA nanoparticles loaded with curcumin recover cognitive impairments in the mouse model of AD [232].

7.3. Acetylcholinesterase Inhibitors (AChE)

This class of drugs is characterized by many side effects due to their action on the peripheral tissues, high doses of administration and hepatic metabolism. These side effects are aggravated by the low pharmacokinetic (half-life) profiles of the drugs [150]. The loading of such preparation into nanocontainers would help to eliminate these side effects and to improve their bioavailability to the brain via an intranasal form.

One of the drugs used to treat AD is rivastigmine, which inhibits both the AChE and butyrylcholinesterase enzymes in brain and boosts the cholinergic function. It improves cognition and memory by increasing the ACh concentration in the brain. Nevertheless, the half-life period of rivastigmine in blood circulation is only 1.5 h, which complicates its therapeutic action. Loading drugs in nanocontainers increases its half-life and decreases the necessary dosage, thereby reducing side effects. For example, it has been already demonstrated for AChE inhibitors represented as naturally derived polyphenols, such as epigallocatechin-3-gallate and catechin placed into the sodium-taurocholate liposomal carrier [192], cholesterol/soy-lecithinated liposomal NP formulation [190], PLGA, PEG and gold NPs [233]. Yang and colleagues have also performed analysis of rivastigmine-liposome and CPP27 modified rivastigmine-loaded liposome for intranasal administration and showed the improvement of drug activity [191]. In particular, it was demonstrated that CPP modification increases the drug diffusion across the BBB by enhanced transcytosis and cell membrane permeability. It was acknowledged by the pharmacokinetic study indicated a significant increase of drug concentration in the various regions of the brain like cortex, hippocampus, and olfactory regional. Additionally, that modification has not exerted any toxic effects in the nasal cavity and in the brain. Improved drug properties were also demonstrated for rivastigmine via various nanoparticles. For example, rivastigmine-loaded mucoadhesive NP developed by Fazil et al., PLGA, PBCA NP by Joshi et al. and chitosan (polysorbate 80-coated) NP by Khemariya et al. showed an increased bioavailability [193–195]. In was also shown that gelling cationic nanostructured lipid carriers enhance brain distribution and pharmacodynamics [188]. Moreover, liposomes with RHN increased half-life, decreased the toxicity and improved memory and neurological deficits in Male albino rat with the model of AD [189].

Another AChE inhibitor using for AD treatment is galantamine. Some studies reported that galantamine could also reduce Aβ aggregation and neurotoxicity. Nevertheless, the application of galantamine is limited by its side effects such as nausea, vomiting, dizziness, drowsiness, loss of appetite, etc. That makes it inconvenient for the long-term oral treatment. In addition, galantamine is not able to cross the BBB efficiently [33]. For this reason, NP can improve response and bioavailability of galantamine. For example, Hanafy and colleagues constructed chitosan nanoparticle and cationic nanoparticles for intranasal drug administration [175]. Li et al. developed liposomal system, as a drug carrier for efficient delivery of galantamine through intranasal administration [173]. Other research groups created PLGA [174] and solid lipid NP [172] with galantamine, which have not only increased its bioavailability but also improved cognitive function and memory in Wistar rats.

Donepezil is another frequently used drug for AD treatment, represented as a centrally acting reversible AChE inhibitor. It is characterized by high pharmacokinetic properties with 100% bioavailable and a biological half-life of 70 h. However, the long-term administration leads to severe side effects, especially when taken in a high dose (>10 mg/day) [234]. The development of chitosan nanosuspension for intranasal administration [178] and the chitosan intranasal form of donepezil [235] promoted the usage of lower drug dose. Along with these nanoparticles LGA-b-PEG by Baysal et al. and liposomes by Al Asmari et al. were constructed for this drug [177,180].

Tacrine is AChE inhibitor acting as a histamine N-methyltransferase inhibitor. This drug produces various side effects including not only nausea, vomiting, dizziness, drowsiness, hallucination, confusion, insomnia and anxiety, but also hepatotoxicity, convulsion, urinary tract infection, bradycardia, depression, hypotension, etc. For the problem solution Qian and colleagues have developed in situ gelling systems for intranasal administration of tacrine [185]. That drug form enhanced the substance retention time in the nasal cavity and improved the nasomucosal absorbance. Wilson et al. have constructed a tacrine loaded chitosan nanoparticle coated with polysorbate 80 and demonstrated the improvement of its biodistribution [197]. Luppi et al. has also developed albumin nanoparticles carrying cyclodextrins for nasal delivery and drug properties advance [186].

Huperzine is another preparation used for AD treatment. For improvement of it bioavailability some research groups also constructed NP. For example, Yang et al. created nanostructured lipid carriers [181]. The treatment with huperzine lipid NP performed by Patel et al. demonstrated behavioral and memory improvement in the mouse model of AD [182].

7.4. Memantine, the NMDA Receptors Antagonist

Memantine hydrochloride (MEM) is the only anti-AD drug used in the US and Europe for the moderate-to-severe form of AD. The labeled formulation for memantine hydrochloride is Namenda, which is prescribed in tablet or capsule form. MEM prevents the aggregation of Aβ1–40 and enhances memory in rodents. Despite the best results in improving cognitive impairments in patients, the clinical applicability of MEM is limited. MEM should be administered daily, which leads to poor compliance with the drug regimen [205]. The development of nanocarriers with memantine can help to solve these problems. Toxicologically safe lipid nanoparticles with lipoyl-memantine have been elaborated and can be used to deliver memantine to the brain [206]. Gothwal et al. (2019) developed memantine-loaded polyamidoamine dendrimers. He used lactoferrin as a targeting ligand. The profile of memantine release from nanoparticles was slow and persisted for up to 48 h. The brain absorption of NPs was significantly higher than that of pure memantine. The in vivo research in an AlCl3-induced AD mice model demonstrated a considerable improving in behavioral tests [205].

7.5. Other Drugs for AD Treatment

Many literature data suggest that various growth factors may have therapeutic potential in the AD treatment. In particular, growth factors such as basic fibroblast growth factor, neurotrophins (nerve growth factors; glial-derived neurotrophic factor and BDNF and insulin-like growth factor (IGF-1/IGF-2)) and bone morphogenetic proteins are promising molecules [236]. In such a way PEG-PLGA nanoparticles loaded with basic fibroblast growth factor have been shown to improve cognitive function in the Morris test in rats exposed to intraventricular administration of β-amyloid 25–35 and ionic acid [221].

Metal chelators are another potential drugs to treat AD because they block the effects of metal ions stimulating the formation of Aβ aggregates and active oxygen forms. However, their use is limited due to non-specific interactions with metal ions and the inability to pass through BBB. Such problems have been solved by using controlled release systems of gold nanoparticles with mesoporous silica based on H_2O_2. Loading metal chelator CQ in these nanocontainers allowed targeted CQ release in the brain areas where the level of H_2O_2 is increased, for example, in Aβ-plaques [201].

Several recent studies have demonstrated that some antidiabetic drugs also have a therapeutic potential in AD patients. For example, Hsieh and colleagues has shown the inhibitory effect of gold nanoparticles on the fibrillogenesis of insulin fibrils [167]. Gold nanoparticles, coincubated with insulin, retarded the structural transformation of insulin fibrils into amyloid-like fibrils for about a week [167]. The neuroprotective effect was also demonstrated for nanoparticles with peptide NAPVSIPQ as a model drug and lactoferrin as a targeting ligand, which improved cognitive function in mice. As lactoferrin is a natural iron binding protein, whose receptor is highly expressed in both respiratory epithelial cells and neurons, its administration facilitates the nose-to-brain drug delivery of neuroprotection peptides like NAPVSIPQ [200].

7.6. Others Methods of AD Treatment

Currently, siRNA gene therapy is a promising method of treating of many brain disorders. Potentially it can also be used for the treatment of AD. An example of such a therapy method is the inhibition of the Beta-Secretase 1 (BACE1), which leads to suppression of disease development.

Nanoparticles of the solid lipid with and without chitosan were used for directed delivery of BACE1 siRNA to the brain. These nanoparticles contained a RVG-9R peptide derived from the rabies virus glycoprotein, which enhanced the transcellular delivery of nanosystems to the brain during their intranasal injection. It was demonstrated that the investigated siRNA permeates the monolayer of the cell culture Caco-2 to a greater extent when released from nanocarriers, primarily from chitosan-coated solid lipid nanoparticles, than from bare siRNA [153].

The same research strategies were developed by other researchers. Wang and colleagues designed siRNA nanocarriers based on PEGylated poly(2-(*N*,*N*-dimethylamino) ethyl methacrylate) (PEG-PDMAEMA) modified with both the CGN peptide for BBB penetration and the Tet1 peptide for neuron-specific binding [154]. These nanocomplexes have been shown to successfully enter the cytoplasm of neurons, effectively suppressing the expression of BACE1 mRNA (by about 50%) and preventing synaptic damage caused by Aβ25-35. These results were also confirmed by studies of transgenic APP/PS1 mice, where the administration of nanoparticles stimulated neurogenesis in the hippocampus, inhibited the formation of amyloid plaques and tau-protein by repression of BACE1 mRNA. The administration of the nanocomplexes restored the cognitive function of the AD transgenic mice to the level of wild-type control without significant adverse effects on myelination [154].

Downregulation of the key enzyme in amyloid-β formation by delivering non-coding RNA plasmid is another potential way of AD treatment. It was shown that simultaneous delivery of the therapeutic peptide into the brain leads to the suppression of neurofibrillary tangles formation. In particular, a multifunctional nanocarrier contained the peptide to achieve the therapeutic gene, based on the PEGylated dendrigraphte of polylysines, has been developed for the treatment of AD [155]. Directional nanoparticle delivery has been investigated in transgenic AD mice [155].

Treatment of AD is extremely difficult because no precise mechanisms have been discovered for its development and pathogenesis. Despite that fact, a large number of different drug forms and therapy methods are being investigated. Among others, many nanocontainer systems have been constructed for different groups of drugs, inducing targeted delivery to pathological brain centers. Various clinical data provide an opportunity to hope that these strategies will bring their results.

8. Conclusions

The development of nanocontainer systems for the treatment of various diseases is a modern, promising and actively evolving field of science. Among other things, nanoparticles also contain agents for the treatment of neuropsychiatric diseases. All mental illnesses require long-term therapy, and patients need constant medication for months or even years. For this reason, it is important that the drug is delivered using nanocontainer systems that facilitate a longer release of the medicine. Various nanocontainers are opening up prospects for new forms of medication, such as subcutaneous transdermal drug delivery systems—"patches". Non-compliance with therapy in patients is a very common and serious problem, which can be solved by prescribing injections of long-acting drugs or implants. Many neuroleptics have low bioavailability when used orally due to liver metabolism and low brain permeability, and drug delivery systems can improve these indicators. Prolonged therapy inevitably leads to side effects. Studies of some combined medications for the treatment of neuropsychiatric diseases have shown a reduction in side effects compared to pure drugs. Thus, the use of nanocontainer systems for the delivery of antidepressants, antipsychotics and drugs for the treatment of neurodegenerative diseases can contribute to more effective therapy and improve patients' quality of life.

Author Contributions: Original draft preparation, Y.Z., O.A., V.U., A.M. (Anna Morozova); review and editing, E.Z.; review and editing of the part about types of nanocarriers P.M.; review and editing of the part about BBB penetration M.V.; supervision, V.C.; project administration, A.M. (Alexander Majouga); funding acquisition, A.M. (Alexander Majouga). All authors have read and agreed to the published version of the manuscript.

Abbreviations

AChE	acetylcholinesterase inhibitors
AD	Alzheimer's disease
BACE1	beta-Secretase 1
BBB	blood–brain barrier
BDNF	brain-derived neurotrophic factor
DOPE	dioleylphosphatidylethanolamine
FDA	U.S. Food and Drug Administration
Lf	lactoferrin
MAOIs	monoamine oxidase inhibitors
MEM	memantine hydrochloride
MRI	magnetic resonance imaging
NMDA	*N*-methyl-D-aspartate
NPs	nanoparticles
PEG	polyethylene glycol
PLA	polylactide acid
PLGA	poly lactic-co-glycolic acid
RES	reticuloendothelial system
SARIs	serotonin antagonists and reuptake inhibitors
SLNs	solid lipid nanoparticles
SNRIs	serotonin and norepinephrine reuptake inhibitors
SPIONs	superparamagnetic iron oxide nanoparticles
SSRIs	selective serotonin reuptake inhibitors
TCAs	tricyclic antidepressants

References

1. James, S.L.; Abate, D.; Abate, K.H.; Abay, S.M.; Abbafati, C.; Abbasi, N.; Abbastabar, H.; Abd-Allah, F.; Abdela, J.; Abdelalim, A.; et al. Global, regional, and national incidence, prevalence, and years lived with disability for 354 diseases and injuries for 195 countries and territories, 1990–2017: A systematic analysis for the Global Burden of Disease Study 2017. *Lancet* **2018**, *392*, 1789–1858. [CrossRef]
2. Agrahari, V. The exciting potential of nanotherapy in brain-tumor targeted drug delivery approaches. *Neural Regen. Res.* **2017**, *12*, 197–200. [CrossRef] [PubMed]
3. Rakotoarisoa, M.; Angelov, B.; Garamus, V.M.; Angelova, A. Curcumin- and fish oil-loaded spongosome and cubosome nanoparticles with neuroprotective potential against H_2O_2-induced oxidative stress in differentiated human SH-SY5Y cells. *ACS Omega* **2019**, *4*, 3061–3073. [CrossRef]
4. Deeken, J.F.; Löscher, W. The blood-brain barrier and cancer: Transporters, treatment, and Trojan horses. *Clin. Cancer Res.* **2007**, *13*, 1663–1674. [CrossRef] [PubMed]
5. Van Tellingen, O.; Yetkin-Arik, B.; De Gooijer, M.; Wesseling, P.; Wurdinger, T.; De Vries, H.E. Overcoming the blood–brain tumor barrier for effective glioblastoma treatment. *Drug Resist. Updates* **2015**, *19*, 1–12. [CrossRef] [PubMed]
6. Villabona-Rueda, A.; Erice, C.; Pardo, C.A.; Stins, M.F. The evolving concept of the blood brain barrier (BBB): From a single static barrier to a heterogeneous and dynamic relay center. *Front. Cell. Neurosci.* **2019**, *13*. [CrossRef]
7. Abbott, N.J.; Patabendige, A.A.K.; Dolman, D.E.M.; Yusof, S.R.; Begley, D.J. Structure and function of the blood–brain barrier. *Neurobiol. Dis.* **2010**, *37*, 13–25. [CrossRef] [PubMed]

8. Weidle, U.H.; Niewöhner, J.; Tiefenthaler, G. The blood-brain barrier challenge for the treatment of brain cancer, secondary brain metastases, and neurological diseases. *Cancer Genom. Proteom.* **2015**, *12*, 167–177.
9. Pardridge, W.M. Drug and gene targeting to the brain with molecular Trojan horses. *Nat. Rev. Drug Discov.* **2002**, *1*, 131–139. [CrossRef]
10. Agarwal, S.; Sane, R.; Oberoi, R.; Ohlfest, J.R.; Elmquist, W.F. Delivery of molecularly targeted therapy to malignant glioma, a disease of the whole brain. *Expert Rev. Mol. Med.* **2011**, *13*, e17. [CrossRef]
11. Lesniak, W.G.; Chu, C.; Jablonska, A.; Du, Y.; Pomper, M.G.; Walczak, P.; Janowski, M. A Distinct advantage to intraarterial delivery of 89Zr-bevacizumab in PET imaging of mice with and without osmotic opening of the blood–brain barrier. *J. Nucl. Med.* **2018**, *60*, 617–622. [CrossRef] [PubMed]
12. Côté, J.; Bovenzi, V.; Savard, M.; Dubuc, C.; Fortier, A.; Neugebauer, W.; Tremblay, L.; Müller-Esterl, W.; Tsanaclis, A.-M.; Lepage, M.; et al. Induction of selective blood-tumor barrier permeability and macromolecular transport by a biostable kinin B1 receptor agonist in a glioma rat model. *PLoS ONE* **2012**, *7*, e37485. [CrossRef] [PubMed]
13. Hendricks, B.K.; Cohen-Gadol, A.A.; Miller, J.C. Novel delivery methods bypassing the blood-brain and blood-tumor barriers. *Neurosurg. Focus* **2015**, *38*, E10. [CrossRef] [PubMed]
14. Hersh, D.S.; Wadajkar, A.S.; Roberts, N.B.; Perez, J.G.; Connolly, N.P.; Frenkel, V.; Winkles, J.A.; Woodworth, G.F.; Kim, A.J. Evolving drug delivery strategies to overcome the blood brain barrier. *Curr. Pharm. Des.* **2016**, *22*, 1177–1193. [CrossRef]
15. Alkhani, A.M.; Al-Shaar, H.A. Intrathecal baclofen therapy for spasticity: A compliance-based study to indicate effectiveness. *Surg. Neurol. Int.* **2016**, *7*, S539–S541. [CrossRef]
16. Lochhead, J.J.; Thorne, R.G. Intranasal delivery of biologics to the central nervous system. *Adv. Drug Deliv. Rev.* **2012**, *64*, 614–628. [CrossRef]
17. Li, X.; Tsibouklis, J.; Weng, T.; Zhang, B.; Yin, G.; Feng, G.; Cui, Y.; Savina, I.N.; Mikhalovska, L.; Sandeman, S.R.; et al. Nano carriers for drug transport across the blood–brain barrier. *J. Drug Target.* **2017**, *25*, 17–28. [CrossRef]
18. Adjei, I.M.; Sharma, B.; Labhasetwar, V. Nanoparticles: Cellular uptake and cytotoxicity. *Atherosclerosis* **2014**, *811*, 73–91. [CrossRef]
19. Zhang, H.; Jiang, Y.; Zhao, S.-G.; Jiang, L.-Q.; Meng, Y.; Liu, P.; Kim, M.O.; Li, S. Selective neuronal targeting, protection and signaling network analysis via dopamine-mediated mesoporous silica nanoparticles. *MedChemComm* **2015**, *6*, 1117–1129. [CrossRef]
20. Alvarez-Erviti, L.; Seow, Y.; Yin, H.; Betts, C.; Lakhal, S.; Wood, M.J. Delivery of siRNA to the mouse brain by systemic injection of targeted exosomes. *Nat. Biotechnol.* **2011**, *29*, 341–345. [CrossRef]
21. Hasadsri, L.; Kreuter, J.; Hattori, H.; Iwasaki, T.; George, J.M. Functional protein delivery into neurons using polymeric nanoparticles. *J. Biol. Chem.* **2009**, *284*, 6972–6981. [CrossRef] [PubMed]
22. Scuderi, C.; Stecca, C.; Iacomino, A.; Steardo, L. Role of astrocytes in major neurological disorders: The evidence and implications. *IUBMB Life* **2013**, *65*, 957–961. [CrossRef] [PubMed]
23. Rittchen, S.; Boyd, A.; Burns, A.; Park, J.; Fahmy, T.M.; Metcalfe, S.; Williams, A. Myelin repair in vivo is increased by targeting oligodendrocyte precursor cells with nanoparticles encapsulating leukaemia inhibitory factor (LIF). *Biomaterials* **2015**, *56*, 78–85. [CrossRef] [PubMed]
24. Hutter, E.; Boridy, S.; Labrecque, S.; Lalancette-Hébert, M.; Kriz, J.; Winnik, F.M.; Maysinger, D. Microglial response to gold nanoparticles. *ACS Nano* **2010**, *4*, 2595–2606. [CrossRef] [PubMed]
25. Patel, S.K.; Janjic, J.M. Macrophage targeted theranostics as personalized nanomedicine strategies for inflammatory diseases. *Theranostics* **2015**, *5*, 150–172. [CrossRef]
26. Papa, S.; Rossi, F.; Ferrari, R.; Mariani, A.; De Paola, M.; Caron, I.; Fiordaliso, F.; Bisighini, C.; Sammali, E.; Colombo, C.; et al. Selective nanovector mediated treatment of activated proinflammatory microglia/macrophages in spinal cord injury. *ACS Nano* **2013**, *7*, 9881–9895. [CrossRef]
27. Kim, Y.-T.; Caldwell, J.-M.; Bellamkonda, R.V. Nanoparticle-mediated local delivery of methylprednisolone after spinal cord injury. *Biomaterials* **2009**, *30*, 2582–2590. [CrossRef]
28. Fan, Y.; Chen, M.; Zhang, J.; Maincent, P.; Xia, X.; Wu, W. Updated progress of nanocarrier-based intranasal drug delivery systems for treatment of brain diseases. *Crit. Rev. Ther. Drug Carr. Syst.* **2018**, *35*, 433–467. [CrossRef]
29. Fonseca-Santos, B.; Chorilli, M.; Gremião, M.P.D. Nanotechnology-based drug delivery systems for the treatment of Alzheimer's disease. *Int. J. Nanomed.* **2015**, *10*, 4981–5003. [CrossRef]

30. Wilczewska, A.Z.; Niemirowicz, K.; Markiewicz, K.H.; Car, H. Nanoparticles as drug delivery systems. *Pharmacol. Rep.* **2012**, *64*, 1020–1037. [CrossRef]
31. Zhou, Y.; Peng, Z.; Seven, E.S.; Leblanc, R.M. Crossing the blood-brain barrier with nanoparticles. *J. Control. Release* **2018**, *270*, 290–303. [CrossRef]
32. Wen, M.M.; El-Salamouni, N.S.; El-Refaie, W.M.; Hazzah, H.A.; Ali, M.M.; Tosi, G.; Farid, R.M.; Blanco-Prieto, M.J.; Billa, N.; Hanafy, A.S. Nanotechnology-based drug delivery systems for Alzheimer's disease management: Technical, industrial, and clinical challenges. *J. Control. Release* **2017**, *245*, 95–107. [CrossRef] [PubMed]
33. Agrawal, M.; Saraf, S.; Saraf, S.K.; Antimisiaris, S.G.; Hamano, N.; Li, S.-D.; Chougule, M.; Shoyele, S.A.; Gupta, U.; Ajazuddin; et al. Recent advancements in the field of nanotechnology for the delivery of anti-Alzheimer drug in the brain region. *Expert Opin. Drug Deliv.* **2018**, *15*, 589–617. [CrossRef] [PubMed]
34. Majumder, J.; Taratula, O.; Minko, T. Nanocarrier-based systems for targeted and site specific therapeutic delivery. *Adv. Drug Deliv. Rev.* **2019**, *144*, 57–77. [CrossRef] [PubMed]
35. Shah, P.; Chavda, K.; Vyas, B.; Patel, S. Formulation development of linagliptin solid lipid nanoparticles for oral bioavailability enhancement: Role of P-gp inhibition. *Drug Deliv. Transl. Res.* **2020**, 1–20. [CrossRef] [PubMed]
36. Mathew, A.; Fukuda, T.; Nagaoka, Y.; Hasumura, T.; Morimoto, H.; Yoshida, Y.; Maekawa, T.; Venugopal, K.; Kumar, D.S. Curcumin loaded-PLGA nanoparticles conjugated with Tet-1 peptide for potential use in Alzheimer's disease. *PLoS ONE* **2012**, *7*, e32616. [CrossRef] [PubMed]
37. Teleanu, D.M.; Chircov, C.; Grumezescu, A.M.; Volceanov, A.; Teleanu, R.I. Blood-brain delivery methods using nanotechnology. *Pharmaceutics* **2018**, *10*, 269. [CrossRef]
38. Igartúa, D.E.; Martinez, C.S.; Temprana, C.F.; Alonso, S.D.V.; Prieto, M.J. PAMAM dendrimers as a carbamazepine delivery system for neurodegenerative diseases: A biophysical and nanotoxicological characterization. *Int. J. Pharm.* **2018**, *544*, 191–202. [CrossRef]
39. Barenholz, Y. Doxil®—The first FDA-approved nano-drug: Lessons learned. *J. Control. Release* **2012**, *160*, 117–134. [CrossRef]
40. Yu, B.; Lee, R.J.; Lee, L.J. Microfluidic methods for production of liposomes. *Methods Enzymol.* **2009**, *465*, 129–141. [CrossRef]
41. Carugo, D.; Bottaro, E.; Owen, J.; Stride, E.; Nastruzzi, C. Liposome production by microfluidics: Potential and limiting factors. *Sci. Rep.* **2016**, *6*, 25876. [CrossRef] [PubMed]
42. Deshpande, P.P.; Biswas, S.; Torchilin, V. Current trends in the use of liposomes for tumor targeting. *Nanomedicine* **2013**, *8*, 1509–1528. [CrossRef] [PubMed]
43. Stenehjem, D.D.; Hartz, A.M.; Bauer, B.; Anderson, G.W. Novel and emerging strategies in drug delivery for overcoming the blood–brain barrier. *Futur. Med. Chem.* **2009**, *1*, 1623–1641. [CrossRef] [PubMed]
44. Hattori, Y.; Suzuki, S.; Kawakami, S.; Yamashita, F.; Hashida, M. The role of dioleoylphosphatidylethanolamine (DOPE) in targeted gene delivery with mannosylated cationic liposomes via intravenous route. *J. Control. Release* **2005**, *108*, 484–495. [CrossRef]
45. Luo, L.; Bian, Y.; Liu, Y.; Zhang, X.; Wang, M.; Xing, S.; Li, L.; Gao, D. Gold nanoshells: Combined near infrared photothermal therapy and chemotherapy using gold nanoshells coated liposomes to enhance antitumor effect (Small 30/2016). *Small* **2016**, *12*, 4102. [CrossRef]
46. Lindqvist, A.; Rip, J.; Van Kregten, J.; Gaillard, P.J.; Hammarlund-Udenaes, M. In vivo functional evaluation of increased brain delivery of the opioid peptide DAMGO by glutathione-PEGylated liposomes. *Pharm. Res.* **2016**, *33*, 177–185. [CrossRef]
47. Tapeinos, C.; Battaglini, M.; Ciofani, G. Advances in the design of solid lipid nanoparticles and nanostructured lipid carriers for targeting brain diseases. *J. Control. Release* **2017**, *264*, 306–332. [CrossRef]
48. Karakoti, A.S.; Das, S.; Thevuthasan, S.; Seal, S. PEGylated inorganic nanoparticles. *Angew. Chem. Int. Ed.* **2011**, *50*, 1980–1994. [CrossRef]
49. Joralemon, M.J.; McRae, S.; Emrick, T. PEGylated polymers for medicine: From conjugation to self-assembled systems. *Chem. Commun.* **2010**, *46*, 1377–1393. [CrossRef]
50. Qiao, R.; Jia, Q.; Hüwel, S.; Xia, R.; Liu, T.; Gao, F.; Galla, H.-J.; Gao, M. Receptor-mediated delivery of magnetic nanoparticles across the blood–brain barrier. *ACS Nano* **2012**, *6*, 3304–3310. [CrossRef]

51. Luo, S.; Ma, C.; Zhu, M.-Q.; Ju, W.-N.; Yang, Y.; Wang, X. Application of iron oxide nanoparticles in the diagnosis and treatment of neurodegenerative diseases with emphasis on Alzheimer's disease. *Front. Cell. Neurosci.* **2020**, *14*, 21. [CrossRef] [PubMed]
52. Frigell, J.; García, I.; Gómez-Vallejo, V.; Llop, J.; Penadés, S. ^{68}Ga-Labeled gold glyconanoparticles for exploring blood–brain barrier permeability: Preparation, biodistribution studies, and improved brain uptake via neuropeptide conjugation. *J. Am. Chem. Soc.* **2013**, *136*, 449–457. [CrossRef] [PubMed]
53. Wang, Q.; Timberlake, M.A., II; Prall, K.; Dwivedi, Y. The recent progress in animal models of depression. *Prog. Neuro-Psychopharmacol. Biol. Psychiatry* **2017**, *77*, 99–109. [CrossRef]
54. McQuaid, R.J.; McInnis, O.A.; Abizaid, A.; Anisman, H. Making room for oxytocin in understanding depression. *Neurosci. Biobehav. Rev.* **2014**, *45*, 305–322. [CrossRef]
55. O'Leary, O.F.; Dinan, T.G.; Cryan, J.F. Faster, better, stronger: Towards new antidepressant therapeutic strategies. *Eur. J. Pharmacol.* **2015**, *753*, 32–50. [CrossRef] [PubMed]
56. Cirri, M.; Maestrini, L.; Maestrelli, F.; Mennini, N.; Mura, P.; Ghelardini, C.; Mannelli, L.D.C. Design, characterization and in vivo evaluation of nanostructured lipid carriers (NLC) as a new drug delivery system for hydrochlorothiazide oral administration in pediatric therapy. *Drug Deliv.* **2018**, *25*, 1910–1921. [CrossRef]
57. Vitorino, C.; Silva, S.; Bicker, J.; Falcão, A.; Fortuna, A. Antidepressants and nose-to-brain delivery: Drivers, restraints, opportunities and challenges. *Drug Discov. Today* **2019**, *24*, 1911–1923. [CrossRef]
58. Jani, P.; Vanza, J.; Pandya, N.; Tandel, H. Formulation of polymeric nanoparticles of antidepressant drug for intranasal delivery. *Ther. Deliv.* **2019**, *10*, 683–696. [CrossRef]
59. Shinde, M.; Bali, N.R.; Rathod, S.; Karemore, M.N.; Salve, P. Effect of binary combinations of solvent systems on permeability profiling of pure agomelatine across rat skin: A comparative study with statistically optimized polymeric nanoparticles. *Drug Dev. Ind. Pharm.* **2020**, *46*, 826–845. [CrossRef]
60. Chen, B.; Luo, M.; Liang, J.; Zhang, C.; Gao, C.; Wang, J.; Wang, J.; Li, Y.; Xu, D.; Liu, L.; et al. Surface modification of PGP for a neutrophil–nanoparticle co-vehicle to enhance the anti-depressant effect of baicalein. *Acta Pharm. Sin. B* **2018**, *8*, 64–73. [CrossRef]
61. Harris, N.M.; Ritzel, R.; Mancini, N.S.; Jiang, Y.; Yi, X.; Manickam, D.S.; Banks, W.A.; Kabanov, A.V.; McCullough, L.D.; Verma, R. Nano-particle delivery of brain derived neurotrophic factor after focal cerebral ischemia reduces tissue injury and enhances behavioral recovery. *Pharmacol. Biochem. Behav.* **2016**, 48–56. [CrossRef] [PubMed]
62. He, X.; Zhu, Y.; Wang, M.; Jing, G.; Zhu, R.; Wang, S. Antidepressant effects of curcumin and HU-211 coencapsulated solid lipid nanoparticles against corticosterone-induced cellular and animal models of major depression. *Int. J. Nanomed.* **2016**, *11*, 4975–4990. [CrossRef] [PubMed]
63. He, X.; Yang, L.; Wang, M.; Zhuang, X.; Huang, R.; Zhu, R.; Wang, S. Targeting the endocannabinoid/CB1 receptor system for treating major depression through antidepressant activities of curcumin and dexanabinol-loaded solid lipid nanoparticles. *Cell Physiol. Biochem.* **2017**, *42*, 2281–2294. [CrossRef] [PubMed]
64. Fidelis, E.M.; Savall, A.S.P.; Abreu, E.D.L.; Carvalho, F.; Teixeira, F.E.G.; Haas, S.E.; Sampaio, T.B.; Pinton, S. Curcumin-loaded nanocapsules reverses the depressant-like behavior and oxidative stress induced by β-amyloid in mice. *Neuroscience* **2019**, *423*, 122–130. [CrossRef]
65. Alam, M.I.; Baboota, S.; Ahuja, A.; Ali, M.; Ali, J.; Sahni, J.K.; Bhatnagar, A. Pharmacoscintigraphic evaluation of potential of lipid nanocarriers for nose-to-brain delivery of antidepressant drug. *Int. J. Pharm.* **2014**, *470*, 99–106. [CrossRef]
66. Ravouru, N.; Kondreddy, P.; Korakanchi, D. Formulation and evaluation of niosomal nasal drug delivery system of folic acid for brain targeting. *Curr. Drug Discov. Technol.* **2013**, *10*, 270–282. [CrossRef]
67. Margret, A.A.; Dhayabaran, V.V.; Kumar, A.G. Nanoparticulated polymeric composites enfolding lithium carbonate as brain drug in persuading depression: An in vivo study. *Prog. Biomater.* **2017**, *6*, 165–173. [CrossRef]
68. Nagpal, K.; Singh, S.K.; Mishra, D. Evaluation of safety and efficacy of brain targeted chitosan nanoparticles of minocycline. *Int. J. Biol. Macromol.* **2013**, *59*, 20–28. [CrossRef]
69. Singh, D.P.; Rashid, M.; Hallan, S.S.; Mehra, N.K.; Prakash, A.; Mishra, N. Pharmacological evaluation of nasal delivery of selegiline hydrochloride-loaded thiolated chitosan nanoparticles for the treatment of depression. *Artif. Cells Nanomed. Biotechnol.* **2015**, *44*, 1–13. [CrossRef]

70. Ashraf, A.; Mahmoud, P.A.; Reda, H.; Mansour, S.; Helal, M.H.; Michel, H.E.; Nasr, M. Silymarin and silymarin nanoparticles guard against chronic unpredictable mild stress induced depressive-like behavior in mice: Involvement of neurogenesis and NLRP3 inflammasome. *J. Psychopharmacol.* **2019**, *33*, 615–631. [CrossRef]
71. Alam, M.; Najmi, A.K.; Ahmad, I.; Ahmad, F.J.; Akhtar, J.; Imam, S.S.; Akhtar, M. Formulation and evaluation of nano lipid formulation containing CNS acting drug: Molecular docking, in-vitro assessment and bioactivity detail in rats. *Artif. Cells Nanomed. Biotechnol.* **2018**, *46*, 46–57. [CrossRef] [PubMed]
72. Kaur, P.; Garg, T.; Vaidya, B.; Prakash, A.; Rath, G.; Goyal, A.K. Brain delivery of intranasalin situgel of nanoparticulated polymeric carriers containing antidepressant drug: Behavioral and biochemical assessment. *J. Drug Target.* **2014**, *23*, 275–286. [CrossRef] [PubMed]
73. Qin, J.; Yang, X.; Zhang, R.-X.; Luo, Y.-X.; Li, J.-L.; Hou, J.; Zhang, C.; Li, Y.-J.; Shi, J.; Lu, L.; et al. Monocyte mediated brain targeting delivery of macromolecular drug for the therapy of depression. *Nanomed. Nanotechnol. Biol. Med.* **2015**, *11*, 391–400. [CrossRef] [PubMed]
74. Haque, S.; Shadab; Fazil, M.; Kumar, M.; Sahni, J.K.; Ali, J.; Baboota, S. Venlafaxine loaded chitosan NPs for brain targeting: Pharmacokinetic and pharmacodynamic evaluation. *Carbohydr. Polym.* **2012**, *89*, 72–79. [CrossRef] [PubMed]
75. Cayero-Otero, M.; Gomes, M.J.; Martins, C.; Álvarez-Fuentes, J.; Fernández-Arévalo, M.; Sarmento, B.; Martín-Banderas, L. In vivo biodistribution of venlafaxine-PLGA nanoparticles for brain delivery: Plain vs. functionalized nanoparticles. *Expert Opin. Drug Deliv.* **2019**, *16*, 1413–1427. [CrossRef]
76. Haque, S.; Shadab; Sahni, J.K.; Ali, J.; Baboota, S. Development and evaluation of brain targeted intranasal alginate nanoparticles for treatment of depression. *J. Psychiatr. Res.* **2014**, *48*, 1–12. [CrossRef]
77. Grabrucker, A.M.; Garner, C.C.; Boeckers, T.M.; Bondioli, L.; Ruozi, B.; Forni, F.; Vandelli, M.A.; Tosi, G. Development of novel Zn^{2+} loaded nanoparticles designed for cell-type targeted drug release in CNS neurons: In vitro evidences. *PLoS ONE* **2011**, *6*, e17851. [CrossRef]
78. Vinzant, N.; Scholl, J.L.; Wu, C.-M.; Kindle, T.; Koodali, R.; Forster, G.L. Iron oxide nanoparticle delivery of peptides to the brain: Reversal of anxiety during drug withdrawal. *Front. Neurosci.* **2017**, *11*, 608. [CrossRef]
79. Bari, N.K.; Fazil, M.; Hassan, Q.; Haider, R.; Gaba, B.; Narang, J.K.; Baboota, S.; Ali, J. Brain delivery of buspirone hydrochloride chitosan nanoparticles for the treatment of general anxiety disorder. *Int. J. Biol. Macromol.* **2015**, *81*, 49–59. [CrossRef]
80. Abdelnabi, D.M.; Abdallah, M.H.; Elghamry, H.A. Buspirone hydrochloride loaded in situ nanovesicular gel as an anxiolytic nasal drug delivery system: In vitro and animal studies. *AAPS PharmSciTech* **2019**, *20*, 134. [CrossRef]
81. Bohrey, S.; Chourasiya, V.; Pandey, A. Polymeric nanoparticles containing diazepam: Preparation, optimization, characterization, in-vitro drug release and release kinetic study. *Nano Converg.* **2016**, *3*, 1–7. [CrossRef]
82. Nagpal, K.; Singh, S.K.; Mishra, D. Optimization of brain targeted gallic acid nanoparticles for improved antianxiety-like activity. *Int. J. Biol. Macromol.* **2013**, *57*, 83–91. [CrossRef]
83. Sinha, S.V. Enhancement of in vivo efficacy and oral bioavailability of aripiprazole with solid lipid nanoparticles. *AAPS PharmSciTech* **2018**, *19*, 1264–1273. [CrossRef]
84. Sawant, K.; Pandey, A.; Patel, S. Aripiprazole loaded poly(caprolactone) nanoparticles: Optimization and in vivo pharmacokinetics. *Mater. Sci. Eng. C* **2016**, *66*, 230–243. [CrossRef]
85. Singh, S.K.; Hidau, M.K.; Gautam, S.; Gupta, K.; Singh, K.P.; Singh, S.K. Glycol chitosan functionalized asenapine nanostructured lipid carriers for targeted brain delivery: Pharmacokinetic and teratogenic assessment. *Int. J. Biol. Macromol.* **2018**, *108*, 1092–1100. [CrossRef]
86. Shreya, A.B.; Managuli, R.S.; Menon, J.; Kondapalli, L.; Hegde, A.R.; Avadhani, K.; Shetty, P.K.; Amirthalingam, M.; Kalthur, G.; Mutalik, S. Nano-transfersomal formulations for transdermal delivery of asenapine maleate: In vitro and in vivo performance evaluations. *J. Liposome Res.* **2015**, *26*, 221–232. [CrossRef]
87. Piazza, J.; Hoare, T.; Molinaro, L.; Terpstra, K.; Bhandari, J.; Selvaganapathy, P.R.; Gupta, B.; Mishra, R.K. Haloperidol-loaded intranasally administered lectin functionalized poly(ethylene glycol)–block-poly(D,L)-lactic -co-glycolic acid (PEG–PLGA) nanoparticles for the treatment of schizophrenia. *Eur. J. Pharm. Biopharm.* **2014**, *87*, 30–39. [CrossRef]
88. Narayan, S. Lithium entrapped chitosan nanoparticles to reduce toxicity and increase cellular uptake of lithium. *Environ. Toxicol. Pharmacol.* **2018**, *61*, 79–86. [CrossRef]

89. Patel, M.H.; Mundada, V.P.; Sawant, K.K. Fabrication of solid lipid nanoparticles of lurasidone HCl for oral delivery: Optimization, in vitro characterization, cell line studies and in vivo efficacy in schizophrenia. *Drug Dev. Ind. Pharm.* **2019**, *45*, 1242–1257. [CrossRef]
90. Jazuli, I.; Nabi, B.; Moolakkadath, T.; Alam, T.; Baboota, S.; Ali, J.; Annu, I.J. Optimization of nanostructured lipid carriers of lurasidone hydrochloride using box-behnken design for brain targeting: In vitro and in vivo studies. *J. Pharm. Sci.* **2019**, *108*, 3082–3090. [CrossRef]
91. Pokharkar, V.; Suryawanshi, S.; Dhapte-Pawar, V. Exploring micellar-based polymeric systems for effective nose-to-brain drug delivery as potential neurotherapeutics. *Drug Deliv. Transl. Res.* **2019**, *10*, 1019–1031. [CrossRef] [PubMed]
92. Natarajan, J.; Baskaran, M.; Humtsoe, L.C.; Vadivelan, R.; Justin, A. Enhanced brain targeting efficacy of Olanzapine through solid lipid nanoparticles. *Artif. Cells Nanomed. Biotechnol.* **2016**, *45*, 1–8. [CrossRef] [PubMed]
93. Gadhave, D.G.; Tagalpallewar, A.A.; Kokare, C.R. Agranulocytosis-protective olanzapine-loaded nanostructured lipid carriers engineered for CNS delivery: Optimization and hematological toxicity studies. *AAPS PharmSciTech* **2019**, *20*, 22. [CrossRef] [PubMed]
94. Abdelbary, G.A.; Tadros, M.I. Brain targeting of olanzapine via intranasal delivery of core–shell difunctional block copolymer mixed nanomicellar carriers: In vitro characterization, ex vivo estimation of nasal toxicity and in vivo biodistribution studies. *Int. J. Pharm.* **2013**, *452*, 300–310. [CrossRef] [PubMed]
95. Fonseca, F.N.; Betti, A.H.; Carvalho, F.C.U.; Gremiao, M.P.D.U.; Dimer, F.A.; Guterres, S.S.; Tebaldi, M.L.; Rates, S.M.K.; Pohlmann, A.R. Mucoadhesive amphiphilic methacrylic copolymer-functionalized poly(ε-caprolactone) nanocapsules for nose-to-brain delivery of olanzapine. *J. Biomed. Nanotechnol.* **2015**, *11*, 1472–1481. [CrossRef] [PubMed]
96. Baltzley, S.; Mohammad, A.; Malkawi, A.H.; Al-Ghananeem, A.M. Intranasal drug delivery of olanzapine-loaded chitosan nanoparticles. *AAPS PharmSciTech* **2014**, *15*, 1598–1602. [CrossRef] [PubMed]
97. Seju, U.; Kumar, A.; Sawant, K. Development and evaluation of olanzapine-loaded PLGA nanoparticles for nose-to-brain delivery: In vitro and in vivo studies. *Acta Biomater.* **2011**, *7*, 4169–4176. [CrossRef]
98. Helal, H.M.; Mortada, S.M.; Sallam, M.A. Paliperidone-loaded nanolipomer system for sustained delivery and enhanced intestinal permeation: Superiority to polymeric and solid lipid nanoparticles. *AAPS PharmSciTech* **2016**, *18*, 1946–1959. [CrossRef]
99. Sherje, A.P.; Londhe, V. Development and evaluation of pH-responsive cyclodextrin-based in situ gel of paliperidone for intranasal delivery. *AAPS PharmSciTech* **2017**, *19*, 384–394. [CrossRef]
100. Muthu, M.S.; Sahu, A.K.; Sonali; Abdulla, A.; Kaklotar, D.; Rajesh, C.V.; Singh, S.; Pandey, B.L. Solubilized delivery of paliperidone palmitate by d-alpha-tocopheryl polyethylene glycol 1000 succinate micelles for improved short-term psychotic management. *Drug Deliv.* **2014**, *23*, 230–237. [CrossRef]
101. Patel, M.R.; Patel, R.B.; Bhatt, K.K.; Patel, B.G.; Gaikwad, R.V. Paliperidone microemulsion for nose-to-brain targeted drug delivery system: Pharmacodynamic and pharmacokinetic evaluation. *Drug Deliv.* **2014**, *23*, 346–354. [CrossRef] [PubMed]
102. Lugasi, L.; Grinberg, I.; Sabag, R.; Madar, R.; Einat, H.; Margel, S. Proteinoid nanocapsules as drug delivery system for improving antipsychotic activity of risperidone. *Molecules* **2020**, *25*, 4013. [CrossRef] [PubMed]
103. Rukmangathen, R.; Yallamalli, I.M.; Yalavarthi, P.R. Formulation and biopharmaceutical evaluation of risperidone-loaded chitosan nanoparticles for intranasal delivery. *Drug Dev. Ind. Pharm.* **2019**, *45*, 1342–1350. [CrossRef] [PubMed]
104. Patel, S.; Chavhan, S.; Soni, H.; Babbar, A.; Mathur, R.; Mishra, A.; Sawant, K. Brain targeting of risperidone-loaded solid lipid nanoparticles by intranasal route. *J. Drug Target.* **2010**, *19*, 468–474. [CrossRef] [PubMed]
105. Kumar, M.; Misra, A.; Mishra, A.K.; Mishra, P.; Pathak, K. Mucoadhesive nanoemulsion-based intranasal drug delivery system of olanzapine for brain targeting. *J. Drug Target.* **2008**, *16*, 806–814. [CrossRef] [PubMed]
106. Narayan, R.; Singh, M.; Ranjan, O.; Nayak, Y.; Garg, S.; Shavi, G.V.; Nayak, U.Y. Development of risperidone liposomes for brain targeting through intranasal route. *Life Sci.* **2016**, *163*, 38–45. [CrossRef]
107. Qureshi, M.; Aqil, M.; Imam, S.S.; Ahad, A.; Sultana, Y. Formulation and evaluation of neuroactive drug loaded chitosan nanoparticle for nose to brain delivery: In-vitro characterization and in-vivo behavior study. *Curr. Drug Deliv.* **2018**, *16*, 123–135. [CrossRef]

108. Li, J.; Zhang, W.-J.; Zhu, J.-X.; Zhu, N.; Zhang, H.-M.; Wang, X.; Zhang, J.; Wang, Q.-Q. Preparation and brain delivery of nasal solid lipid nanoparticles of quetiapine fumarate in situ gel in rat model of schizophrenia. *Int. J. Clin. Exp. Med.* **2015**, *8*, 17590–17600.
109. Boche, M.; Pokharkar, V.B. Quetiapine nanoemulsion for intranasal drug delivery: Evaluation of brain-targeting efficiency. *AAPS PharmSciTech* **2016**, *18*, 686–696. [CrossRef]
110. Upadhyay, P.; Trivedi, J.; Pundarikakshudu, K.; Sheth, N. Direct and enhanced delivery of nanoliposomes of anti schizophrenic agent to the brain through nasal route. *Saudi Pharm. J.* **2017**, *25*, 346–358. [CrossRef]
111. Shah, B.; Khunt, D.; Misra, M.; Padh, H. Non-invasive intranasal delivery of quetiapine fumarate loaded microemulsion for brain targeting: Formulation, physicochemical and pharmacokinetic consideration. *Eur. J. Pharm. Sci.* **2016**, *91*, 196–207. [CrossRef] [PubMed]
112. Shah, B.; Khunt, D.; Misra, M.; Padh, H. Application of box-behnken design for optimization and development of quetiapine fumarate loaded chitosan nanoparticles for brain delivery via intranasal route. *Int. J. Biol. Macromol.* **2016**, *89*, 206–218. [CrossRef] [PubMed]
113. Naik, A.; Nair, H. Formulation and evaluation of thermosensitive biogels for nose to brain delivery of doxepin. *BioMed Res. Int.* **2014**, *2014*, 1–10. [CrossRef] [PubMed]
114. Pandey, Y.R.; Kumar, S.; Gupta, B.K.; Ali, J.; Baboota, S. Intranasal delivery of paroxetine nanoemulsion via the olfactory region for the management of depression: Formulation, behavioural and biochemical estimation. *Nanotechnology* **2016**, *27*, 25102. [CrossRef] [PubMed]
115. Pathan, I.B.; Mene, H.; Bairagi, S. Quality by design (QbD) approach to formulate in situ gelling system for nose to brain delivery of Fluoxetine hydrochloride: Ex-vivo and In-vivo study. *ARS Pharm.* **2017**, *58*, 107–114.
116. Kamel, R.; Abbas, H.; El-Naa, M. Composite carbohydrate interpenetrating polyelectrolyte nano-complexes (IPNC) as a controlled oral delivery system of citalopram HCl for pediatric use: In-vitro/in-vivo evaluation and histopathological examination. *Drug Deliv. Transl. Res.* **2018**, *8*, 657–669. [CrossRef]
117. Rahman, M.A.; Harwansh, R.K.; Iqbal, Z. Systematic development of sertraline loaded solid lipid nanoparticle (SLN) by emulsification-ultrasonication method and pharmacokinetic study in sprague-dawley rats. *Pharm. Nanotechnol.* **2019**, *7*, 162–176. [CrossRef]
118. Bhandwalkar, M.J.; Avachat, A.M. Thermoreversible nasal in situ gel of venlafaxine hydrochloride: Formulation, characterization, and pharmacodynamic evaluation. *AAPS PharmSciTech* **2012**, *14*, 101–110. [CrossRef]
119. Aranaz, I.; Paños, I.; Peniche, C.; Heras, A.; Acosta, N. Chitosan spray-dried microparticles for controlled delivery of venlafaxine hydrochloride. *Molecules* **2017**, *22*, 1980. [CrossRef]
120. Tong, G.-F.; Qin, N.; Sun, L.-W. Development and evaluation of Desvenlafaxine loaded PLGA-chitosan nanoparticles for brain delivery. *Saudi Pharm. J.* **2016**, *25*, 844–851. [CrossRef]
121. Casolaro, M.; Casolaro, I. Controlled release of antidepressant drugs by multiple stimuli-sensitive hydrogels based on α-aminoacid residues. *J. Drug Deliv. Sci. Technol.* **2015**, *30*, 82–89. [CrossRef]
122. Mitroshina, E.V.; Mishchenko, T.A.; Usenko, A.V.; Epifanova, E.A.; Yarkov, R.S.; Gavrish, M.S.; Babaev, A.A.; Vedunova, M.V. AAV-Syn-BDNF-EGFP virus construct exerts neuroprotective action on the hippocampal neural network during hypoxia in vitro. *Int. J. Mol. Sci.* **2018**, *19*, 2295. [CrossRef]
123. Ma, X.-C.; Liu, P.; Zhang, X.-L.; Jiang, W.-H.; Jia, M.; Wang, C.-X.; Dong, Y.-Y.; Dang, Y.-H.; Gao, C.-G. intranasal delivery of recombinant AAV containing BDNF fused with HA2TAT: A potential promising therapy strategy for major depressive disorder. *Sci. Rep.* **2016**, *6*, 22404. [CrossRef]
124. Mill, J.; Petronis, A. Molecular studies of major depressive disorder: The epigenetic perspective. *Mol. Psychiatry* **2007**, *12*, 799–814. [CrossRef]
125. Bandelow, B.; Michaelis, S.; Wedekind, D. Treatment of anxiety disorders. *Dialogues Clin. Neurosci.* **2017**, *19*, 93–107.
126. Pollack, M.; Otto, M.W.; Roy-Byrne, P.P.; Coplan, J.D.; Rothbaum, B.O.; Simon, N.M.; Gorman, J.M. Novel treatment approaches for refractory anxiety disorders. *Depression Anxiety* **2008**, *25*, 467–476. [CrossRef]
127. Loane, C.; Politis, M. Buspirone: What is it all about? *Brain Res.* **2012**, *1461*, 111–118. [CrossRef] [PubMed]
128. Mendrek, A.; Mancini-Marïe, A. Sex/gender differences in the brain and cognition in schizophrenia. *Neurosci. Biobehav. Rev.* **2016**, *67*, 57–78. [CrossRef] [PubMed]
129. Clark, C.T.; Wisner, K.L. Treatment of peripartum bipolar disorder. *Obstet. Gynecol. Clin. N. Am.* **2018**, *45*, 403–417. [CrossRef]

130. Rabin, C.R.; Siegel, S.J. Antipsychotic dosing and drug delivery. In *Behavioral Neurobiology of Schizophrenia and Its Treatment*; Swerdlow, N., Ed.; Springer: Berlin/Heidelberg, Germany, 2010; Volume 4, pp. 141–177.
131. Cheng, Y.-H.; Illum, L.; Davis, S.S. Schizophrenia and drug delivery systems. *J. Drug Target.* **2000**, *8*, 107–117. [CrossRef]
132. Kane, J.M.; García-Ribera, C. Clinical guideline recommendations for antipsychotic long-acting injections. *Br. J. Psychiatry* **2009**, *195*, s63–s67. [CrossRef] [PubMed]
133. Joseph, E.; Reddi, S.; Rinwa, V.; Balwani, G.; Saha, R. Design and in vivo evaluation of solid lipid nanoparticulate systems of Olanzapine for acute phase schizophrenia treatment: Investigations on antipsychotic potential and adverse effects. *Eur. J. Pharm. Sci.* **2017**, *104*, 315–325. [CrossRef] [PubMed]
134. Jawahar, N.; Hingarh, P.K.; Arun, R.; Selvaraj, J.; Anbarasan, A.; Sathianarayanan, S.; Nagaraju, G. Enhanced oral bioavailability of an antipsychotic drug through nanostructured lipid carriers. *Int. J. Biol. Macromol.* **2018**, *110*, 269–275. [CrossRef] [PubMed]
135. Pervaiz, F.; Ahmad, M.; Hussain, T.; Idrees, A.; Yaqoob, A.; Abbas, K. Development of olanzapine loaded PNA microgels for depot drug delivery in treatment of schizophrenia: In vitro an in vivo release profile. *Acta Pol. Pharm. Drug Res.* **2016**, *73*, 175–181.
136. De Freitas, M.R.; Rolim, L.A.; Soares, M.F.D.L.R.; Rolim-Neto, P.J.; De Albuquerque, M.M.; Soares-Sobrinho, J.L. Inclusion complex of methyl-β-cyclodextrin and olanzapine as potential drug delivery system for schizophrenia. *Carbohydr. Polym.* **2012**, *89*, 1095–1100. [CrossRef]
137. Venkateswarlu, V.; Manjunath, K. Preparation, characterization and in vitro release kinetics of clozapine solid lipid nanoparticles. *J. Control. Release* **2004**, *95*, 627–638. [CrossRef]
138. Shafaat, K.; Kumar, B.; Das, S.K.; Hasan, R.U.; Prajapati, S.K. Novel nanoemulsion as vehicles for transdermal delivery of clozapine, in vitro in vivo studies. *Int. J. Pharm. Pharm. Sci.* **2013**, *5*, 126–134.
139. Iqbal, N.; Vitorino, C.; Taylor, K.M.G. How can lipid nanocarriers improve transdermal delivery of olanzapine? *Pharm. Dev. Technol.* **2017**, *22*, 587–596. [CrossRef]
140. Dimer, F.A.; Ortiz, M.; Pase, C.S.; Roversi, K.; Friedrich, R.B.; Pohlmann, A.R.; Burger, M.E.; Guterres, S.S. Nanoencapsulation of olanzapine increases its efficacy in antipsychotic treatment and reduces adverse effects. *J. Biomed. Nanotechnol.* **2014**, *10*, 1137–1145. [CrossRef]
141. Joseph, E.; Reddi, S.; Rinwa, V.; Balwani, G.; Saha, R. DoE based Olanzapine loaded poly-caprolactone nanoparticles decreases extrapyramidal effects in rodent model. *Int. J. Pharm.* **2018**, *541*, 198–205. [CrossRef]
142. Al-Dhubiab, B.E. Aripiprazole nanocrystal impregnated buccoadhesive films for schizophrenia. *J. Nanosci. Nanotechnol.* **2017**, *17*, 2345–2352. [CrossRef] [PubMed]
143. Çelik, B. Risperidone mucoadhesive buccal tablets: Formulation design, optimization and evaluation. *Drug Des. Dev. Ther.* **2017**, *11*, 3355–3365. [CrossRef] [PubMed]
144. Silva, A.C.; Kumar, A.; Wild, W.; Ferreira, D.; Santos, D.; Forbes, B. Long-term stability, biocompatibility and oral delivery potential of risperidone-loaded solid lipid nanoparticles. *Int. J. Pharm.* **2012**, *436*, 798–805. [CrossRef] [PubMed]
145. Alzubaidi, A.F.A.; El-Helw, A.-R.M.; Ahmed, T.A.; Ahmed, O.A.A. The use of experimental design in the optimization of risperidone biodegradable nanoparticles: In vitro and in vivo study. *Artif. Cells Nanomed. Biotechnol.* **2016**, *45*, 1–8. [CrossRef] [PubMed]
146. Mandpe, L.; Pokharkar, V. Targeted brain delivery of iloperidone nanostructured lipid carriers following intranasal administration: In vivo pharmacokinetics and brain distribution studies. *J. Nanopharm. Drug Deliv.* **2013**, *1*, 212–225. [CrossRef]
147. Đorđević, S.M.; Santrač, A.; Cekić, N.D.; Markovic, B.D.; Divović, B.; Ilić, T.M.; Savić, M.M.; Savic, S. Parenteral nanoemulsions of risperidone for enhanced brain delivery in acute psychosis: Physicochemical and in vivo performances. *Int. J. Pharm.* **2017**, *533*, 421–430. [CrossRef]
148. Shan, G.W.; Makmor-Bakry, M.; Omar, M.S. Long term use of lithium and factors associated with treatment response among patients with bipolar disorder. *Psychiatr. Danub.* **2016**, *28*, 146–153.
149. Won, E.; Kim, Y.-K. An oldie but goodie: Lithium in the treatment of bipolar disorder through neuroprotective and neurotrophic mechanisms. *Int. J. Mol. Sci.* **2017**, *18*, 2679. [CrossRef]
150. Karthivashan, G.; Ganesan, P.; Park, S.-Y.; Kim, J.-S.; Choi, D.-K. Therapeutic strategies and nano-drug delivery applications in management of ageing Alzheimer's disease. *Drug Deliv.* **2018**, *25*, 307–320. [CrossRef]
151. Swerdlow, R.H.; Burns, J.M.; Khan, S.M. The Alzheimer's disease mitochondrial cascade hypothesis: Progress and perspectives. *Biochim. Biophys. Acta (BBA) Mol. Basis Dis.* **2014**, *1842*, 1219–1231. [CrossRef]

152. Jojo, G.M.; Kuppusamy, G.; De, A.; Karri, V.V.S.N.R. Formulation and optimization of intranasal nanolipid carriers of pioglitazone for the repurposing in Alzheimer's disease using Box-Behnken design. *Drug Dev. Ind. Pharm.* **2019**, *45*, 1061–1072. [CrossRef] [PubMed]
153. Rassu, G.; Soddu, E.; Posadino, A.M.; Pintus, G.; Sarmento, B.; Giunchedi, P.; Gavini, E. Nose-to-brain delivery of BACE1 siRNA loaded in solid lipid nanoparticles for Alzheimer's therapy. *Colloids Surf. B Biointerfaces* **2017**, *152*, 296–301. [CrossRef] [PubMed]
154. Wang, P.; Zheng, X.; Guo, Q.; Yang, P.; Pang, X.; Qian, K.; Lu, W.; Zhang, Q.; Jiang, X. Systemic delivery of BACE1 siRNA through neuron-targeted nanocomplexes for treatment of Alzheimer's disease. *J. Control. Release* **2018**, *279*, 220–233. [CrossRef] [PubMed]
155. Liu, Y.; An, S.; Li, J.; Kuang, Y.; He, X.; Guo, Y.; Ma, H.; Zhang, Y.; Ji, B.; Jiang, C. Brain-targeted co-delivery of therapeutic gene and peptide by multifunctional nanoparticles in Alzheimer's disease mice. *Biomaterials* **2016**, *80*, 33–45. [CrossRef] [PubMed]
156. Zhang, C.; Gu, Z.; Shen, L.; Liu, X.; Lin, H. A dual targeting drug delivery system for penetrating blood-brain barrier and selectively delivering siRNA to neurons for Alzheimer's disease treatment. *Curr. Pharm. Biotechnol.* **2018**, *18*, 1124–1131. [CrossRef] [PubMed]
157. Agyare, E.; Jaruszewski, K.M.; Curran, G.L.; Rosenberg, J.T.; Grant, S.C.; Lowe, V.J.; Ramakrishnan, S.; Paravastu, A.K.; Poduslo, J.F.; Kandimalla, K.K. Engineering theranostic nanovehicles capable of targeting cerebrovascular amyloid deposits. *J. Control. Release* **2014**, *185*, 121–129. [CrossRef] [PubMed]
158. Loureiro, J.A.; Gomes, B.; Fricker, G.; Coelho, M.A.; Rocha, S.; Pereira, M.C. Cellular uptake of PLGA nanoparticles targeted with anti-amyloid and anti-transferrin receptor antibodies for Alzheimer's disease treatment. *Colloids Surf. B Biointerfaces* **2016**, *145*, 8–13. [CrossRef]
159. Zhang, C.; Zheng, X.; Wan, X.; Shao, X.; Liu, Q.; Zhang, Q.; Zhang, Q. The potential use of H102 peptide-loaded dual-functional nanoparticles in the treatment of Alzheimer's disease. *J. Control. Release* **2014**, *192*, 317–324. [CrossRef]
160. Gobbi, M.; Re, F.; Canovi, M.; Beeg, M.; Gregori, M.F.; Sesana, S.; Sonnino, S.; Brogioli, D.; Musicanti, C.; Gasco, P.; et al. Lipid-based nanoparticles with high binding affinity for amyloid-β1–42 peptide. *Biomaterials* **2010**, *31*, 6519–6529. [CrossRef]
161. Balducci, C.; Mancini, S.; Minniti, S.; La Vitola, P.; Zotti, M.; Sancini, G.; Mauri, M.; Cagnotto, A.; Colombo, L.; Fiordaliso, F.; et al. Multifunctional liposomes reduce brain—amyloid burden and ameliorate memory impairment in Alzheimer's disease mouse models. *J. Neurosci.* **2014**, *34*, 14022–14031. [CrossRef]
162. Tanifum, E.A.; Dasgupta, I.; Srivastava, M.; Bhavane, R.C.; Sun, L.; Berridge, J.; Pourgarzham, H.; Kamath, R.; Espinosa, G.; Cook, S.C.; et al. Intravenous delivery of targeted liposomes to amyloid-β pathology in APP/PSEN1 transgenic mice. *PLoS ONE* **2012**, *7*, e48515. [CrossRef] [PubMed]
163. Song, Q.; Huang, M.; Yao, L.; Wang, X.; Gu, X.; Chen, J.; Huang, J.; Hu, Q.; Kang, T.; Rong, Z.; et al. Lipoprotein-based nanoparticles rescue the memory loss of mice with Alzheimer's disease by accelerating the clearance of amyloid-beta. *ACS Nano* **2014**, *8*, 2345–2359. [CrossRef]
164. Poduslo, J.F.; Hultman, K.L.; Curran, G.L.; Preboske, G.M.; Chamberlain, R.; Marjańska, M.; Garwood, M.; Jack, C.R., Jr.; Wengenack, T.M. Targeting vascular amyloid in arterioles of Alzheimer disease transgenic mice with amyloid β protein antibody-coated nanoparticles. *J. Neuropathol. Exp. Neurol.* **2011**, *70*, 653–661. [CrossRef] [PubMed]
165. Prades, R.; Guerrero, S.; Araya, E.; Molina, C.; Salas, E.; Zurita, E.; Selva, J.; Egea, G.; López-Iglesias, C.; Teixidó, M.; et al. Delivery of gold nanoparticles to the brain by conjugation with a peptide that recognizes the transferrin receptor. *Biomaterials* **2012**, *33*, 7194–7205. [CrossRef] [PubMed]
166. Gao, N.; Sun, H.; Dong, K.; Ren, J.; Qu, X. Gold-nanoparticle-based multifunctional amyloid-β inhibitor against Alzheimer's disease. *Chem. A Eur. J.* **2015**, *21*, 829–835. [CrossRef] [PubMed]
167. Hsieh, S.; Chang, C.-W.; Chou, H.-H. Gold nanoparticles as amyloid-like fibrillogenesis inhibitors. *Colloids Surf. B Biointerfaces* **2013**, *112*, 525–529. [CrossRef]
168. Cimini, A.; D'Angelo, B.; Das, S.; Gentile, R.; Benedetti, E.; Singh, V.; Monaco, A.; Santucci, S.; Seal, S. Antibody-conjugated PEGylated cerium oxide nanoparticles for specific targeting of Aβ aggregates modulate neuronal survival pathways. *Acta Biomater.* **2012**, *8*, 2056–2067. [CrossRef]
169. Vakilinezhad, M.A.; Amini, A.; Javar, H.A.; Zarandi, B.F.B.B.; Montaseri, H.; Dinarvand, R. Nicotinamide loaded functionalized solid lipid nanoparticles improves cognition in Alzheimer's disease animal model by reducing Tau hyperphosphorylation. *DARU J. Pharm. Sci.* **2018**, *26*, 165–177. [CrossRef]

170. Jinwal, U.K.; Groshev, A.; Zhang, J.; Grover, A.; Sutariya, V.B. Preparation and characterization of methylene blue nanoparticles for Alzheimer's disease and other tauopathies. *Curr. Drug Deliv.* **2014**, *11*, 541–550. [CrossRef]
171. Sonawane, S.K.; Ahmad, A.; Chinnathambi, S. Protein-capped metal nanoparticles inhibit Tau aggregation in Alzheimer's disease. *ACS Omega* **2019**, *4*, 12833–12840. [CrossRef]
172. Misra, S.; Chopra, K.; Sinha, V.R.; Medhi, B. Galantamine-loaded solid–lipid nanoparticles for enhanced brain delivery: Preparation, characterization, in vitro and in vivo evaluations. *Drug Deliv.* **2015**, *23*, 1434–1443. [CrossRef] [PubMed]
173. Li, W.; Zhou, Y.-Q.; Zhao, N.; Hao, B.; Wang, X.; Kong, P. Pharmacokinetic behavior and efficiency of acetylcholinesterase inhibition in rat brain after intranasal administration of galanthamine hydrobromide loaded flexible liposomes. *Environ. Toxicol. Pharmacol.* **2012**, *34*, 272–279. [CrossRef] [PubMed]
174. Fornaguera, C.; Feiner-Gracia, N.; Calderó, G.; García-Celma, M.J.; Solans, C. Galantamine-loaded PLGA nanoparticles, from nano-emulsion templating, as novel advanced drug delivery systems to treat neurodegenerative diseases. *Nanoscale* **2015**, *7*, 12076–12084. [CrossRef] [PubMed]
175. Hanafy, A.S.; Farid, R.M.; Helmy, M.W.; Elgamal, S.S. Pharmacological, toxicological and neuronal localization assessment of galantamine/chitosan complex nanoparticles in rats: Future potential contribution in Alzheimer's disease management. *Drug Deliv.* **2016**, *23*, 3111–3122. [CrossRef] [PubMed]
176. Hanafy, A.S.; Farid, R.M.; Elgamal, S.S. Complexation as an approach to entrap cationic drugs into cationic nanoparticles administered intranasally for Alzheimer's disease management: Preparation and detection in rat brain. *Drug Dev. Ind. Pharm.* **2015**, *41*, 2055–2068. [CrossRef]
177. Ullah, Z.; Al Asmari, A.K.; Tariq, M.; Fatani, A. Preparation, characterization, and in vivo evaluation of intranasally administered liposomal formulation of donepezil. *Drug Des. Dev. Ther.* **2016**, 205–215. [CrossRef]
178. Bhavna, M.D.S.; Ali, M.; Ali, R.; Bhatnagar, A.; Baboota, S.; Ali, J. Donepezil nanosuspension intended for nose to brain targeting: In vitro and in vivo safety evaluation. *Int. J. Biol. Macromol.* **2014**, *67*, 418–425. [CrossRef]
179. Jakki, S.L.; Ramesh, Y.V.; Gowthamarajan, K.; Senthil, V.; Jain, K.; Sood, S.; Pathak, D. Novel anionic polymer as a carrier for CNS delivery of anti-Alzheimer drug. *Drug Deliv.* **2016**, *23*, 3471–3479. [CrossRef]
180. Baysal, I.; Ucar, G.; Gultekinoglu, M.; Ulubayram, K.; Yabanoglu-Ciftci, S. Donepezil loaded PLGA-b-PEG nanoparticles: Their ability to induce destabilization of amyloid fibrils and to cross blood brain barrier in vitro. *J. Neural Transm.* **2017**, *124*, 33–45. [CrossRef]
181. Yang, C.-R.; Zhao, X.-L.; Hu, H.-Y.; Li, K.-X.; Sun, X.; Li, L.; Chen, D.-W. Preparation, optimization and characteristic of huperzine a loaded nanostructured lipid carriers. *Chem. Pharm. Bull.* **2010**, *58*, 656–661. [CrossRef]
182. Patel, P.A.; Patil, S.C.; Kalaria, D.R.; Kalia, Y.N.; Patravale, V. Comparative in vitro and in vivo evaluation of lipid based nanocarriers of Huperzine A. *Int. J. Pharm.* **2013**, *446*, 16–23. [CrossRef] [PubMed]
183. Jiang, Y.; Liu, C.; Zhai, W.; Zhuang, N.; Han, T.; Ding, Z. The optimization design of lactoferrin loaded hupa nanoemulsion for targeted drug transport via intranasal route. *Int. J. Nanomed.* **2019**, *14*, 9217–9234. [CrossRef] [PubMed]
184. Meng, Q.; Wang, A.; Hua, H.; Jiang, Y.; Wang, Y.; Mu, H.; Wu, Z.; Sun, K. Intranasal delivery of Huperzine A to the brain using lactoferrin-conjugated *N*-trimethylated chitosan surface-modified PLGA nanoparticles for treatment of Alzheimer's disease. *Int. J. Nanomed.* **2018**, *13*, 705–718. [CrossRef] [PubMed]
185. Qian, S.; Wong, Y.C.; Zuo, Z. Development, characterization and application of in situ gel systems for intranasal delivery of tacrine. *Int. J. Pharm.* **2014**, *468*, 272–282. [CrossRef]
186. Luppi, B.; Bigucci, F.; Corace, G.; Delucca, A.; Cerchiara, T.; Sorrenti, M.; Catenacci, L.; Di Pietra, A.M.; Zecchi, V. Albumin nanoparticles carrying cyclodextrins for nasal delivery of the anti-Alzheimer drug tacrine. *Eur. J. Pharm. Sci.* **2011**, *44*, 559–565. [CrossRef]
187. Wilson, B.; Samanta, M.K.; Santhi, K.; Kumar, K.S.; Ramasamy, M.; Suresh, B. Chitosan nanoparticles as a new delivery system for the anti-Alzheimer drug tacrine. *Nanomed. Nanotechnol. Biol. Med.* **2010**, *6*, 144–152. [CrossRef]
188. Wavikar, P.; Pai, R.; Vavia, P. Nose to brain delivery of rivastigmine by in situ gelling cationic nanostructured lipid carriers: Enhanced brain distribution and pharmacodynamics. *J. Pharm. Sci.* **2017**, *106*, 3613–3622. [CrossRef]
189. Ismail, M.F.; ElMeshad, A.N.; Salem, N.A.-H. Potential therapeutic effect of nanobased formulation of rivastigmine on rat model of Alzheimer's disease. *Int. J. Nanomed.* **2013**, *8*, 393–406. [CrossRef]

190. Arumugam, K.; Subramanian, G.S.; Mallayasamy, S.R.; Averineni, R.K.; Reddy, M.S.; Udupa, N. A study of rivastigmine liposomes for delivery into the brain through intranasal route. *Acta Pharm.* **2008**, *58*, 287–297. [CrossRef]
191. Yang, Z.-Z.; Zhang, Y.-Q.; Wang, Z.-Z.; Wu, K.; Lou, J.-N.; Qi, X.-R. Enhanced brain distribution and pharmacodynamics of rivastigmine by liposomes following intranasal administration. *Int. J. Pharm.* **2013**, *452*, 344–354. [CrossRef]
192. Mutlu, N.B.; Değim, Z.; Yilmaz, Ş.; Eşsiz, D.; Nacar, A. New perspective for the treatment of Alzheimer diseases: Liposomal rivastigmine formulations. *Drug Dev. Ind. Pharm.* **2011**, *37*, 775–789. [CrossRef] [PubMed]
193. Joshi, S.; Chavhan, S.S.; Sawant, K.K. Rivastigmine-loaded PLGA and PBCA nanoparticles: Preparation, optimization, characterization, in vitro and pharmacodynamic studies. *Eur. J. Pharm. Biopharm.* **2010**, *76*, 189–199. [CrossRef] [PubMed]
194. Khemariya, R.P.; Khemariya, P.S. New-fangled approach in the management of Alzheimer by formulation of polysorbate 80 coated chitosan nanoparticles of rivastigmine for brain delivery and their in vivo evaluation. *Int. J. Cur. Res. Med. Sci.* **2016**, *2*, 18–29.
195. Fazil, M.; Md, S.; Haque, S.; Kumar, M.; Baboota, S.; Sahni, J.K.; Ali, J. Development and evaluation of rivastigmine loaded chitosan nanoparticles for brain targeting. *Eur. J. Pharm. Sci.* **2012**, *47*, 6–15. [CrossRef]
196. Casadomé-Perales, Á.; De Matteis, L.; Alleva, M.; Infantes-Rodríguez, C.; Palomares-Pérez, I.; Saito, T.; Saido, T.C.; Esteban, J.A.; Nebreda, A.R.; De La Fuente, J.M.; et al. Inhibition of p38 MAPK in the brain through nasal administration of p38 inhibitor loaded in chitosan nanocapsules. *Nanomedicine* **2019**, *14*, 2409–2422. [CrossRef]
197. Dara, T.; Vatanara, A.; Sharifzadeh, M.; Khani, S.; Vakilinezhad, M.A.; Vakhshiteh, F.; Meybodi, M.N.; Malvajerd, S.S.; Hassani, S.; Mosaddegh, M.H. Improvement of memory deficits in the rat model of Alzheimer's disease by erythropoietin-loaded solid lipid nanoparticles. *Neurobiol. Learn. Mem.* **2019**, *166*, 107082. [CrossRef]
198. Elnaggar, Y.S.R.; Etman, S.M.; Abdelmonsif, D.A.; Abdallah, O.Y. Novel piperine-loaded Tween-integrated monoolein cubosomes as brain-targeted oral nanomedicine in Alzheimer's disease: Pharmaceutical, biological, and toxicological studies. *Int. J. Nanomed.* **2015**, *10*, 5459–5473. [CrossRef]
199. Huang, M.; Hu, M.; Song, Q.; Song, H.; Huang, J.; Gu, X.; Wang, X.; Chen, J.; Kang, T.; Feng, X.; et al. GM1-modified lipoprotein-like nanoparticle: Multifunctional nanoplatform for the combination therapy of Alzheimer's disease. *ACS Nano* **2015**, *9*, 10801–10816. [CrossRef]
200. Liu, Z.; Jiang, M.; Kang, T.; Miao, D.; Gu, G.; Song, Q.; Yao, L.; Hu, Q.; Tu, Y.; Pang, Z.; et al. Lactoferrin-modified PEG-co-PCL nanoparticles for enhanced brain delivery of NAP peptide following intranasal administration. *Biomaterials* **2013**, *34*, 3870–3881. [CrossRef]
201. Yang, L.; Yin, T.; Liu, Y.; Sun, J.; Zhou, Y.; Liu, J. Gold nanoparticle-capped mesoporous silica-based H2O2-responsive controlled release system for Alzheimer's disease treatment. *Acta Biomater.* **2016**, *46*, 177–190. [CrossRef]
202. Yin, T.; Yang, L.; Liu, Y.; Zhou, X.; Sun, J.; Liu, J. Sialic acid (SA)-modified selenium nanoparticles coated with a high blood–brain barrier permeability peptide-B6 peptide for potential use in Alzheimer's disease. *Acta Biomater.* **2015**, *25*, 172–183. [CrossRef] [PubMed]
203. Loureiro, J.A.; Andrade, S.; Duarte, A.; Neves, A.; Queiroz, J.F.; Nunes, C.; Sevin, E.; Fenart, L.; Gosselet, F.; Coelho, M.A.; et al. Resveratrol and grape extract-loaded solid lipid nanoparticles for the treatment of Alzheimer's disease. *Molecules* **2017**, *22*, 277. [CrossRef] [PubMed]
204. Sun, J.; Wei, C.; Liu, Y.; Xie, W.; Xu, M.; Zhou, H.; Liu, J. Progressive release of mesoporous nano-selenium delivery system for the multi-channel synergistic treatment of Alzheimer's disease. *Biomaterials* **2019**, *197*, 417–431. [CrossRef]
205. Gothwal, A.; Kumar, H.; Nakhate, K.T.; Ajazuddin; Dutta, A.; Borah, A.; Gupta, U. Lactoferrin coupled lower generation PAMAM dendrimers for brain targeted delivery of memantine in aluminum-chloride-induced Alzheimer's disease in mice. *Bioconjugate Chem.* **2019**, *30*, 2573–2583. [CrossRef] [PubMed]
206. Laserra, S.; Basit, A.; Sozio, P.; Marinelli, L.; Fornasari, E.; Cacciatore, I.; Ciulla, M.; Turkez, H.; Geyikoğglu, F.; Di Stefano, A. Solid lipid nanoparticles loaded with lipoyl–memantine codrug: Preparation and characterization. *Int. J. Pharm.* **2015**, *485*, 183–191. [CrossRef]

207. Alawdi, S.H.; Eidi, H.; Safar, M.M.; Abdel-Wahhab, M.A. Loading amlodipine on diamond nanoparticles: A novel drug delivery system. *Nanotechnol. Sci. Appl.* **2019**, *12*, 47–53. [CrossRef]
208. Meng, F.; Asghar, S.; Gao, S.; Su, Z.; Song, J.; Huo, M.; Meng, W.; Ping, Q.; Xiao, Y. A novel LDL-mimic nanocarrier for the targeted delivery of curcumin into the brain to treat Alzheimer's disease. *Colloids Surf. B Biointerfaces* **2015**, *134*, 88–97. [CrossRef]
209. Gao, C.; Wang, Y.; Sun, J.; Han, Y.; Gong, W.; Li, Y.; Feng, Y.; Wang, H.; Yang, M.; Li, Z.; et al. Neuronal mitochondria-targeted delivery of curcumin by biomimetic engineered nanosystems in Alzheimer's disease mice. *Acta Biomater.* **2020**, *108*, 285–299. [CrossRef]
210. Kuo, Y.-C.; Lin, C.-Y.; Li, J.-S.; Lou, Y.-I. Wheat germ agglutinin-conjugated liposomes incorporated with cardiolipin to improve neuronal survival in Alzheimer's disease treatment. *Int. J. Nanomed.* **2017**, *12*, 1757–1774. [CrossRef]
211. Huo, X.; Zhang, Y.; Jin, X.; Li, Y.; Zhang, L. A novel synthesis of selenium nanoparticles encapsulated PLGA nanospheres with curcumin molecules for the inhibition of amyloid β aggregation in Alzheimer's disease. *J. Photochem. Photobiol. B Biol.* **2019**, *190*, 98–102. [CrossRef]
212. Jaruszewski, K.M.; Curran, G.L.; Swaminathan, S.K.; Rosenberg, J.T.; Grant, S.C.; Ramakrishnan, S.; Lowe, V.J.; Poduslo, J.F.; Kandimalla, K.K. Multimodal nanoprobes to target cerebrovascular amyloid in Alzheimer's disease brain. *Biomaterials* **2013**, *35*, 1967–1976. [CrossRef] [PubMed]
213. Bilia, A.R.; Nardiello, P.; Piazzini, V.; Leri, M.; Bergonzi, M.C.; Bucciantini, M.; Casamenti, F. Successful brain delivery of andrographolide loaded in human albumin nanoparticles to TgCRND8 mice, an Alzheimer's disease mouse model. *Front. Pharmacol.* **2019**, *10*, 910. [CrossRef] [PubMed]
214. Al-Azzawi, S.; Masheta, D.; Guildford, A.; Phillips, G.; Santin, M. Dendrimeric poly(epsilon-lysine) delivery systems for the enhanced permeability of flurbiprofen across the blood-brain barrier in Alzheimer's disease. *Int. J. Mol. Sci.* **2018**, *19*, 3224. [CrossRef] [PubMed]
215. Muntimadugu, E.; Dhommati, R.; Jain, A.; Challa, V.G.S.; Shaheen, M.; Khan, W. Intranasal delivery of nanoparticle encapsulated tarenflurbil: A potential brain targeting strategy for Alzheimer's disease. *Eur. J. Pharm. Sci.* **2016**, *92*, 224–234. [CrossRef]
216. Saffari, P.M.; Alijanpour, S.; Takzaree, N.; Sahebgharani, M.; Etemad-Moghadam, S.; Noorbakhsh, F.; Partoazar, A. Metformin loaded phosphatidylserine nanoliposomes improve memory deficit and reduce neuroinflammation in streptozotocin-induced Alzheimer's disease model. *Life Sci.* **2020**, *255*, 117861. [CrossRef]
217. Fernandes, J.; Ghate, V.M.; Mallik, S.B.; Lewis, S. Amino acid conjugated chitosan nanoparticles for the brain targeting of a model dipeptidyl peptidase-4 inhibitor. *Int. J. Pharm.* **2018**, *547*, 563–571. [CrossRef]
218. Kuo, Y.-C.; Wang, C.-T. Protection of SK-N-MC cells against β-amyloid peptide-induced degeneration using neuron growth factor-loaded liposomes with surface lactoferrin. *Biomaterials* **2014**, *35*, 5954–5964. [CrossRef]
219. Kuo, Y.-C.; Lin, C.-Y. Targeting delivery of liposomes with conjugated p-aminophenyl-α-D-manno-pyranoside and apolipoprotein E for inhibiting neuronal degeneration insulted with β-amyloid peptide. *J. Drug Target.* **2014**, *23*, 147–158. [CrossRef]
220. Kuo, Y.-C.; Chou, P.-R. Neuroprotection against degeneration of SK-N-MC cells using neuron growth factor-encapsulated liposomes with surface cereport and transferrin. *J. Pharm. Sci.* **2014**, *103*, 2484–2497. [CrossRef]
221. Zhang, C.; Chen, J.; Feng, C.; Shao, X.; Liu, Q.; Zhang, Q.; Pang, Z.; Jiang, X. Intranasal nanoparticles of basic fibroblast growth factor for brain delivery to treat Alzheimer's disease. *Int. J. Pharm.* **2014**, *461*, 192–202. [CrossRef]
222. Angelova, A.; Drechsler, M.; Garamus, V.M.; Angelov, B. Pep-lipid cubosomes and vesicles compartmentalized by micelles from self-assembly of multiple neuroprotective building blocks including a large peptide hormone PACAP-DHA. *ChemNanoMat* **2019**, *5*, 1381–1389. [CrossRef]
223. Leblanc, R.M.; Liyanage, P.Y.; Devadoss, D.; Guevara, L.R.R.; Cheng, L.; Graham, R.M.; Chand, H.S.; Al-Youbi, A.O.; Bashammakh, A.S.; El-Shahawi, M.S.; et al. Nontoxic amphiphilic carbon dots as promising drug nanocarriers across the blood–brain barrier and inhibitors of β-amyloid. *Nanoscale* **2019**, *11*, 22387–22397. [CrossRef]
224. Chen, Y.; Fan, H.; Xu, C.; Hu, W.; Yu, B. Efficient cholera toxin B subunit-based nanoparticles with MRI capability for drug delivery to the brain following intranasal administration. *Macromol. Biosci.* **2018**, *19*, e1800340. [CrossRef]

225. Cui, N.; Lu, H.; Li, M. Magnetic nanoparticles associated PEG/PLGA block copolymer targeted with anti-transferrin receptor antibodies for Alzheimer's disease. *J. Biomed. Nanotechnol.* **2018**, *14*, 1017–1024. [CrossRef] [PubMed]
226. Do, T.D.; Amin, F.U.; Noh, Y.; Kim, M.O.; Yoon, J.; Duc, D.T.; Ul, A.F.; YeongIl, N.; Ok, K.M.; Jungwon, Y. Guidance of magnetic nanocontainers for treating Alzheimer's disease using an electromagnetic, targeted drug-delivery actuator. *J. Biomed. Nanotechnol.* **2016**, *12*, 569–574. [CrossRef] [PubMed]
227. Sanati, M.; Khodagholi, F.; Aminyavari, S.; Ghasemi, F.; Gholami, M.; Kebriaeezadeh, A.; Sabzevari, O.; Hajipour, M.J.; Imani, M.; Mahmoudi, M.; et al. Impact of gold nanoparticles on amyloid β-induced Alzheimer's disease in a rat animal model: Involvement of STIM proteins. *ACS Chem. Neurosci.* **2019**, *10*, 2299–2309. [CrossRef]
228. Pardridge, W.M. Blood–brain barrier drug delivery of IgG fusion proteins with a transferrin receptor monoclonal antibody. *Expert Opin. Drug Deliv.* **2014**, *12*, 207–222. [CrossRef]
229. Liu, W.; Sun, F.; Wan, M.; Jiang, F.; Bo, X.; Lin, L.; Tang, H.; Xu, S. β-Sheet breaker peptide-HPYD for the treatment of Alzheimer's disease: Primary studies on behavioral test and transcriptional profiling. *Front. Pharmacol.* **2018**, *8*, 969. [CrossRef]
230. Zheng, X.; Shao, X.; Zhang, C.; Tan, Y.; Liu, Q.; Wan, X.; Zhang, Q.; Xu, S.; Jiang, X. Intranasal H102 peptide-loaded liposomes for brain delivery to treat Alzheimer's disease. *Pharm. Res.* **2015**, *32*, 3837–3849. [CrossRef]
231. Hu, B.; Dai, F.; Fan, Z.; Ma, G.; Tang, Q.; Zhang, X. Nanotheranostics: Congo Red/Rutin-MNPs with enhanced magnetic resonance imaging and H2O2-responsive therapy of alzheimer's disease in APPswe/PS1dE9 transgenic mice. *Adv. Mater.* **2015**, *27*, 5499–5505. [CrossRef]
232. Gao, C.; Chu, X.; Gong, W.; Zheng, J.; Xie, X.; Wang, Y.; Yang, M.; Li, Z.; Gao, C.; Yang, Y. Neuron tau-targeting biomimetic nanoparticles for curcumin delivery to delay progression of Alzheimer's disease. *J. Nanobiotechnol.* **2020**, *18*, 1–23. [CrossRef] [PubMed]
233. Singh, N.A.; Mandal, A.K.A.; Khan, Z.A. Potential neuroprotective properties of epigallocatechin-3-gallate (EGCG). *Nutr. J.* **2015**, *15*, 1–17. [CrossRef] [PubMed]
234. Agrawal, M.; Saraf, S.; Saraf, S.; Antimisiaris, S.G.; Chougule, M.B.; Shoyele, S.A.; Alexander, A. Nose-to-brain drug delivery: An update on clinical challenges and progress towards approval of anti-Alzheimer drugs. *J. Control. Release* **2018**, *281*, 139–177. [CrossRef] [PubMed]
235. Md, S.; Haque, S.; Fazil, M.; Kumar, M.; Baboota, S.; Narang, J.K.; Ali, J. Optimised nanoformulation of bromocriptine for direct nose-to-brain delivery: Biodistribution, pharmacokinetic and dopamine estimation by ultra-HPLC/mass spectrometry method. *Expert Opin. Drug Deliv.* **2014**, *11*, 827–842. [CrossRef]
236. Lauzon, M.-A.; Daviau, A.; Marcos, B.; Faucheux, N. Nanoparticle-mediated growth factor delivery systems: A new way to treat Alzheimer's disease. *J. Control. Release* **2015**, *206*, 187–205. [CrossRef]

2

Mesoporous Silica Nanoparticles: A Comprehensive Review on Synthesis and Recent Advances

Reema Narayan [1], Usha Y. Nayak [1,*], Ashok M. Raichur [2] and Sanjay Garg [3]

1 Department of Pharmaceutics, Manipal College of Pharmaceutical Sciences, Manipal Academy of Higher Education, Manipal 576104, India; nsreema@gmail.com
2 Department of Materials Engineering, Indian Institute of Science, Bengaluru 560012, India; amr@iisc.ac.in
3 School of Pharmacy and Medical Science, University of South Australia, Adelaide, SA 5000, Australia; Sanjay.Garg@unisa.edu.au
* Correspondence: usha.nayak@manipal.edu;

Abstract: Recent advancements in drug delivery technologies utilizing a variety of carriers have resulted in a path-breaking revolution in the approach towards diagnosis and therapy alike in the current times. Need for materials with high thermal, chemical and mechanical properties have led to the development of mesoporous silica nanoparticles (MSNs). These ordered porous materials have garnered immense attention as drug carriers owing to their distinctive features over the others. They can be synthesized using a relatively simple process, thus making it cost effective. Moreover, by controlling the parameters during the synthesis; the morphology, pore size and volume and particle size can be transformed accordingly. Over the last few years, a rapid increase in research on MSNs as drug carriers for the treatment of various diseases has been observed indicating its potential benefits in drug delivery. Their widespread application for the loading of small molecules as well as macromolecules such as proteins, siRNA and so forth, has made it a versatile carrier. In the recent times, researchers have sorted to several modifications in the framework of MSNs to explore its potential in drug resistant chemotherapy, antimicrobial therapy. In this review, we have discussed the synthesis of these multitalented nanoparticles and the factors influencing the size and morphology of this wonder carrier. The second part of this review emphasizes on the applications and the advances made in the MSNs to broaden the spectrum of its use especially in the field of biomedicine. We have also touched upon the lacunae in the thorough understanding of its interaction with a biological system which poses a major hurdle in the passage of this carrier to the clinical level. In the final part of this review, we have discussed some of the major patents filed in the field of MSNs for therapeutic purpose.

Keywords: mesoporous silica nanoparticles; MCM-41; protocells; SBA-15; Stober's synthesis; tetraethyl orthosilicate

---

1. Introduction

Modern nanotechnology has evolved as the principal component of science in the current century. Over the years, diagnosis of diseases and its therapy is constantly leaping milestones due to the application of nanotechnology in the field of biomedicine. The evolution of nanomedicine and green technology for its production have been a great boon and have shifted paradigms in therapy and tissue engineering, owing to the advantages of nanocarriers such as a high surface area to volume ratio, unique features of surface modification and engineering to obtain particles of various sizes, shapes and different chemical characteristics. These have proven to be biocompatible, biodegradable and non-toxic which adds to its advantages [1–5]. Lipid-based nanocarriers [6–8], polymeric nanoparticles [9–11], dendrimers [12] have revolutionized the therapy for various conditions especially cancer and infectious diseases. Many of these products have been approved and are commercially available. Table 1 enlists some of the marketed nanomedicines.

Table 1. List of some marketed products containing nanoparticles.

Marketed Product	Formulation	Drug	Use	References
AmBisome®	Liposome	Amphotericin B	Antifungal	[13]
DaunoXome®	Liposome	Daunorubicin	Kaposi's sarcoma associated with HIV	[14]
Doxil®	Liposome	Doxorubicin	Kaposi's sarcoma associated with HIV, breast cancer, ovarian cancer	[15]
Myocet®	Liposome	Doxorubicin	Breast cancer	[16]
Emend®	Nanocrystals	Aprepitant	Antiemetic	[17]
Megace ES®	Nanocrystals	Megestrol acetate	Anorexia	[17]
Tricor®	Nanocrystals	Fenofibrate	In hypercholesterolemia	[17]

Apart from the above mentioned organic nanoparticles, inorganic nanoparticles have also been widely explored for their application in biomedicine. Out of them, quantum dots, iron oxide nanoparticles have been approved and are commercially available. Carbon dots, nanoparticles of gold, silver, various other metal oxides, layered double hydroxide nanoparticles and silica nanoparticles have been widely used for various diagnostic and therapeutic purposes [2,18–20]. Of these, silica nanoparticles comprising of organic dyes and radioactive iodide known as Cornell dots (C dots) has successfully attained an important benchmark of safety by its approval for Phase I human trials which is vital for any substance requiring Investigational New Drug (IND) approval. C dots are core-shell silica nanoparticles containing fluorescent molecules within the silica core surrounded with silica shell which is further coated with polyethylene glycol (PEG). C dots were first developed by the Spencer T. Olin Professor of Engineering, Ulrich Wiesner from Department of Materials Science and Engineering at Cornell University [21,22].

Silica nanoparticles with mesopores–referred to as mesoporous silica nanoparticles (MSNs)–have gained wide popularity over the recent years. Its advantages of uniform and tunable pore size, easy independent functionalization of the surface, internal and external pores and the gating mechanism of the pore opening make it a distinctive and promising drug carrier. Scientists have successfully worked on the utilization of these carriers for loading variety of cargo ranging from drugs to macromolecules such as proteins [23,24], DNA [25,26] and RNA [27,28]. An exhaustive set of literatures are available and research is still underway in evaluating new avenues for the use of MSNs in drug delivery. Several reviews pertaining to MSNs in improving the solubility of the drug [29,30], as controlled/sustained drug delivery system [31], applications in biomedicine [32,33] have been published. The present review focuses on literatures published on a broad perspective of MSNs ranging from synthesis to the patents filed. In doing so, we realize that all the reported papers in each of the areas could not be discussed in detail. We have detailed and overviewed the recent research and patents applied for MSNs specifically on Mobil Crystalline Materials (MCM-41) and Santa Barbara Amorphous type material (SBA-15). An overview of the synthesis and theory behind the formation of MSNs is provided to discuss the factors affecting the shape and size of MSNs. The major research in the field of MSNs related to the biomedical applications for therapy based on small molecules and the related patents literature are included.

2. Origin of Mesoporous Silica Materials

Although the synthesis of mesoscopic materials dates back to 1970s, Mobil Research and Development Corporation was the first to synthesize mesoporous solids from aluminosilicate gels using liquid crystal template mechanism in the year 1992. They designated it as (Mobil Crystalline Materials or Mobil Composition of Matter) MCM-41. As per IUPAC, mesoporous materials are defined as the one having a pore size in the range of 2–50 nm and an ordered arrangement of pores giving an ordered structure to it [34–36]. The pore size of these could be varied and tuned through the choice of surfactants used. Generally, MCM-41 is hexagonal with a pore diameter of 2.5 to 6 nm wherein cationic surfactants were used as templates. MCM-41 is one of the most widely explored materials for drug delivery. Apart from this, various other materials of mesoporous nature have also been synthesized by varying the starting precursors and reaction conditions. These may vary in their structural arrangement or the pore size. MCM-48 has a cubic arrangement whereas MCM-50 has a lamella-like arrangement [37]. Non-ionic triblock copolymers like alkyl poly(ethylene oxide) (PEO) oligomeric surfactants and poly(alkylene oxide) block copolymers have also been used as a template which has been designated as SBA-11 (cubic), SBA-12 (3-*d* hexagonal), SBA-15 (hexagonal) and SBA-16 (cubic cage-structured) based on the symmetry of the mesoporous structure and the triblock polymers used. The ratio of ethylene oxide to propylene oxide was varied to achieve the desired symmetry of mesoporous materials. Highly ordered mesoporous structure of SBA-15 has also been widely used for the biomedical purpose. This was first synthesized by University of California, Santa Barbara and hence named Santa Barbara Amorphous type material (SBA). This is different from MCM in that they possess larger pores of 4.6–30 nm and thicker silica walls [38]. FSM-16, that is, folded sheets of mesoporous materials are another type of mesoporous materials, which are synthesized using quaternary ammonium surfactant as a template and layered polysilicate kanemite. Tozuka et al. demonstrated that FSM-16 could be used for pharmaceutical applications other than as an adsorbent and for catalysis [39]. Various other MSNs coined Technical Delft University (TUD-1), Hiroshima Mesoporous Material-33 (HMM-33), Centrum voor Oppervlaktechemie en Katalyse/Centre for Research Chemistry and Catalysis (COK-12) have been synthesized which vary in their pore symmetry and shape [40,41]. The structural characteristics of some mesoporous materials have been listed in Table 2. Figure 1 shows the representation of some MSNs. Of these, MCM-41, MCM-48, SBA-15, SBA-16 are widely employed for drug delivery. In addition, they have also been explored as adsorbents, catalysis and as biosensors. MCM-50, SBA-11 and SBA-12 have been reported to behave as excellent adsorbents and in catalysis.

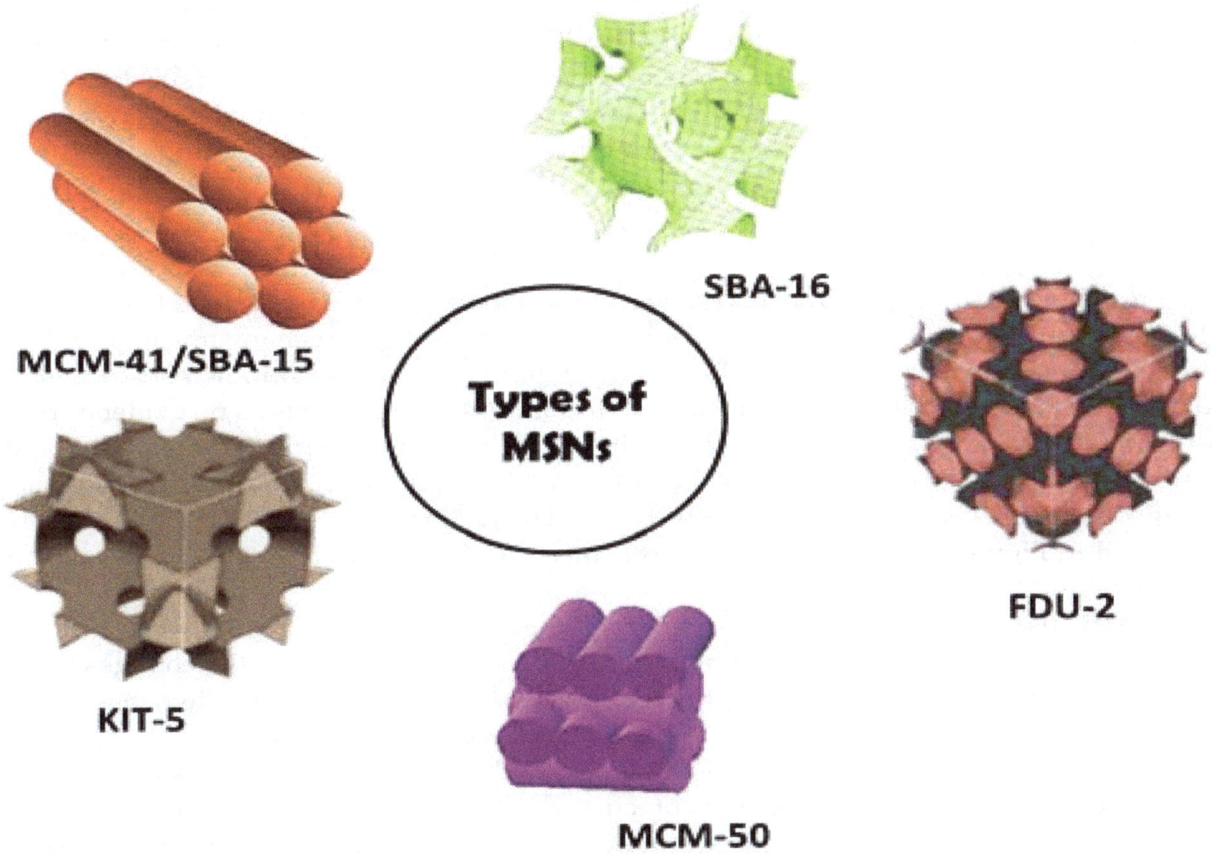

Figure 1. Representation of different types of mesoporous silica nanoparticles (MSNs).

Table 2. List of some of the types of mesoporous silica nanoparticles (MSNs) and their characteristics.

MSN Family	MSN Type	Pore Symmetry	Pore Size (nm)	Pore Volume (cm^3/g)	References
M41S	MCM-41	2D hexagonal *P6mm*	1.5–8	>1.0	[42,43]
	MCM-48	3D cubic I*a*3*d*	2–5	>1.0	[42,43]
	MCM-50	Lamellar *p*2	2–5	>1.0	[44,45]
SBA	SBA-11	3D cubic *Pm*3*m*	2.1–3.6	0.68	[45–47]
	SBA-12	3D hexagonal $P6_3/mmc$	3.1	0.83	[48–50]
	SBA-15	2D hexagonal *p6mm*	6–0	1.17	[43,51]
	SBA-16	Cubic I*m*3*m*	5–15	0.91	[43,52]
KIT	KIT-5	Cubic F*m*3*m*	9.3	0.45	[53,54]
COK	COK-12	Hexagonal *P6m*	5.8	0.45	[55,56]

MCM-Mobil Crystalline Materials; SBA- Santa Barbara Amorphous; KIT- Korea Advanced Institute of Science and Technology, COK- Centre for Research Chemistry and Catalysis.

3. Synthesis of MSNs

Stober was the pioneer in developing a system of chemical reactions for the synthesis of spherical monodisperse micron size silica particles [57]. From then on, the method is known as Stober synthesis. Many modifications have constantly been made to the Stober's synthesis to yield monodisperse, ordered, nanosized silica particles. The synthesis of MSNs can be accomplished in basic, acidic and neutral conditions. Manipulating the reaction parameters resulted in particles with different shapes and sizes. The Stober's method of synthesis was first modified by Grun et al. where they introduced a cationic surfactant as a template to yield a spherical rather than a hexagonal MCM-41 structure. They were successful in generating spherical MCM-41 with similar properties as that generated by other methods [58]. Constant research has led to a lot of variations in the synthesis conditions and methods to yield stable, monodisperse MSNs.

For MSNs to be an ideal carrier for drug delivery the particle size needs to be uniform; pore volume has to be large to enhance loading capacity. These parameters can be controlled during the synthesis by varying the pH of the reaction mixture, temperature, concentration of surfactant and silica source. The synthesis of MSNs occurs by liquid crystal template mechanism wherein hydrolysis and condensation of silica on the surface of surfactant micelles takes place. The liquid silica (tetraethyl orthosilicate) transforms to solid silica [59–61].

3.1. Mechanism of Formation of MSNs

A thorough understanding of the mechanism of formation of MSNs is essential to obtain particles with desired properties for drug delivery. The early reports on the mechanism suggested that the silica network gets built throughout the liquid–crystalline phases of non-ionic surfactants. This is particularly true for materials prepared from a dilute solution of surfactants as no evidence of regular mesostructured materials was observed [62]. The literature has shown that either the hydrolysed silica gets adsorbed around the micelles or in the case of SBA-15, the surfactant and the silica interact at the initial stage and form a core shell-like structure [63]. The mechanism for the formation of MCM-41 is represented in Figure 2. Efforts have been on since then by research groups to unveil the exact mechanism behind the formation of MSNs.

The in-situ usage of time-resolved small-angle neutron scattering (SANS) has been used to study the formation of MSNs. Using this method, they were able to predict the changes happening concurrently with the formation process. It was observed that during the early hydrolysis (~40 s) of silica source tetramethyl orthosilicate (TMOS), the silicate ions tend to adsorb around the surfactant micelles during the growth phase. As the charge around the surfactant reduces due to the initial hydrolysis and the condensation of the silica precursor, the intermicellar repulsion reduces, allowing the further formation of small aggregates of silica. After ~400 s, the reaction mixture contained sufficiently discrete hexagonally ordered mesopores of silica which was confirmed by transmission electron microscopy (TEM) studies. This is in accordance with the previously proposed 'current bun model' for the mechanism of formation of MSNs [64,65].

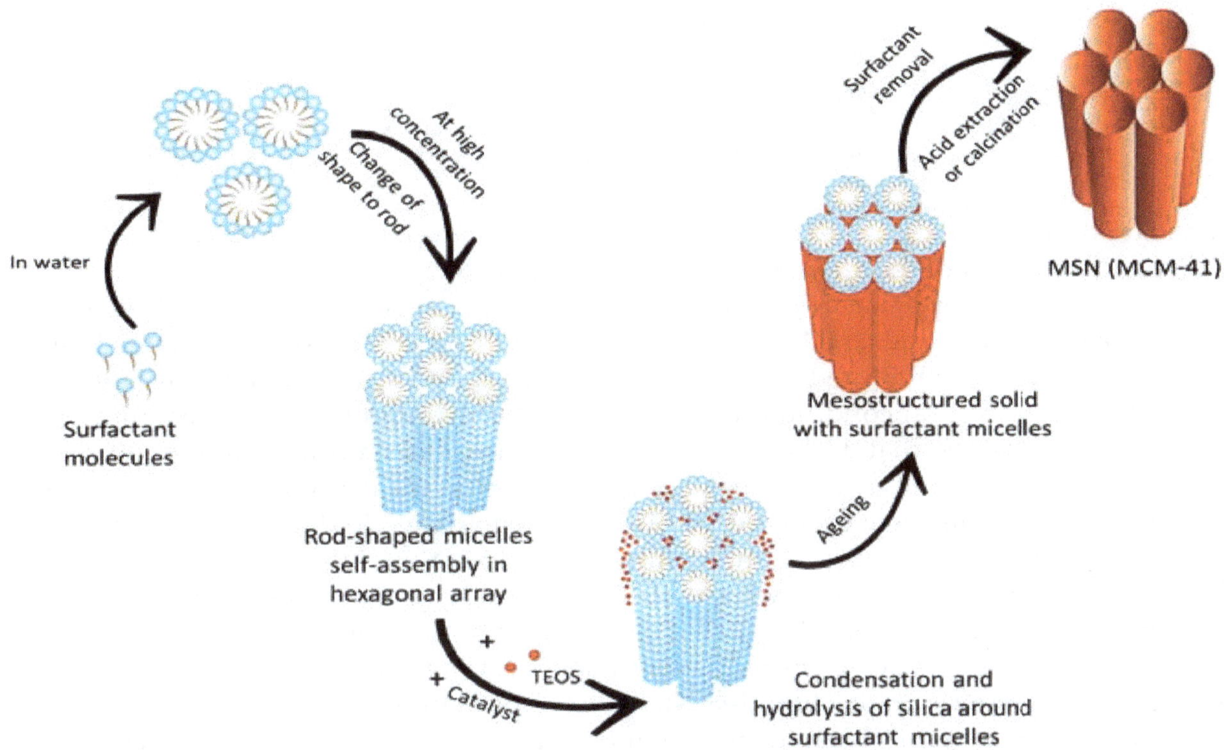

Figure 2. Mechanism of formation of Mobil Crystalline Materials No.41 (MCM-41).

Another mechanism named 'swelling-shrinking mechanism' was proposed for the formation of MSNs utilizing the technique of time-resolved synchrotron small-angle X-ray scattering (SAXS). This mechanism holds well when tetraethyl orthosilicate (TEOS) alone is used as the precursor in the absence of any other solvent like ethanol. TEOS being oil-like monomer showed phase separation under static condition, whereas, under vigorous stirring, an emulsion-like system was obtained. Initially, cetyltrimethylammonium bromide (CTAB) forms ellipsoidal micelles with an inner core consisting of the hydrophobic tail. When TEOS is added, it gets solubilized in the hydrophobic core, thus enlarging the micelles and resulting in the transformation of micelle shape from ellipsoidal to spherical. On hydrolysis of TEOS, the monomers become hydrophilic and are released into the aqueous surroundings. The negatively charged hydrolysed monomers of TEOS get adsorbed onto positively charged CTAB micelles via electrostatic attraction. On complete consumption of the TEOS within the hydrophobic core, the micelles shrink and become smaller in size. As this process of hydrolysis and condensation occurs simultaneously, the micelles shrink continuously until all the TEOS gets hydrolysed and form silica shell around the micelles. The neighbouring micelles aggregate, resulting in particle growth forming a mesoporous structure [66].

3.2. Approaches for the Synthesis of MSNs

Majority of the MSNs are fabricated by modified Stober's method otherwise popularly known as a sol-gel process. Sol-gel chemistry is a widely explored process for the synthesis of many inorganic materials. It involves the hydrolysis and condensation of the alkoxide monomers into a colloidal solution (sol), which acts as a precursor to form an ordered network (gel) of polymer or discrete particles. A typical sol-gel process takes place in the presence of an acid or a base catalyst. Depending on the reaction conditions and the molar ratio of Si/H_2O, the alkoxide group gets hydrolysed. The rate of hydrolysis proceeds faster in basic conditions compared to acidic. Condensation succeeds the hydrolysis step and the effective condensation depends on the hydrolysis step. Multiple condensation results in a chain-like structure in the sol and network-like structure in gel form [67]. The schematic representation of the reaction is shown in Equation (1).

$$\begin{array}{l} \equiv\text{Si-OH} + \text{OH-Si}\equiv \;\leftrightarrow\; \equiv\text{Si-O-Si}\equiv + \text{HOH} \\ \equiv\text{Si-OH} + \text{RO-Si}\equiv \;\leftrightarrow\; \equiv\text{Si-O-Si}\equiv + \text{ROH} \\ \cdots\cdots\cdots\cdots \longrightarrow \text{polysilicates} \end{array} \quad (1)$$

"R' may be methyl, ethyl, propyl, butyl etc.

To yield particles of the desired size and to enhance the properties of MSNs, the sol-gel process has been modified. Some of the approaches are discussed below:

A simple quenching approach was adopted by Mann et al. to synthesize small sized and ordered MSNs. The reaction was quenched after 40 s by the addition of an excess of water followed by neutralization to pH 7 with dilute hydrochloric acid after a delay time ranging from 60 s to 220 s. The rest of the experimental condition and reagents were maintained the same as in the routine procedure. It was observed that dilution reduces coalescence, and neutralization reduces the rate of silica condensation. The results showed that greater the delay in the neutralization, larger the particle size [68,69]. Similar results were observed by Moller group. The colloidal suspension obtained was found to be stable for long periods of time. However, the MSNs produced by this technique were found to be less ordered in a structure which could be due to scale-up issues during dilution [70].

Evaporation-induced self-assembly (EISA) is another approach for the synthesis of MSNs. In this technique, all the reactants undergo concentration changes during evaporation throughout the process. This results in the organization of a liquid-crystal like template of the silica precursor. In this method, the required concentration of precursor formulations was prepared in ethanol/water solvent with a surfactant. This was converted to monodisperse droplets via injection into an aerosol generator. The droplet size can be controlled by altering its orifice. The alcohol evaporation during drying induces micelle formation and the co-assembly of silica-surfactant into liquid-crystal mesophases [71]. Fontecave et al. modified the EISA method by incorporating different amphiphilic drugs (stearoyl choline, sophorolipid and glucosyl-resveratrol) which behave both as a structure directing agent as well as an active cargo. Sol compositions containing TEOS, drug, water, ethanol and HCl were prepared and injected into an aerosol apparatus. A spray dryer with sufficient air flow and pressure was provided to convert the droplets into solid particles. Characterization of the particles for its pore size and structure using TEM revealed similar results to those with CTAB as surfactant template. Even though the mesostructure formation was not that good, the drug loading was found to be high in all the three cases with complete elimination of burst release. This method would be an ideal strategy for hydrophilic drugs functionalized with hydrophobic tails. Due to the absence of the surfactant template, intrinsic toxicity can be reduced [72].

A recent widely used modification to the synthesis of parent MSNs is encapsulating drugs in hollow mesoporous silica nanoparticles (HMSNs). Their large hollow cavity inside each MSN has garnered tremendous attention. These hollow cavities are capable of holding a high amount of drug compared to its non-hollow counterparts. This unique property of HMSNs makes it widely useful in cancer therapy and imaging [73,74]. Shi et al. were one of the first groups to report the synthesis of HMSNs [75,76]. Preliminary studies to ascertain its enhanced loading capacity was performed using ibuprofen as the model drug wherein, HMSNs showed an enhanced drug loading of 744.5 mg/g, as compared to 358.6 mg/g of MCM-41 [75]. The frequently used method for the synthesis of HMSNs includes the 'core-templating method'. In this approach, many soft/hard templates are used to form the core followed by coating with desired substance at different concentrations to obtain a shell around the substrate with a desired thickness. Subsequently, the core template can be eliminated by calcination or treatment with a suitable solvent leaving behind the shell with a hollow core [77]. She et al. synthesized HMSNs using eudragit S-100 and Triton X-100 as the core-shell template [78]. HMSNs using SiO_2@CTAB-SiO_2 nanoparticles as templates were synthesized by selective etching process [79]. Ghasemi et al. synthesized HMSNs using poly tert-butyl acrylate (PtBA) nanospheres as core-forming hard templates in the presence of CTAB as soft templates [80].

Many hard/soft templates like vesicles, polymeric micelles [81,82], gold [83] or silica nanoparticles were used to construct templates [84,85]. Lin and collaborators proposed a new technique for the synthesis of MSNs using water-in-oil microemulsion as a template. The advantages of this method were the uniformly sized particles obtained compared to other methods. Also, the microemulsion is said to be thermodynamically stable [86].

As the commonly used sol-gel process is a laborious, time consuming process, many different fast methods were used for the synthesis of MSNs. Ling and Su proposed a low-cost electrochemistry assisted approach to synthesize MSNs in large-scale. The formation of MSNs was accomplished by the production of hydroxide at the stainless steel substrate/solution interface which resulted in the self-assembly of surfactant micelles and the polycondensation of silica precursors [87]. Microwave assisted technique for the synthesis of MSNs could be another low-cost approach for the synthesis of MSNs. Various reports show that MSNs with ordered pore size and arrangement could be rapidly synthesized by this method [88,89]. Another rapid, cost effective method for the fabrication of MSNs is sonochemcial synthesis. The use of photoacoustic cavitations during the process was found to generate ordered MSNs, giving scope for the fine tuning of the process in a shorter duration of time [90,91].

3.3. Raw Materials Used and Factors Affecting the Characteristics of MSNs

The three main elements that form the heart of MSN includes a silica precursor (tetraethyl orthosilicate-TEOS, tetramethyl orthosilicate-TMOS, tetramethoxyvinylsilane- TMVS, sodium meta-silicate and tetrakis(2-hydroxyethyl) orthosilicate- THEOS), a surfactant (non-ionic or cationic surfactant) as a structure directing agent (SDA) and a catalyst. Other additives like cosolvents, compounds to prevent aggregation may also be incorporated based on the requirements. In order to ensure the scale-up of MSNs at reasonable cost, natural perlite materials like pumice rock, rice husk, and renewable biomass could also be explored for the synthesis of MSNs [92,93]. The common chemical constituents explored so far are listed in Table 3.

Table 3. List of commonly used chemicals in the synthesis of MSNs.

Chemical Constituents	Function	References
Cetyltrimethylammonium bromide (CTAB)	Structure directing agent/template	[94,95]
Cetyltrimethylammonium chloride (CTAC)	Structure directing agent/template	[96,97]
Pluronic F123, F127	Surfactant template	[38,98]
Brij-76	Surfactant template	[99,100]
Triton X-100	Surfactant	[101,102]
Tween 20, 40, 60, 80	Surfactant	[103]
Tetraethyl orthosilicate (TEOS)	Inorganic silica source	[94,95]
Tetramethoxy silane (TMOS)	Inorganic silica source	[104,105]
Tetrakis(2-hydroxyethyl) orthosilicate (THEOS)	Inorganic silica source	[106]
Trimethoxyvinylsilane (TMVS)	Inorganic silica source	[107]
Sodium silicate	Inorganic silica source	[108]
Ethanol	Cosolvent to solubilize TEOS	[97,109]
Sodium hydroxide (NaOH)	Base catalyst	[95]
Ammonium hydroxide (NH_4OH)	Base catalyst	[94]
Triethanolamine (TEA)	Base catalyst, complexing agent and growth inhibitor	[96]
Diethanolamine (DEA)	Base catalyst	[96,109]
Disodium hydrogen phosphate-sodium dihydrogen phosphate buffer solution	Reaction medium	[109]
Triisopropylbenzene (TIPB)	Pore-expanding agent	[110,111]
Tetrapropoxysilane (TPOS)	Pore- expanding agent	[111]
Pluronic polymer P103	Pore-expanding agent	[112]

The particle size, pore size and morphology of MSNs can be successfully modulated as required by varying the reaction conditions (relative amounts of alkoxysilane, water, catalyst) and temperature.

3.3.1. Control of Particle Size

Particle size is a very important feature for the biomedical application of MSNs as drug carriers. Hence careful tuning of particle size is essential for effective drug delivery. pH of the reaction medium plays a pivotal role in governing the size of MSNs. The particle size can be effectively controlled by adding suitable additive agents like alcohols, amine, inorganic bases and inorganic salts. These agents alter the hydrolysis and condensation of silica precursor. They accelerate the reaction kinetics thus resulting in particles of smaller size. Moller et al. replaced the often used base catalyst sodium hydroxide (NaOH) and ammonium hydroxide (NH_4OH) with triethanolamine (TEA). In addition to conferring a basic pH, it also acts a complexing agent to obtain discrete nanoparticles. When the molar ratio of TEOS: TEA was changed from 1:1 to 1:4, the largest particle size was observed with the ratio 1:4 [97]. Qiao [96] suggested that the initial pH value of the system greatly affects the particle size of MSNs. When they provided Na_2HPO_4-NaH_2PO_4 as a source of OH^- ions, particle size was found to increase with an increase in the initial pH of the solution. El-Toni et al. observed that on increasing the concentration of ammonia beyond a certain level, the agglomeration of silica particles takes place due to the increase in the ionic strength of the reaction medium [113]. Bouchoucha et al. also reported the efficiency of TEA in producing well-dispersed nanoparticles [114]. Use of L-lysine as a base catalyst was found to hinder the growth of silica particles, thus resulting in sub-nanometre size particles. This may be due to the electrostatic interaction between the protonated amine groups of L-lysine and a deprotonated hydroxyl group on silica surface further delaying the condensation process [115]. PEG-silane capping on the surface of silica particles was also found to effectively attenuate the particle growth process by steric stabilization. When PEG-silane was added immediately after addition of TMOS, the particle size was found to be 5 nm but when it was added at a delay of 50 min after addition of TMOS, the particle diameter increased to >13 nm [115]. A change from monodisperse to heterogeneous particle size distribution was observed when the amount of silica precursor TEOS was increased, which may be attributed to the secondary condensation reactions taking place due to the presence of excess silica precursor which starts producing new nuclei amongst the already existing silica particles [107,116]. A similar trend of results was obtained by Chiang et al. who found that particle size was found to increase with an increase in the amount of TEOS [117]. An increase in the particle size was observed by using different tetraalkoxysilane with different alkoxy groups ($Si(OR)_4$, R = Me, Et, Pr and Bu). Along with this, the addition of alcohols also influenced the particle size of the MSNs. This may be due to the alteration in the hydrolysis rate [118]. Low concentration of CTAB as surfactant yielded a homogenous spherical particle size distribution. On investigating the effect of CTAB on the particle size, it was observed that transformation from discrete spherical to agglomerates was observed due to variation in the hydrolysis and micellization of CTAB [119]. By tuning the concentration of F127 polymer, the particle size could be controlled. An increase of particle size up to 300 nm was reported with an increase in the triblock copolymer Pluronic F127 concentration. Reports state that a balance between the molar composition of various reactants was necessary to obtain MSNs with desired size and quality [120]. The reaction parameters equally influenced the mean particle size of MSNs. On increasing the temperature of the reaction from 30 to 70 °C, an increase in the particle size from 28.91 nm to 113.22 nm was observed. This may be due to the increase in the rate of reaction leading to polycondensation of the silica monomers resulting in a dense silica structure and a larger size [107].

3.3.2. Control of Pore Size, Pore Volume and Mesostructural Ordering

Depending on the type of surfactant, the pore size of MSNs can be varied. The longer chain length of surfactant results in MSNs with larger pores and those with short chain length gives MSNs with smaller pores [121–124]. The concentration of TEOS influenced the mesostructural ordering of the particles. The higher amount of TEOS showed a disordered mesostructure whereas lesser amount was not sufficient to form a mesoporous structure [117]. The concentration of surfactant CTAB was also found to have a profound impact on the mesostructural arrangement of the particles. A lower concentration of surfactant fails to form micelles and hence the resulting nanoparticles will be template deficient whereas the too high concentration of CTAB may result in a disordered structure [35]. Hence an optimum balance has to be struck between various reagents used. Moreover, mesostructural ordering takes place in dilute aqueous solutions [125]. Addition of N, *N*-dimethylhexadecylamine (DMHA) behaves as a pore size mediator and thus helps with efficient control of pore size as per requirements [126]. Pore size was also found to have a profound influence on the release rate of the drugs as observed using ibuprofen [127,128]. The selection of surfactant species greatly influences the mesostructural ordering of the nanoparticles and the pore size. Effect of the templating agent due to change in the counterions present in cetyltrimethylammonium was studied. Cetyltrimethylammonium chloride (CTAC) as pore generating template produced MSNs with the wormhole-like arrangement. On changing the counter ion to a much larger tosylate ion (CTATOS), the pore radius was found to increase and the pore morphology changed from wormlike to stellate [129]. Of late, novel strategies have been adopted by scientists to bring about modifications in the properties of the MSNs in order to overcome the drawbacks of the traditional MSNs such as small pore size and poor particle size uniformity. In this regard, Huang et al. [130], synthesized highly monodisperse silica nanoparticles having a large pore size with dendritic morphology using a novel dual templating sol-gel reaction by mixing partially fluorinated short chain anionic fluorocarbon surfactant, Capstone FS-66 and CTAB. An interesting observation was made by them showing that an increase in the amount of Capstone FS-66 incorporated resulted in a change in the morphology. The particle size was larger with a dendritic channel pore structure. As the amount of Capstone is further increased, the morphology transforms into a flower-like large dendritic structure. The same strategy was used by Yu et al., who synthesized dendritic MSNs with particle size of less than 200 nm using imidazolium ionic liquids with different alkyl lengths as cosurfactants and Pluronic F127 as a particle growth inhibitor. They observed that neither the reaction temperature nor the time showed any influence on the particle size of MSNs [131].

3.3.3. Control of Shape

The shape of the MSNs greatly affects the cellular uptake and biodistribution of MSNs. Hence stringent control of the shape of MSNs is important to regulate its excretion and other effects in vivo [132]. A clear picture of the relationship between particle shape and cellular responses was demonstrated in the paper by Huang et al. [133]. Till date, spherical MSNs have been widely explored for their drug delivery potential. However, the non-spherical MSNs are seldom used. By carefully controlling the reaction conditions, non-spherical materials with rod, ellipsoid, film, platelet, sheet and cube shapes could be generated. The molar concentration of surfactant, water, base catalyst and TEOS was found to have an impact on the morphology of the MSNs. Cai et al. generated MSNs with different shapes like spherical, silica rods and micrometre-sized oblate silica by manipulating the concentration of TEOS, $NaOH/NH_4OH$ and CTAB [134]. By regulating the amount of dodecanol as a soft template and the temperature of synthesis, a broad range of silica particles could be realized varying from sphere to shell, rugby, peanut, hollow and yolk shell-like structures. The six different particles fabricated had controlled size, porosity, interior spaces and shell structure. Their results showed that inclusion of dodecanol as a soft template resulted in particles with different morphologies [135]. This indicates that any changes in the micelle structure at the initial stage leads to a change in the particle morphologies. MSNs of various shapes can be obtained with a wide range of aspect-ratio. Rod-shaped MSNs are widely exploited counterparts of spherical MSNs. These can be obtained by varying the reaction parameters in a typical sol-gel reaction. An increase in the amount of catalyst and addition of co-solvent like heptane, change in temperature, varying the molar composition of reactants yield rod-shaped MSNs [133,136,137]. Ellipsoidal shaped MSNs also form a part of drug delivery carrier. Inability to retain its shape due to minimization of surface free energy leading to spherical particles poses a major challenge. These MSNs can be synthesized by the introduction of a co-surfactant [138], the addition of potassium chloride and ethanol [139]. Platelet-shaped MSNs with high pore accessibility can be synthesized by addition of low amounts of ammonium fluoride and heptane [137], the presence of non-ionic block copolymer P104 [140], using a ternary surfactant system of cetyltrimethylammonium bromide–sodium dodecyl sulfate–Pluronic123 [141].

Apart from the silica precursors, certain organosilanes were incorporated, which performed the dual function of shape transformation and surface functionalization. Morphological variants of MSNs could be synthesized by the co-condensation method of incorporation of organosilanes. The particle morphology depends on the type and amount of the organoalkoxysilane precursors introduced [36,142]. Various shapes of MSNs such as spheres, rods and hexagonal tubes could be generated using 3-aminopropyltrimethoxysilane (APTMS), *N*-(2-aminoethyl)-3-aminopropyltrimethoxysilane (AAPTMS), 3-[2-(2-aminoethyl amino) ethylamino] propyltrimethoxysilane (AEPTMS), ureidopropyltrimethoxysilane (UDPTMS), 3-isocyanatopropyltriethoxysilane (ICPTES), 3-cyanopropyltriethoxysilane (CPTES) and allyltrimethoxysilane (ALTMS) as organoalkoxysilanes. The transformation in shape of the MSNs may be attributed to the different types of interaction such as hydrogen bonding, hydrophobic interactions between the organoalkoxysilane and the surfactant template.

4. Drug Loading and Release of Drugs from MSNs

The unique feature of MSNs which makes it a widely exploited carrier for drug delivery is its high loading capacity due to the large pore volume and surface engineering properties both on the external and internal surface for better drug targeting.

4.1. Drug Loading

The drug loading is mainly based on the adsorptive properties of MSNs. Both hydrophilic and hydrophobic cargos can be incorporated into the pores of MSNs. Owing to their large pore volume, MSNs inherently possess greater loading capacity compared to other carriers. Nevertheless, extensive work has been carried out to further enhance the loading of the drugs. Synthesis of HMSNs is one such approach to enhance the loading of MSNs (explained in Section 3.2). She et al. attempted to increase the loading of 5-fluorouracil (5-FU) into hollow MSNs by functionalizing the surface silanol groups with different silanes *viz*, octadecyltrimethoxysilane (OTMS), (3-aminopropyl) triethoxysilane (APTES), 3-cyanopropyltriethoxysilane (CPTES). An improved loading of 28.89% was observed for amine functionalized HMSNs compared to plain HMSNs with 18.34%. This may be via the electrostatic interactions between the negatively charged 5-FU and positively charged amino modified HMSNs. A similar strategy could be used for improving the loading capacity of drugs by electrostatic attractions by varying the type of functionalization [78]. However, a contrasting theory was put forth by Wang et al. whose paper suggested that loading of a drug prior to surface grafting yielded a carrier with high loading as compared to grafting followed by loading of the drug [143,144]. Compared to MSNs, HMSNs proved to be a better carrier in terms of loading capacity due to their hollow cavities. 3–15 times higher loading of drugs was observed in HMSNs when compared to MSNs. In addition, dual loading of drugs was also achieved using the same carrier [74,75,145]. The loading capacity of MSNs could be further enhanced by utilizing polymer gatekeeping for the entrapment of hydrophobic drugs [146]. Consecutive drug loading process which increases the intermolecular interactions can also lead to improved loading of the drugs [147]. An increase in the drug feeding ratio was also found to have a profound influence on the loading capacity of MSNs [145,148]. The pore volume of MSNs is the major factor which dictates the loading of the drug. Hence pore expansion strategy can be adopted to introduce and hold a large amount of cargo. Pore swelling agents such as alkanes/ethanol, triisopropyl benzene (TIPB), trioctylamine (TOA), decane and *N*,*N*-dimethylhexadecylamine (DMHA) aid pore expansion [129,149,150]. Table 4 gives a comparison of the drug loading capacity of various MSNs.

Table 4. Comparison of loading in MSNs.

Carrier	Drug	Loading (wt %)	References
MCM-41 HMSNs	Ibuprofen	35.9 74.5	[75]
MCM-41 HMSNs	Doxorubicin	48.16 112.12	[74]
HMSNs HMSNs-NH_2 HMSNs-COOH HMSNs-CN HMSNs-CH_3	5-fluorouracil	18.54 28.89 20.73 22.54 12.13	[78]
MCM-$41_{(C12)}$ MCM-$41_{(C16)}$ SBA-15	Captopril	23.6 34 22.6	[151]
MCM-41 SBA-15 SBA-15 (C8) SBA-15 (C18)	Erythromycin	29 34 13 18	[152]
MCM-41 MCM-41-NH_2 SBA-15 SBA-15-NH_2	Alendronate	14 37 8 22	[153]
MSN-C0 MSN-C10	Lysozyme	34 42	[149]

HMSNs—Hollow mesoporous silica nanoparticles.

4.2. Release of Drugs from MSNs

The release profile of drugs from MSNs mainly depends on its diffusion from the pores which can be tailored by modifying the surface of the MSNs to suit the biological needs. The decisive factor responsible for controlling the release is the interaction between the surface groups on pores and the drug molecule [154]. It was observed that drug loading followed by surface functionalization with amine groups played a significant role in sustaining the drug release as compared to the systems which were functionalized first and then loaded with the drug. This could be attributed to the loading of the drugs within the pores and the capping with APTES which prevents the drug release. If the surface was first functionalized and then loaded, there are possibilities that the drug will get adsorbed on the surface of MSNs resulting in burst release. The role of APTES concentration in drug release was studied, the results of which revealed that a change in the APTES concentration played a vital role in controlling the drug release from the pores [143]. Aspirin loading and release from the MSNs were studied by post-synthetic grafting as well as co-condensation method. It was observed that co-condensation method showed a greater drug loading compared to the other method. In case of plain MCM-41, weak interaction between aspirin and silanol groups resulted in faster drug release following Fick's diffusion. With amino functionalized MCM-41, the strong interaction between the amine group and aspirin resulted in slow drug release especially for the co-condensed MCM-41 [155]. Echoing similar results, the release of ibuprofen from SBA-15 was found to be greatly influenced by the surface modification. In case of amino-functionalized SBA-15 by one-pot synthesis, complete drug release was observed at the end of 10 h whereas the release from that of post-synthetically modified SBA-15, the release of ibuprofen up to 3 days was observed [156]. Table 5 presents the comparison of release rates of different MSNs.

Table 5. Comparison of release rate of MSNs.

Carrier	Drug	Release Rate	References
MCM-41 (C12) MCM-41 (C16) SBA-15	Captopril	45 wt % within 2 h, total drug release over 16 h 47.47 wt % within 2 h, total drug release >30 h 60 wt % within 0.5 h, total drug release over 16 h	[151]
SBA-15 SBA-15 (C8) SBA-15 (C18)	Erythromycin	60% release within 5 h, total drug release within 14 h	[152]
SBA-15 unmodified (PS0) SBA-15-NH_2 by post synthesis (PS2) SBA-15-NH_2 by one pot synthesis (OPS2)	Ibuprofen	Complete release in 10 h Initial burst release of 50% in 10 h followed by 100% release in 3 days Complete release in 10 h	[156]
MSN (grafting-loading approach) MSN (loading-grafting approach)	Doxorubicin	40% in 8 h and stagnant release beyond 8 h 10% in first 24 h, sustained beyond 160 h	[143]

5. Applications of MSNs in Drug Delivery

MSNs have been widely utilized for a variety of purposes ranging from its use in medicine, as a catalyst in chemical synthesis, adsorbents to adsorb wastes, toxic substances and also as sensors. One of the advantages of MSNs is the ease with which it can be functionalized based on the requirements for a wide variety of applications to control the release of drugs. Figure 3 shows a pictorial representation depicting the versatility of MSN carrier. Vast research is being conducted in utilizing these carriers for drug delivery. In the following section, the major applications of MSNs for drug delivery are discussed. Table 6 provides a list of few of the diseases for which MSNs have been exploited.

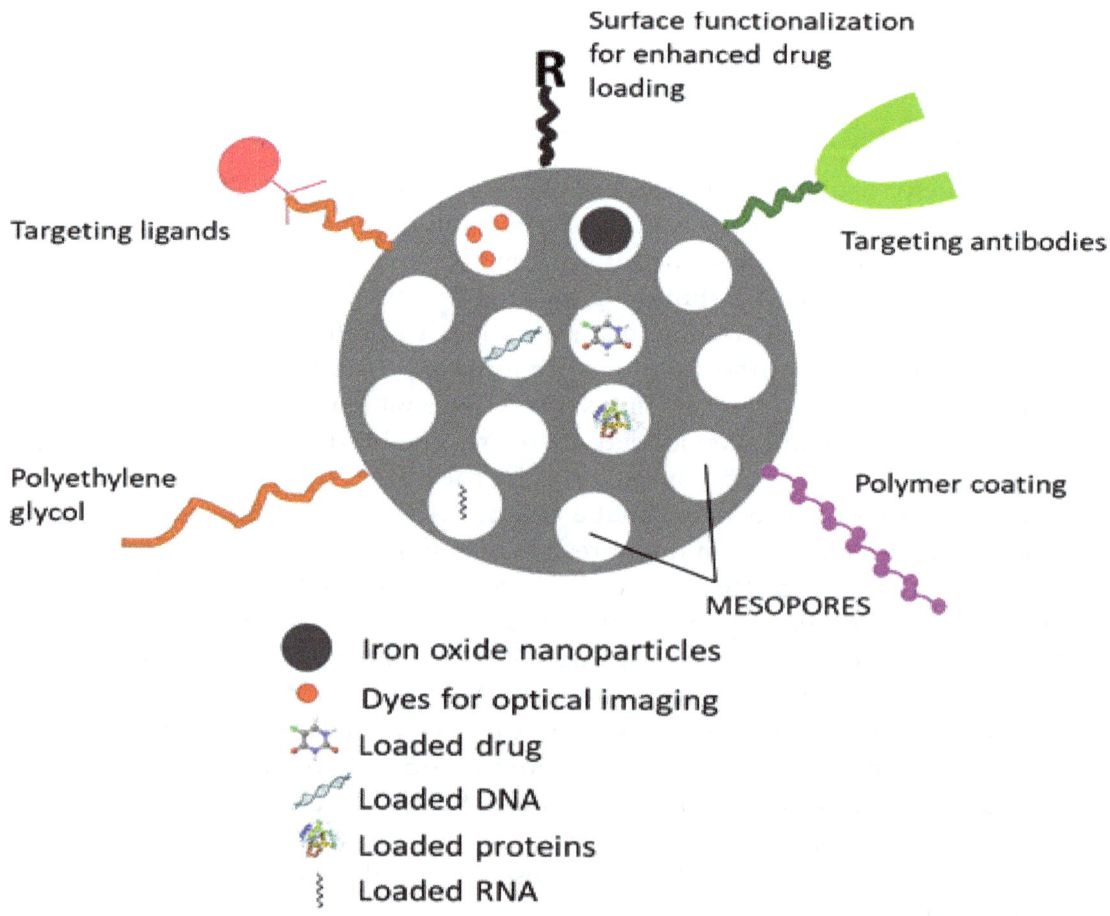

Figure 3. Illustration of versatility of MSN as a carrier in loading variety of drugs.

Table 6. List of some biomedical applications of MSNs.

Category	Drug	Carrier	PS, D_p (nm)	Activity Testing	References
Anticancer	Doxorubicin	Hollow MSNs	120, 2.7	HeLa cells	[157]
		Lipid-coated MSNs	295, 2.3	MCF-7 human breast cancer cells	[158]
	Topotecan	MCM-41	72.9, 2.7	Female athymic nude mice injected with MDA-MB-231 human epithelial breast cancer cells s.c.	[159]
	Quercetin	MCM-41			[159]
	Curcumin	SLN-silica microcapsules	305, 7.8	Caco-2 cells	[160]
	Paclitaxel	MSNs	100, 2.3	PK studies in peritoneal MIA-PaCa-2 (human pancreatic cancer cell) tumour bearing nude mice	[161]
	5-fluorouracil	MCM-41	135, 2.9	Human colonic HT-29 cells	[162]
	Etoposide	MCM-41-PAA	142.85, 3.69	PC-3 and LNCaP human prostate cancer cells	[163]
	16-hydroxy-cleroda-3,13-dien-16,15-olide (HCD)	Eudragit S100-HCD-Cu-MSN	514, 4.3	Athymic male nude mice injected with C6 Glioma cells s.c.	[164]
Antidepressant	Duloxetine hydrochloride	MSNs	PS not reported, 2.6–7.2	Not reported	[165]
Anti-tuberculosis	Rifampicin	MCM-41	218, 2.4	Not reported	[166]
Anti-inflammatory	Ibuprofen	MSNs	PS not reported, 3.6–4.1	Not reported	[101]
	Ketoprofen	MCM-41 SBA-15	1500, 3.4 970, 6.24	Not reported	[167]
	Budesonide	MCM-41	100, 2.7	Coculture of HT-29 cells and PMA treated human EOL-1 (acute myeloid eosinophilic leukemia) cells	[168]
Antibacterial	Ciprofloxacin	Lipid-coated MSNs	80–100, D_p not reported	*Salmonella typhimurium* administered mice	[169]
	Ciprofloxacin	Arg-MSN	75, 7.2	*Salmonella* infected BALB/*c* mice	[170]
	Tetracycline	MCM-41	41 and 406, D_p not reported	In vitro against *Escherichia coli*	[171]
Antihypertensive	Captopril	SBA-15	PS not reported, 7.15	Not reported	[172]
	Aliskiren	SBA-15			[172]
	Hydrochlorothiazide, Losartan potassium, Amlodipine besylate, Simvastatin	MCM-41 polypill	150, 4.64	Not reported	[173]
Hypoglycemic drugs	Gluconated insulin Rosiglitazone maleate	Alizarin complexone-MSNs	60–100, ~2.3	In vitro monitoring of drug release in human serum	[174]
	16-hydroxycleroda-3,13-dine-16,15-olide (HCD)	MSNs	259, 3.9	Diet-induced ICR male diabetic mice	[175]
Osteogenic	Alendronate	MCM-41 SBA-15	PS not reported, 3.8 PS not reported, 9.0	Not reported	[153]
	Alendronate	HA-AL-MS-PLGA microspheres	245–258 μm	In vitro on synovium-derived mesenchymal stem cells (MSCs)	[176]
	Dexamethasone	MCM-41	265, D_p not reported	Male Sprague−Dawley rats	[177]
Antioxidant	Morin	MSNs	150, 3	In vitro	[178]

PS—Particle size; D_p—Pore diameter; SLN—Solid lipid nanoparticles; HA-AL-MS-PLGA-Hydroxyapatite-Alendronate-Mesoporous silica-poly(lactic-co-glycolic acid); Arg-MSN—Arginine coated MSN; MCF- Michigan Cancer Foundation; MDA-MB- M.D. Anderson- Metastasis breast cancer; MIA- Melanoma inhibitory activity; PK—Pharmacokinetics; PMA—phorbol myristate acetate ester; PAA—Polyacrylic acid.

5.1. Targeted Antitumor Therapy Using MSNs

The property of surface functionalization of MSNs is widely explored to enhance the site-specific delivery of drugs and avoid side effects. It is a versatile carrier where drugs with different physicochemical properties can be loaded and further functionalized for effective therapy. They can accumulate significantly in the tumour due to the enhanced permeation and retention (EPR) effect [179]. Active targeting aids in maximizing the uptake of actives into the cells. Based on the difference between the normal and tumour cells, suitable receptors overexpressed on tumour cells are selected and ligands specific to those receptors are conjugated on the surface of the MSNs. Specific drug delivery can be achieved by anchoring MSNs with targeting ligands. Folic acid (FA) is a well-known ligand which complements the folate receptors overexpressed on tumour cells. The FA conjugation on the surface of MSNs is brought about by an amide linkage between the carboxyl group of FA and amine group of aminopropyltriethoxysilane (APTES). Ma et al. [180] delivered 5-aminolevulinic acid for photodynamic therapy by conjugating folic acid on the surface of HMSNs against B16F 10 skin cancer cells. The developed formulation was observed to show a high photocytotoxicity to the cancer cells. Similar reports were presented wherein the presence of amine functionalization on the surface aids in the binding of folic acid covalently on the surface of the receptors to ensure selective uptake of doxorubicin (DOX) in breast cancer cells. The apoptosis and cellular uptake studies revealed that FA-MSN-NH_2-DOX showed higher internalization into the cells as compared to MSN-NH_2-DOX [181]. Hyaluronic acid (HA) is another widely explored ligand for targeting CD44 receptors overexpressed on cancer cells. Zhang et al. reported an HA functionalized DOX-MSN which behaved both as enzyme responsive and receptor-mediated delivery system. The increased uptake by colon cancer cells and low in vivo toxicity to the body was proved by in vivo tumour growth inhibition and biodistribution studies. In addition to receptor-mediated uptake, the release of DOX was triggered by hyaluronidase enzyme present in tumour microenvironment [182]. Similar results were reported by Gary-Bobo et al. [183] who fabricated HA-MSNs for photodynamic therapy against colon cancer. The experiments were conducted on HCT-116 colon cancer cell lines which showed the higher efficiency of HA-MSNs owing to their CD44 receptor targeted action as compared to that of plain MSNs. Another novel approach for active targeting of hepatoma cells was reported wherein lactosaminated (Lac) MSNs were designed. These novel delivery systems showed a promising outcome as it had the ability to be endocytosed by asialoglycoprotein (ASGPR) receptors present on the surface of hepatocytes. The findings were supported by the results from cellular uptake studies in ASGPR-positive cells (HepG2 and SMMC7721) wherein Lac-MSNs showed improved cellular uptake when compared to that of plain MSNs. The results also highlighted an interesting point wherein the ligand lactose was recognized only when conjugated with MSNs and not in its free form [184]. Analogues for targeting mannose-6-phosphate receptor overexpressed in cancer cells were grafted onto MSNs to enhance the uptake by tumour cells. These were found to show positive results for the treatment of prostate and colon cancers [185,186]. Arginine-glycine-aspartic acid (RGD) was demonstrated to be selectively engulfed by $\alpha v\beta 3$ and $\alpha v\beta 5$ integrin receptors, which are overexpressed in diverse tumours. The drug-loaded surface engineered RGD-MSNs were thwarted by the normal cells and taken up by the liver cancer cells thus improving the treatment efficacy [187]. In addition to molecular targeting, efforts were also made to club positron-emission tomography (PET) imaging and chemotherapy into a single carrier. Sunitinib as a model anticancer drug was loaded onto the MSNs and surface engineered with cyclo-(Arg-Gly-Asp-D-Tyr-Lys) peptide (cRGDyK) and polyethylene glycol. The efficacy of the receptor uptake was confirmed by flow cytometry studies, PET imaging and histopathological studies. The studies were carried out in U87MG human glioblastoma cells and athymic nude mice were used for in vivo experiments. The tumour uptake of the nanoconjugates was found to be lower in the case of plain HMSNs as compared to that of cRGDyK conjugated HMSNs [188]. Numerous positive outcomes have been demonstrated using a plethora of ligands which are grafted onto the surface of MSNs rendering it target specific. Table 7 lists a few of the ligands which have been explored for cancer drug delivery using MSNs.

Table 7. List of some functionalized MSNs explored for tumour targeting.

Drugs	Application	Targeting Ligand	Receptor	References
5-fluorouracil	Colorectal cancer	Hyaluronic acid	CD44	[189]
5-fluorouracil	Colorectal cancer	EGF	EGF	[190]
Curcumin	Cervical cancer	Chondroitin sulphate	CD44	[191]
Docetaxel	Breast cancer	Folic acid	Folate	[181]
Docetaxel	Hepatoma	Lactose	Asialoglycoprotein	[184]
Doxorubicin	Hepatic cancer	Transferrin	Transferrin	[192]
Doxorubicin	Colon cancer	Aptamer	(EpCAM)	[193]
Photosensitizer merocyanine	Breast cancer	Mannose	Mannose	[194]
Quercetin	Triple negative breast cancer	cRGD peptide	Integrin receptor $\alpha v\beta 3$	[159]
Quercetin	Breast cancer	Folic acid	Folate	[195]
Sunitinib	Glioblastoma	$VEGF_{121}$	VEGF	[196]
Topotecan	Triple-negative breast cancer	cRGD peptide	Integrin receptor $\alpha v\beta 3$	[159]

EGF—Epidermal growth factor; VEGF—Vascular endothelial growth factor; EpCAM—Epithelial cell adhesion molecule.

The surface functionalization of MSNs is not limited to just one ligand. Multiple ligands can be anchored onto the surface of MSNs for receptor targeting. For example, the surface of MSNs loaded with chlorambucil was functionalized with HA and RGD peptide for a synergistic effect. The in vitro cell line studies on human ovarian cancer (SKOV-3) cells showed a significant improvement in the uptake of the MSNs by CD44 and integrin receptors as compared to that of single ligand or plain MSNs [197].

In the recent times, a novel chemotherapeutic strategy utilizing copper impregnated MSNs (Cu-MSNs) have been explored for their potential reactive oxygen species (ROS) mediated apoptosis of cancer cells. Kankala et al. developed a novel Cu-MSN loaded with a catalase inhibitor, 3-amino-1,2,4-triazole (AT) for ROS mediated killing of cancer cells. On uptake by cells and delivery to the endosomal compartment (pH 5.0), the binding between copper and AT breaks off which releases AT to inhibit catalase activity. This in turn, leads to an increase in the ROS production induced by catalysis of copper on MSNs which aids in the cancer cell apoptosis. Positive results were obtained by them when evaluated in HT-29 cells [198]. An effort to overcome the multidrug resistance observed in chemotherapy was made utilizing Cu-MSNs loaded with DOX as model drug. In this system, DOX was conjugated to copper metal through a pH sensitive coordination link susceptible to acidic tumour environment (pH 5.0–6.0). This entire system was further coated with liposomes comprising of cholesterol, D-α-tocopheryl polyethylene glycol 1000 succinate (TPGS), MPEG-2000-DSPE (1,2-Distearoyl-phosphatidylethanolamine-methyl-polyethyleneglycol conjugate-2000), a P-gp inhibitor. Copper ions play a synergistic role in enhancing the intracellular ROS levels which results in killing of cancer cells efficiently. Positive results were obtained by the group when the delivery system was tested in DOX-resistant tumour (MES-SA-DX-5 derived from human uterine sarcoma) and HT-29 cell lines. The antitumor activity of Liposomes-Cu-MSN-DOX was found to be higher when compared to that of pure DOX. The antiproliferative activity of the optimized formulation was found to be profoundly higher in drug resistant cells than the sensitive cells [199].

5.2. MSNs for Anti-Inflammatory Activities

The unique properties of MSNs have been used to accommodate various anti-inflammatory drugs and control their release rate. MCM-41 and SBA-15 are the two widely used silica drug carriers. Ibuprofen was loaded onto multimodal pore channels and the effect on its release was studied. On analysing the release data, it was observed that the release of the drug occurs in three stages *viz,* initial rapid release of the drug adsorbed on the surface of MSNs followed by prolonged release of the drug entrapped in the small pores present in the periphery of the particles having a different pore structural orientation compared to the inner mesopores. The final prolonged release stage occurs by the drug embedded deep in the long length pores of the particles [200]. The bulk of the research work on MSNs for effective delivery of anti-inflammatory drugs has been carried out using ibuprofen as a model drug. Efforts were made to modulate the release rate of the drug by various organic modifications of the surface silanol groups. Surface functionalization was found to alter and also stabilize the drug release rates [127,201]. SBA-15 has also been used to precisely deliver ibuprofen and other anti-inflammatory agents. One such work by Ahmadi et al. demonstrated a change in the release rate of ibuprofen when the surface of the carrier was modified with aminopropyl groups. Plain SBA-15 was not able to sustain the release of the drug due to weak interaction between the surface silanol group and the carboxyl group of ibuprofen. However, on amino functionalization, a relatively prolonged release of the drug was observed due to the strong interaction between the amino groups of silica surface and carboxyl groups of ibuprofen [202]. Other similar studies were carried out to successfully deliver aspirin [155] and indomethacin [203] using MSNs with high drug loading and slow release profile.

5.3. Gated Drug Release/Controlled Drug Delivery

Although the length and the pore structure altered the drug release rate, efforts are constantly underway to achieve smart, zero-release of the drugs by capping the surface of the pores. Controlled and intelligent delivery of drugs to the target site through MSNs is possible due to gated release. The gates of the pores open only in response to certain stimuli like pH, temperature, enzyme, redox and so forth. The principle of gated drug release is very effective when toxic side effects of drugs to other organs are to be avoided [204]. Numerous reports in this regard have been published, a few of which we have discussed in the following section.

5.3.1. pH-Responsive Drug Release

pH is the widely explored stimuli to trigger the drug release as the body has a wide range of pH. MCM-48 particles loaded with prednisolone were coated with succinylated ε-polylysine (SPL) to ensure the pH-dependent release of the drug in the colon region. The in vitro release experiments showed a delay in the release of drug which indicated the successful approach of pH-responsive drug delivery. At acidic pH of the stomach, SPL prevents drug release due to its unionized form whereas, at colonic pH, SPL gets converted to its ionized form facilitating drug diffusion out of the MSNs. The developed nanoparticles could be an alternative for the treatment of diseases of the colon (inflammatory bowel disease and cancer) [205]. The promising outcome of pH-responsive MSNs was observed for tumour-targeted therapy and another disease where the pH of the affected area is slightly acidic than the normal tissues. This pH-responsive drug release can be realized by capping the pores of MSN using acid degradable polymers, polyelectrolytes, some pH-sensitive linkers and so forth. pH sensitive polysaccharide, chitosan was coated onto the MSNs to achieve controlled delivery of curcumin for the treatment of cancer. In vitro drug release studies proved the pH-sensitive nature of chitosan by sustained drug release. The release of curcumin improved when moving from pH 7.4 to pH 5.5. Cell uptake studies in U87MG glioblastoma cancer cell-line showed a decrease in the half maximal inhibitory concentration (IC50) values indicating an improved accumulation of curcumin in cancer cells when encapsulated within chitosan loaded MSNs [206]. Similar studies using chitosan as the pH-triggered cap was carried out by Hu et al. for the release of doxorubicin on MCF-7 breast cancer cells. At acidic pH, the amino groups of chitosan become protonated resulting in swelling of the polymer chains. This opens up the pores of MSNs releasing the drugs [207]. Modulation of doxorubicin via pH-responsive stimuli was also achieved using polymers such as poly(acrylic acid) [208] and polydopamine [209]. Both these reports suggested an enhanced uptake by cancer cells and a sustained release of the drugs. Reports with different polyelectrolytes as pH motifs have shown promising outcomes [208,210]. Tannins as pH motifs were proved by the work of Hu and collaborators. Tannins, by the formation of boronate esters were found to modulate the release of the dye rhodamine at acidic pH [211].

Macromolecular compounds like cyclodextrin (CD) has also been explored for its pH-sensitive property [212]. Tan et al. used a stalk of p-anisidine, loaded the cargo and finally capped the pores with β-CD. The pH sensitivity of the resulting MSNs was evaluated over a pH range of 7.4 to 5.5. A pH-dependent release was observed with a greater release at pH 5.5. When the pH fell below the pKa of the stalk, the interaction between p-anisidine and β-CD reduced thus resulting in the release of the drug. An optimum density of the stalk was the key to control the pH-triggered release. In addition, the effect of both α and β-CD capping on the release of drug was studied. It was observed that the percentage release with α-CD was comparatively lesser that β-CD. This could be due to the different formation constants between CD and p-anisidine stalks [213]. Figure 4 illustrates the release of drug from β-CD capped MSNs in response to stimuli.

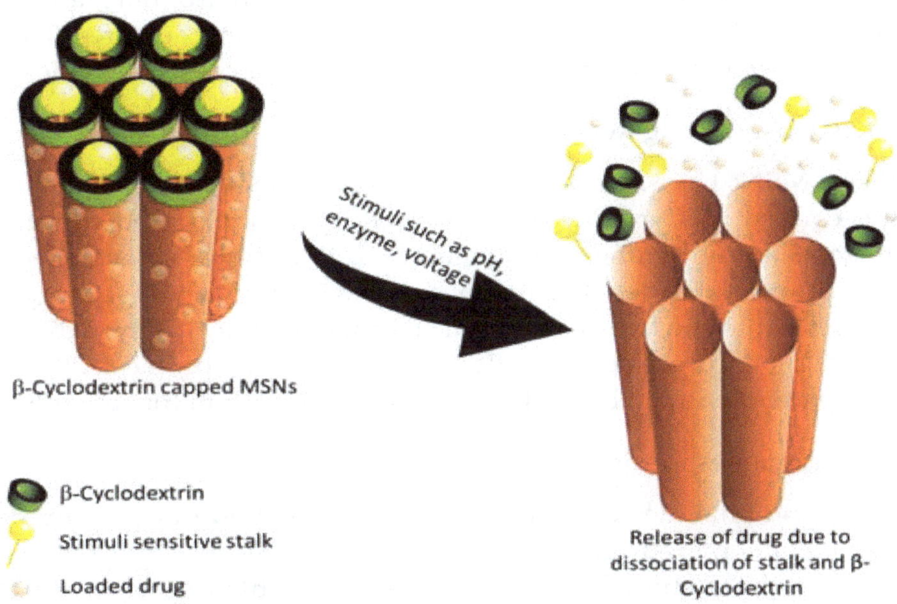

Figure 4. Schematic illustration of the release of drug from β-CD capped MSNs in response to stimuli.

Kuthati et al. devised a strategy to ensure the efficient delivery of antimicrobial agent by modifying the MSN framework via pH sensitive MSNs. Institute of Bioengineering and Nanotechnology-4 (IBN-4) nanoparticles, a type of MSNs was used as a carrier. This was immobilized with silver-indole-3-acetic acid hydrazide (IAAH-Ag) via a pH sensitive hydrazine bond. When exposed to the acidic environment of the site of bacterial infection (pH 5.0), the silver ions are preferentially released up to 12 h to ensure controlled release of the model drug by the cleavage of IAAH-Ag coordination bond. The antibacterial efficacy was investigated on two drug resistant strains of gram negative and gram positive bacteria namely *Escherichia coli* and *Staphylococcus aureus* respectively. In addition to this, the effect of IBN-4-IAAH-Ag NPs on inhibiting the formation of biofilms by four strains of bacteria *viz, Escherichia coli, Bacillus subtilis, Staphylococcus aureus* and *Staphylococcus epidermidis* revealed promising results. The in vitro results were substantiated by in vivo experiments on *Escherichia coli* infected C57BL6 mice. A remarkable reduction in *Escherichia coli* was observed in the formulation treated group of mice. Hence the developed system could be a plausible alternative to the antibiotics used currently [214].

5.3.2. Redox Responsive Drug Release

Redox triggering is another widely used strategy to control the release of cargo from carriers. This technique is being used to deliver anticancer drugs making use of endogenously present reducing agents. Redox cleavable disulfide bonds are often utilized for this kind of drug release. Wang et al. synthesized a disulfide-linked polyethylene glycol (PEG) tethered to MSN for redox responsive drug release. The efficiency of the synthesized MSNs was evaluated by in vitro release studies using Rhodamine B (RhB) as the model drug. Glutathione (GSH) equivalent to intracellular concentration was added to the release media. It was observed that in the absence of GSH, the release of RhB was negligible signifying the efficiency of the cap in blocking the drug release. In addition, the PEG surface modification conferred on the nanoparticles a significant biocompatibility [215]. Dual responsive stalks with β-CD caps were synthesized to control the release of multiple drugs. HMSNs with acetal and ferrocene carboxylic acid units were obtained by selective functionalization. The redox responsiveness of the carrier was confirmed by in vitro experiments using hydrogen peroxide as stimuli. On increasing the concentration of hydrogen peroxide, an increase in the release rate of the drug was observed due to the oxidation of the ferrocenyl moiety. The mechanism behind the release is the strong electrostatic repulsion between β-CD and the oxidized hydrophilic ferrocenyl moiety which results in the dissociation of β-CD caps thus releasing the drug from the pores. The same carrier was also made pH-responsive by introducing an acetal linker to develop a synergistic effect [216].

5.3.3. Temperature Responsive Drug Release

Thermoresponsive MSNs have also been widely been studied as a possible means of controlling drug release. In this context, PEO-b-poly (*N*-isopropylacrylamide) based copolymeric micelles as structure directing agents for the synthesis of functionalized MSNs was developed by Bathfield et al. Ibuprofen as a model drug was loaded into the mesopores using one-pot strategy wherein the drug was incorporated directly into the hybrid material. Ultimately, the structure directing agent in this formulation was the drug-loaded polymer micelles. The drug release profile at 20 and 45 °C revealed a temperature sensitive pattern with a higher drug release at 45 °C than that at 20 °C [217].

5.3.4. Chemical and Enzyme Responsive Drug Release

Several chemicals and enzymes present inherently in the body or produced during diseased conditions have also been explored for the possibility of triggering drug release from the MSNs. Glucose as a chemical has been studied by scientists as a possible trigger to release drugs and has been a boon for diabetes management [218]. In one of the studies, MSNs functionalized with a signal reporter, alizarin complexone (ALC) was developed. Gluconated insulin was then introduced within the pores by benzene-1,4-diboronic acid (BA) mediated esterification reaction. This behaved both as a hypoglycaemic agent as well as pore blocker. In addition, rosiglitazone maleate was also introduced into the pores to form multifunctional MSN. In the presence of glucose, competitive binding between ALC and BA occurs which leads to opening of the pores and release of the drug [174]. Similar work for controlling the drug release using two stimuli that is, glucose and pH was carried out by Tan et al. They fabricated glucosamine-poly(acrylic acid) conjugated MSNs. The pores were capped by the crosslinking of the poly(acrylic acid) chains by the formation of boronate esters. The drug release was governed by pH or the presence of glucose. At mild acidic conditions of pH 6.0 and the presence of 10 mM glucose, the drug release was found to be higher by around 65%. These results suggested that at pH 6.0, combined stimuli showed a sufficiently enhanced release of the drug [219]. Another novel chemical sensitive MSN was with that using thrombin. The MSNs were loaded with an anticoagulant drug (acenocoumarol) and the pores were capped with peptide LVPRGSGGLVPRGSGGLVPRGSK-pentanoic acid (P) which is a substrate for proteolytic α-human thrombin. The results demonstrated that the release of drug was highly specific to the presence of thrombin. Thrombin results in the hydrolysis of the capping peptide releasing the drug [220].

Tailoring the drug release in response to the presence of certain enzymes is another new avenue for modifying the MSN as a carrier. NAD(P)H: quinone oxidoreductase 1 (NQO1) enzyme as stimuli for the release of doxorubicin was demonstrated by Gayam et al. They synthesized MSNs surface functionalized successively with alkyne followed by drug loading. To avoid premature drug release, the mesopores were blocked with rotaxane followed by tethering it to benzoquinone. In the presence of NQO1 enzyme which is upregulated in several tumours, the benzoquinone gets reduced leading to the opening of the pores and the release of doxorubicin. In vivo experiments in nude mice bearing tumour (lung) showed promising results with a significant reduction in tumour volume in the mice treated with MSN-NQO1 compared to those treated with saline and free doxorubicin [221]. Matrix metalloproteinase (MMP-2) triggered drug release for the treatment of liver cancer is another possible line of therapy. Many tumours have shown to overexpress MMP-2, the advantage of which could be explored to target drugs to tumour sites. A two-component that is, a cell penetrating peptide polyarginine and PVGLIG which is a substrate for MMP-2 cleaving based polypeptide was linked with phenylboronic acid-human serum albumin (PBA-HSA) onto the MSNs to render it target specific. Doxorubicin (DOX) was used as the model drug. Human serum albumin was used to cap the pores and phenylboronic acid behaved as the targeting moiety specific to sialic acid overexpressed in liver tumours. The enzyme responsive behaviour of the carrier was studied in vitro where around 73% of the drug released in the presence of MMP-2 as compared to only 15% of release in the absence of MMP-2. In vivo studies in HepG2 cells injected nude mice were performed which revealed encouraging results with DOX-loaded MSN-HSA-PBA showing significant tumour growth inhibition compared to non-functionalized MSN loaded with DOX [222]. An experiment along similar line was performed by Radhakrishnan et al. who explored the use of protamine, a peptide drug as a capping agent to prevent the premature release of diclofenac from MSNs. The protamine cap was found to get hydrolysed in the presence of trypsin enzyme which cleaves the L-arginine residues in protamine thereby releasing the drug. This concept was evaluated by studies on COLO 205 cells. The results showed that about 87% of the drug released within 120 min in COLO 205 cells as compared to 13% in healthy cells. This shows the selective drug release in colon cancer cells as compared to normal cells [223]. Radhakrishnan et al. also demonstrated the use of chondroitin sulphate (CHD) as a gate to the pores of MSNs which would trigger the release of drug in the presence of hyaluronidase enzyme. In addition, CHD also acts as a ligand which gets specifically uptaken by cells overexpressing CD44 receptors. CHD behaves as a cap which prevents the outward diffusion of the drug in the absence of hyaluronidase enzyme [191].

In one of the studies, controlled release of drug was achieved by surface functionalization of MSNs with ferrocenyl moiety β-cyclodextrin complex (Fc-β-CD) to prevent premature release of the drug. The experiments suggested that on stimulation by heme protein (horse-radish peroxidase and hydrogen peroxide) and the production of hydrogen peroxide via the oxidation of glucose by glucose oxidase or +1.5 V stimuli, the ferrocenyl moiety gets dissociated resulting in the opening of the nanovalves and thus releasing the drug. In vitro studies conducted to assess the release property of the carrier revealed that on stimulation with heme protein, a greater amount of drug was released as compared to that with glucose stimulation and without stimuli [224].

5.3.5. External Stimuli for Drug Release

Various other stimuli have also been investigated in modulating the drug delivery from MSNs such as light [225–227], magnetic [227,228], ultrasound [229–231], electroresponsive [224,232] systems. Figure 5 depicts the release of drug from gated MSNs in response to stimuli.

Use of light as an activating mechanism of drug delivery has garnered attention due to its advantages of spatial and temporal control of release of drugs. Febvay et al. [225] combined the advantages of light triggering with a high loading of MSNs in their study to enable the delivery of a model molecule, a fluorescent dye–Alexa546–which is impermeable to the cytosolic compartment. The MSNs were prepared using secondary surfactant pluronic F127 and further tagged with biotin or streptavidin. Following endocytosis, the LN-229 cells (human glioma, ATCC) were exposed to green excitation light for 3 to 120 s which resulted in the dye being released into the cytosol. This could be attributed to the cell membrane damage induced by the light irradiation. Liu et al. [226] explored the potential of deeper tissue penetration potential of near infrared (NIR) radiations to control the release of the drugs. They developed MSNs with gold nanorods forming the inner core and phase changing molecule, 1-tetradecanol as gatekeepers. DOX was chosen as the model drug molecule. These nanoparticles were further functionalized with folate moieties to target KB cells. The system was able to release DOX due to heating induced by near IR radiation generated by a gold nanorod core. The successful release of the drug on IR radiation was ascertained by first subjecting it to external heating which did not show any release at 37 °C. On NIR irradiation of 802 nm for 10 min, the temperature increased to 45 °C which resulted in the release of DOX which may be attributed to the change in the fluid state of tetradecanol molecules above T_m. In vitro studies on KB cells showed preferential uptake by the cell owing to the surface functionalization. The combined effect of phototherapy (NIR irradiation), chemotherapy (DOX) and targeted therapy resulted in remarkable killing of cancer cells. Hence the developed nanoparticulate system could be efficiently used for multimodal therapy. Li et al. [227] worked on similar lines where they explored the potential of MSNs as multimodal carriers using MRI monitored magnetic targeting and NIR mediated phototherapy. In their work, they developed iron oxide (Fe_3O_4) nanoparticles coated with trisoctahedral gold (Au) shell which were loaded with DOX. These were further coated with silica shell capped with oligonucleotides. Au shell here acted as NIR responsive material whereas Fe_3O_4 facilitated magnetically triggered release of drug. The controlled release property of the carrier was confirmed via in vitro studies on HeLa cell lines which showed DOX release upon NIR irradiation at 808 nm and magnetic attraction for a brief period of 2 h. These results were further supported by in vivo studies on nude mice. HeLa cells were transplanted to the nude mice for the development of tumour after which the nanoparticles were injected. On exposure to magnetic attraction for 30 min and laser exposure at 3 W/cm^2 for 30 min, a complete disappearance of tumour was observed after 14 days. These findings suggest the plausible use of these carriers to enable efficient combination therapy options for tumours.

Another novel strategy to induce visible light irradiated delivery of drugs using MSNs as drug carriers was put forth by Kuthati et al. They developed a silver nanoparticle (SNPs) decorated copper impregnated MSNs (Cu-MSNs) to aid in the photodynamic inactivation of antibiotic resistant *Escherichia coli*. Curcumin (Cur), a phototherapeutic agent was loaded into the MSNs. They explored the plasmonic resonance coupling between curcumin and silver nanoparticles to enhance the transfer of silver nanoparticle to photosensitizer to effectively kill gram negative *Escherichia coli*. They hypothesized that curcumin would produce large amounts of ROS under light irradiation which will enhance the release of silver ions. SNP+Cur behaves as a positively charged nanocomposite which improves the binding ability of Cur to the bacterial membrane. The antibacterial efficacy against *Escherichia coli* was studied by constant illumination using LED array at 470 nm at a fluence of 72 J/cm^2. The study yielded promising results revealing that Cur-Cu-MSN-SNP efficiently killed bacteria in light conditions with very mild toxicity in dark conditions. The successful eradication of bacterial cells may be attributed to three factors, namely, improved solubility and local concentration of Cur loaded into MSNs, improved binding of positively charged nanoparticle to bacterial membrane, enhanced ROS production due to Cu-MSN-SNPs. Similar strategy can be used for the development of wide variety of photobactericidal systems [233].

The release of drugs from MSNs can also be triggered via magnetic attraction. Baeza et al. [228] reported the synthesis of a hybrid polymer which responded to both thermal and magnetic stimuli. They incorporated superparamagnetic iron-oxide nanocrystals into the mesopores which was capable of providing a sufficient heating capacity for hypothermia cancer therapy. To enable thermoresponsive release of the drug molecule, poly(*N*-isopropylacrylamide) was tethered to the surface of MSNs. Fluorescein and soybean trypsin inhibitor type II was loaded into the pores of the MSNs to model the release property. In response to an alternating magnetic field of 24 kA/m and 100 kHz inside a thermostatic chamber maintained at 20 °C, a higher release of fluorescein was observed which may be due to the heat energy and enlargement of the pores leading to greater release of the drugs.

Among the non-invasive routes to enhance the spatio-temporal delivery of drugs, ultrasound is slowly gaining popularity owing to its advantages of lower cost, absence of ionizing radiations and ease of tissue penetration regulation by tuning the frequency of the cycles and exposure time. They are capable of inducing thermal/mechanical effects which can trigger the release of the drugs. Several efforts are underway to utilize this technology for the therapy of diseases especially cancer. Paris et al. formulated an ultrasound responsive MSNs capped with the copolymer, poly(2-(2-methoxyethoxy) ethyl methacrylate-co-2-tetrahydropyranyl methacrylate), with two functional ends and a monomer ratio 90:10 (MEO_2MA:THPMA). They utilized fluorescein as the model molecule to monitor the developed system. Ultrasound irradiation resulted in the cleavage of the hydrophobic tetrahydropyranyl moiety of the cap leading to a change in its conformation allowing the drug to be released. They studied this concept further by surface functionalization of the MSNs with biotin and RGD peptide to enable selective uptake by tumour cells (HeLa cell lines). DOX was loaded as the cargo within the mesopores. They successfully proved the efficiency of the developed nanoparticulate system in enhancing the efficiency of the DOX in killing cancer cells [229,231]. Studies on similar line was reported by Kim et al. [230] using ibuprofen as a model drug which were loaded into MSNs and covered with poly(dimethylsiloxane) as the implantable body. On exposure to ultrasound of 28 kHz with a power of 1.5 W/cm^2, an increase in the diffusion of ibuprofen was observed. In addition, negligible damage was observed to the polymer material on subjecting it to ultrasound frequency. These results suggest the possible use of this stimulus in enabling controlled release of drug to the diseased sites.

Another interesting approach to non-invasive drug therapy could be the use of a mild electric field that aids in controlling the release of the cargo by activating certain mechanisms, *viz*, electrochemical reduction-oxidation and movement of a charged molecule. Xiao et al. [224] developed a novel controlled release MSNs sensitive to enzyme or voltage. These were functionalized with ferrocene and further loaded with rhodamine and capped with β-cyclodextrin (β-CD). Voltage ranging from 0.5 V to 1.5 V was applied to trigger the release of the cargo from the pores. Both the enzyme and voltage triggered release was based on the presence of ferrocenyl (Fc) and β-CD valve. The release is based on the conversion of Fc to Fc^+ which dissociates from the surface of the pores under a standard potential of +0.32 V. They observed that at a higher voltage, the release rate was higher and vice versa. Wang et al. [232] also utilized the potential of ferrocene functionalized β-CD as nanovalves to modulate the drug release from MSNs. They loaded two drugs that is, gemcitabine and doxorubicin and evaluated the potential of ferrocene in controlling the drug release. On applying a voltage of +1.5 V, a controlled release of 23% of gemcitabine was observed over 15 min. Thereafter −1.5 V was applied, which ceased the release of the drug. Hence, this approach can be effectively used for controlling the drug release from MSNs and thus avoiding side effects.

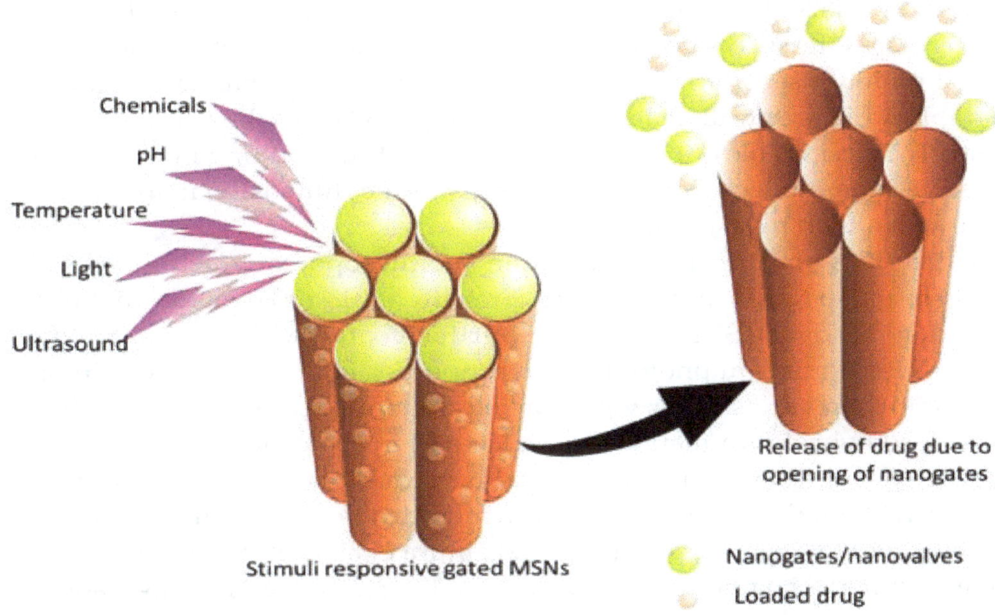

Figure 5. Schematic illustration of the release of drug from gated MSNs in response to stimuli.

5.4. MSNs for Improvement of Solubility of Drugs

MSNs owing to their modifiable surface chemistry can act as carriers for poorly soluble drugs and tackle their solubility issues [234]. Bukara et al. [235] proved this potential of MSNs by loading the poorly soluble drug fenofibrate and assessing them in healthy human volunteers. The volunteers were monitored for a period of 96 h post dosing and their plasma samples were collected and assessed for the pharmacologically active metabolite fenofibric acid. A significant increase in C_{max} with a point estimate of 177% and a reduction in t_{max} were observed for fenofibrate formulation following single oral administration. No serious adverse events were reported and none of the volunteers discontinued the study. This demonstrates that the MSNs could also be used as a possible alternative to other carriers to improve the solubility and bioavailability of drugs. Enhanced oral bioavailability of telmisartan (TEL) was achieved by loading it into MSNs. Based on the results obtained by the study on beagle dogs, Zhang et al. set forth a basis to use MSNs as a drug carrier for poorly soluble drugs. In vitro cellular uptake studies showed that TEL-MSN showed an enhanced uptake in Caco-2 cells resulting in accumulation in the cell membrane as compared to TEL-mesoporous silica microparticles. The uptake mechanism of these MSNs occurred in three major steps: first, binding of MSNs to intestinal cell membrane followed by nonspecific cellular uptake and merging with endosomes and finally, release from endosomes and enters the cytoplasm. In vivo absorption studies of TEL-MSN in beagle dogs revealed a 1.29 times increase in $AUC_{0\rightarrow 72h}$ as compared to that of marketed tablet and MSN [236]. Thomas et al. synthesized MSNs loaded with BSC-II antiepileptic drugs, carbamazepine (CBZ), oxcarbazepine (OXC) and rufinamide (RFN). The dissolution profile of the drugs in phosphate buffer, showed faster release for CBZ and OXC whereas RFN showed a slower release of drugs after an initial burst release. The profile resembled a first order release mechanism related to the drug diffusion process. This could be widely exploited for the improvement in drug absorption and bioavailability of poorly soluble drugs by further proving this concept via in vivo studies [237].

5.5. MSNs in Biomedical Imaging and Theranostic Purpose

The versatile features of MSNs such as ability to incorporate wide variety and large number of compounds within them, their stability and controllable size, makes it an ideal platform for biomedical imaging and theranostic applications. Many of the fluorophores face certain drawbacks such as poor solubility and stability especially those for near infrared (NIR) imaging. These compounds can be incorporated within the MSNs to improve their photophysical and photochemical properties. Various literatures have suggested the successful utilization of this carrier for imaging and theranostic purposes.

MSNs can be widely used for optical imaging, magnetic resonance imaging (MRI), positron emission tomography (PET). Optical imaging is a technique wherein the specific probes are excited by incident light usually in the visible or near infrared regions, thus emitting light at a lower energy. MRI is a powerful in vivo imaging technique which gives a three dimensional anatomical picture of the region of interest with a high resolution.

Most often, the dyes are incorporated within the mesopores which gives sufficient stability and protection from the external environment. Sreejith et al. developed a novel hybrid material constituting squaraine loaded MSNs which were further coated with thin sheets of graphene oxide. Squaraine dyes possess significant photophysical properties in the NIR region. In order to ascertain their bioimaging ability, in vitro studies were carried out on HeLa cell lines which showed positive results. The developed hybrid formulation was successful in protecting the dye as well as preventing its leakage from the system showing a potential platform for bioimaging [238]. Moreover, these MSNs can also be tagged with surface active moieties which can be preferentially directed to abnormal tissues for diagnostic and therapeutic purposes. Nakamura et al. reported the synthesis of multimodal MSNs possessing features of imaging as well as drug delivery. The carrier was loaded with ^{19}F, a MRI contrast reagent. These nanoparticles were further labeled with fluorescent dyes and tethered with folic acid to ensure adequate uptake by tumour cells. The developed nanoparticles demonstrated positive results in vitro exhibiting sufficient cellular uptake by folate expressing cancer cells which was observed via ^{19}F MRI and fluorescence microscopy [239]. Jun et al. reported the use of silica nanoparticles embedded with quantum dots (QDs) and constituting a core-shell of CdSe@ZnS for bioimaging purposes (Si@QDs@Si NPs). They observed that the system showed superior fluorescence as compared to single quantum dots when studied in HeLa cells. The same was confirmed via in vivo testing wherein the mice were injected with Si@QDs@Si NPs mixed with HeLa cells. The nanoparticles exhibited enhanced fluorescence and hence can be effectively used for bioimaging which requires minute cell tracking with high sensitivity [240]. Helle et al. explored the potential of cyanine 7-doped silica nanoparticles for lymph node mapping using NIR imaging. They were able to map the lymph nodes for the diagnosis of possible metastatic and draining nodes. In addition, the developed platform were found to be excreted via hepatobiliary route and was found to be safe when tested in mice up to a period of three months showing an efficient hepatobiliary excretion [241].

5.6. MSNs for Bone Tissue Engineering and Repair

MSNs have found a special place in the field of tissue engineering. Most of the research in this area revolves around bone tissue differentiation and osteogenesis. The surface silanol groups present on MSNs react with the body fluids to generate carbonated apatite which can further lead to bone generation. In addition to this, the MSNs can be loaded with osteogenic agents to augment the bone tissue engineering process [242,243]. For instance, bone morphogenetic protein-2 (BMP2) derived peptide functionalized dexamethasone loaded MSNs were formulated to evaluate its efficacy for the osteogenic differentiation. The evaluation was carried out using cell line studies to study the endocytosis and uptake of the functionalized MSNs. The ectopic bone formation was studied in vivo, the results of which indicated that the BMP2-pep functionalized MSNs held great promise in bone repair. The addition of dexamethasone synergized the bone differentiation effect [177]. Similar results were reported by Luo et al. for bone forming peptide incorporated MSNs [244]. Incorporation of bioactive glasses into mesoporous silica is another interesting application of MSN in bone repair. Increased bone tissue regeneration was observed with these materials containing SiO_2-CaO-P_2O_5 as composition. Readers are directed to references [245,246] for a detailed review of these materials.

6. Biodistribution and Biocompatibility of MSNs

The safety and toxicity of nanoparticles are a cause of major concern owing to their high surface-to-volume ratio compared to its counterparts. The biocompatibility of any carrier is a prerequisite property for any pharmaceutical product to ascertain that these products do not accumulate in the body over a period of time causing untoward effects.

Many of the formulations containing conventional nanocarriers have been approved by US FDA (Table 1). Biomaterials such as lipids and polymers constitute these conventional nanocarriers. Due to its inherent biodegradability and biocompatibility, these nanocarriers have been constantly exploited for further research to enhance its biomedical applicability. Liposomes are one such carrier which comprises of phospholipid bilayer within which both hydrophobic and hydrophilic drug can be encapsulated. Liposomes have proven to be capable of being used for site specific drug targeting in a variety of diseases [247,248]. These carriers have been found to be safe which may be attributed to the biocompatible nature of phospholipids used [249]. Another nanocarrier that shares a similar importance to that of liposomes is the polymeric nanocarrier. In this regard, poly(lactic-co-glycolic acid) (PLGA) is one of the renowned polymer-based carriers. This is a part of an FDA approved device [249,250]. Although these encouraging results have been obtained regarding their safety for human use, there are certain drawbacks such as stability related issues, lack of control over drug release and difficulty in overcoming certain biological barriers associated with these carriers. Nevertheless, these are still the most widely explored carriers due to their non-toxic property.

Inorganic nanocarriers with robust characteristics, MSNs, although has shown positive in vitro results, studies are still being carried out extensively due to the age-old toxicity-related issues of silicon dioxide, especially silicosis. Efforts are underway in identifying the major routes of toxicity of silica in both its crystalline as well as amorphous forms. In this section, we have focused on the current data available on the biodistribution and biocompatibility of MSNs. Control over the size, shape, pore order and surface chemistry is crucial in deciding the fate of MSNs.

6.1. Effect of Surface Chemistry, Shape, and Size of MSNs

As per the reports, the major pathway of toxicity associated with silica is due to its surface chemistry (silanol groups) which can interact with the membrane components leading to the lysis of the cells and leaking of the cellular components [251,252]. Mesoporous silica exhibited lower hemolytic effect compared to non-porous silica. This could be attributed to the lower density of silanol groups on the surface of mesoporous structures [94]. Surface properties of MSNs also have a great impact on the biodistribution and biocompatibility of MSNs. Altering the surface features by functionalization with polyethylene glycol (PEG) helps the MSNs to escape from being captured by liver, spleen and lung tissues. This could be attributed to the longer circulation time of PEG-MSNs [253]. Yu et al. studied the impact of pore size, shape and surface features of silica nanoparticles on the cellular toxicity. The cellular toxicity was evaluated on macrophages (RAW 264.7) and cancer epithelial (A549) cells. Post 72 h exposure, they observed that A549 cells were resistant to the nanoparticles even at the concentration of 500 μg/mL. However, at a concentration of 1000 μg/mL, observable toxicity was seen. The IC50 value for the nanoparticles when tested on macrophages was found to be between 50 and 100 μg/mL. The cellular level of association was determined using inductively coupled plasma mass spectrometry (ICP-MS). Interestingly; it was observed that amino modified MSNs showed a higher level of cellular association which is contradictory to literature which report that increase in surface silanol groups are responsible for higher cellular association [251,252]. The plausible explanation for this higher interaction between amino MSNs and cells could be that a particular surface threshold exists beyond which cell interaction is facilitated. The observations from the above study suggest that toxicity depends on the type of cells, concentration of nanoparticles treated and pore size and surface charge of nanoparticles [254].

An interesting experiment to identify the effect of the spatial arrangement of MSN surface amine groups on its interaction pattern with cells was performed by Townson et al. MSNs with the same size, porosity and charge were modified with suitable reagents (trimethoxysilylpropyl modified polyethyleneimine, 2-[methoxy(polyethyleneoxy)propyl]trimethoxysilane, *N*-trimethoxysilylpropyl-*N*,*N*,*N*-trimethyl ammonium chloride) resulting in PEG-PEI and PEG-NMe_3^+ MSNs to ensure exposed polyamines and distributed, obstructed amine groups respectively. Both in vitro and in vivo experiments were performed to determine the toxicity effects. The synthesized nanoparticles were subjected to cytotoxicity studies on a wide range of cell lines such as A549 (human lung carcinoma), A431 (human epithelial cancer), Hep3B (human hepatocellular carcinoma) and human hepatocytes. PEG-PEI MSNs were found to bind to all the cells whereas PEG-NMe_3^+ MSNs showed limited binding. To confirm these results and to ascertain if the same effects will be observed in a biological system as well, 50 μg was injected into the veins of ex vivo chick embryos which helped in real-time imaging of particles. The results showed a similar trend as that observed in in vitro studies. PEG-PEI MSNs were found to bind endothelial cells and stationary and circulating white blood cells (WBCs) whereas PEG-NMe_3^+ MSNs remained in circulation for >6 h. In order to verify the importance of amine groups in binding, the MSNs were subjected to acetylation thereby shielding the amine groups. This reduces the binding affinity of the MSNs. From the study, it was concluded that exposure to charged particles and its effect on the formation of protein corona in vivo should also be considered when designing MSNs for biomedical applications [255].

The biodegradation and toxicity of MSNs also depend on the shape of the MSNs. The effect of shape on in vivo toxicity of MSNs after oral administration was studied by Li et al. for MSNs with different aspect ratios of 1, 1.75 and 5. These MSNs were administered at a dose of 40 mg/kg. Two hours post administration, a significant number of MSNs were observed in the liver and spleen. The number of spherical nanoparticles showed a marked increase in the liver compared to its rod-shaped counterparts. It was observed that MSNs showed a rapid excretion from the body via faeces while some of the unchanged MSNs or their degradation products could be absorbed and later excreted via urine. The in vitro results of degradation showed that spherical nanoparticles showed rapid degradation while long rods have slow degradation rate, especially in intestinal fluid. These results suggest that degradation of MSNs depends on the shape and biological environment. No abnormalities were observed in liver, spleen, lung and heart. However, spherical nanoparticles induced renal tubular necrosis and haemorrhage which may be due to the degradation products. Contrasting results were obtained for MSNs administered via an intravenous route where no major abnormality in kidney was detected [132,256]. However, there is a lack of clear picture of the degradation pathway and pharmacokinetics of MSNs. With this regard, efforts were made by Zhao et al. to study the pharmacokinetics and biodistribution of different shapes of MSNs namely, long rod, short rod and spherical particles following oral administration. The retention of the nanoparticles in the gastrointestinal tract was determined by ex vivo optical imaging method. In vitro cytotoxicity study revealed that all the three nanoparticles were nearly non-toxic in nature which can be attributed to the conversion of nanoparticles to non-toxic silicate ions. To predict the biodistribution of the nanoparticles, Si content in different organs was determined by inductively coupled plasma optical emission spectrometry (ICP-OES). On examining the Si content in different organs, Zhao et al. also arrived at the same conclusion as that by Li [256], that majority of the MSNs accumulate in the liver. The synthesized MSNs did not show any visible histopathological changes when compared with that of the control indicating that the particles did not produce any gastrointestinal toxicity or inflammation [257].

Size of the nanoparticles also has a profound influence on the biodistribution and excretion of MSNs. MSNs with a varying particle size from 80 to 360 nm was prepared and their biodistribution was assessed in ICR mice. An increase in particle size led to an increase in its accumulation in the liver and spleen following intravenous (i.v.) administration. However, no pathological abnormalities were observed at the end of 1 month. Smaller sized MSNs undergo slower degradation as it can escape the degradation by liver and spleen [253]. Different types of MSNs (MCM-41, SBA-15) were injected subcutaneously (s.c.) and intraperitoneally (i.p.) to mice. Intraperitoneal injection resulted in the death of animals which may be attributed to the rapid systemic distribution following i.p. injection as compared to s.c. [258]. Acute and sub-acute toxicity profiling of fluorescent mesoporous silica nanoparticles (FMSNs) were performed in female nude mice. 1 mg/mouse/day was administered via the intravenous route. No observable toxicity was seen in the animals. Long-term toxicity study following intraperitoneal injection of FMSNs at a dose of 1 mg/mouse/day twice per week for 2 months was conducted to assess the long-term effects of MSNs. The histopathological examination of body tissues, haematological parameters displayed no apparent changes compared to control. In addition, the FMSNs also showed an enhanced tumour uptake property resulting in a reduction in tumour volume [259]. Single dose toxicity studies by Tang et al. revealed that the nanoparticles exhibited a size-dependent toxicity [260]. Zhang et al. synthesized DOX-loaded MSNs functionalized with folic acid of varying sizes of 48, 72 and 100 nm and investigated the effect of particle size on its in vivo distribution in MDA-MB-231 tumour-bearing Balb/c mice. The animals were sacrificed at the end of 24, 48 and 72 h post injection and their organs were harvested. The amount of Si content in each of the organs was determined by inductively coupled plasma mass spectrometry (ICP-MS). It was observed that MSNs with size of 48 nm showed the highest accumulation in the tumour tissues. The results suggest that particle size and surface modification alters the biodistribution of MSNs [261].

The data generated from various literatures suggest that careful control of particle size and shape is the determinant factor in ascertaining the biodistribution and toxicity of MSNs. In addition, the safety and toxicity of MSNs also depend on the dosage of the MSNs administered at which no observable biological effects are detected.

Recently, Shen et al. [262] reported that the novel 3D-dendritic MSNs synthesized by them showed a rapid biodegradation in simulated body fluid within 24 h as compared to two weeks for that of plain MSNs reported earlier. In yet another effort to prepare biodegradable MSNs, He et al. [263] synthesized a novel pH responsive mesoporous silica–calcium phosphate (MSN-CAP) hybrid nanoparticles. The MSNs were doped with calcium phosphate during synthesis process which yielded pH responsive MSNs. The in vitro degradation behaviour of MSN-CAP was observed in simulated fluids. The results showed that the complete degradation of the nanoparticles took place in 24 h. Both these novel MSNs could be an alternative prospect for clinical use. However, their in vivo degradation behaviour has to be ascertained.

6.2. In Vivo Safety and Toxicity of MSNs

Determining the safety and biocompatibility of MSNs is crucial owing to its variable characteristics. Over the last few years, the number of literature on the study of the safety of MSNs has drastically increased. The toxicity of the carriers depends on its various characteristics and the conclusions derived from the studies were found to vary. Nevertheless, most of the reports showed that the MSNs get preferentially accumulated in the liver and spleen following administration.

Liu and collaborators made an attempt to study the single and repeated dose toxicity of HMSNs following intravenous administration in mice. LD_{50} of HMSNs was found to be higher than 1000 mg/kg. In single dose toxicity studies, mice were injected with HMSNs at a low dose and high dose. At the higher dose of 1280 mg/kg, mice did not survive. In contrast, the groups treated with low dose HMSNs did not show any behavioural changes nor any haematology or pathological changes. To carry out the detailed repeated dose toxicity studies, intravenous administration of HMSNs were given to mice continuously for 14 days and observed for a month. During the 1 month observation period, no mortality was observed. Moreover, no remarkable changes in pathology or blood parameters were observed. In order to assess the fate of the nanoparticles, HMSNs were injected intravenously at a dose of 80 mg/kg. Following administration, the majority of the nanoparticles were found to localize in the liver and spleen. Analysis of the silicon content using ICP-OES revealed that highest amount of silica was present in the spleen and liver which gradually reduced over a period of 4 weeks [264].

In order to assess the fate of MSNs after different administration routes, Fu and collaborators tested MSNs with a particle size of 110 nm in ICR mice. Following administration via hypodermic, intramuscular and intravenous injection as well as oral administration, the in vivo distribution of fluorescent-tagged MSNs was tracked. It was observed that of all the exposure routes, the oral route was found to be well tolerated even when the dose was increased to 5000 mg/kg and intravenous route seemed to have the least threshold. MSNs administered via intravenous route were found to preferentially accumulate in the liver and spleen at the end of 24 h and 7 days whereas those administered by other routes did not show any fluorescence in these organs. It was observed that a portion of the MSNs administered via intramuscular and hypodermic route could cross different biological barriers with a slow absorption rate. The major routes of excretion of MSNs were found to be via urine and faeces with the highest values after oral administration as compared to other routes. No histopathological changes were observed in liver, spleen, kidney and lung at the end of 24 h and 7 days by different exposure routes. Nonetheless, a low degree of inflammation was seen in the mice which were treated with MSNs via the hypodermic and intramuscular route. The results suggested that MSNs were found to be safe and well tolerated when administered by oral and intravenous routes [265]. For an extensive review on the biocompatibility of MSNs and silica NPs, the readers are directed to references [260,266,267].

6.3. MSNs v/s Silica Nanoparticles

Different forms of silica *viz,* fumed silica, porous silica and non-porous silica can be used as drug carriers. These carriers have shown encouraging results in preclinical studies. However, to translate these materials to the bedside, a clear understanding of the fate and the inherent toxicity of these carriers in vivo is essential. Silica nanoparticles used for biomedical applications are usually amorphous in nature belonging to either porous or non-porous category. The rapid clearance of amorphous silica from the lung compared to the crystalline forms is responsible for its lower toxicity potential [268]. MSNs are found to dissolve rapidly when it is sufficiently below the saturation levels. As per the reports of Martin [269], silica dissolves in the body fluids which subsequently gets absorbed or excreted as silicic acid in the urine. The silica nanoparticles undergo degradation to silicic acid which is non-toxic via three different processes *viz*, hydration, hydrolysis and ion-exchange. This process of degradation was found to depend on the degradation medium and the concentration of nanoparticles. Various strategies have been explored which can manipulate the degradation kinetics of silica nanoparticles. Some of the approaches are noncovalent doping of organic moieties to accelerate the hydrolytic degradation, covalent binding of organically bridged silsesquioxanes- based NPs, and incorporation of cleavable organically bridged silsesquioxanes into silica NPs to enhance the degradation by the biological trigger. The degradation of MSNs is much more complicated than other silica NPs owing to its varying matrix. This is attributed to the difference in the rate and degree of condensation of silica matrices between the various sol-gel procedures of MSN synthesis. As per the review by Croissant et al., partially condensed MSNs degrade in a few days, well condensed MSNs tend to degrade in weeks and calcined MSNs takes months for its degradation [270].

In order to assess the impact of porous structures on the in vivo immunotoxicity, Lee et al. performed repeated-dose toxicity studies on BALB/c mice. MSNs and colloidal silica NPs were injected intraperitoneally into mice for 4 weeks. At the end of the study period, the animals were sacrificed and organs were harvested to study the effects of the particles. The animals treated with MSNs showed an increase in the relative weight of liver and spleen and an increased response to lymphocyte mitogens, concanavalin A (Con A) or lipopolysaccharide (LPS). In addition, a decrease in the $CD4^+/CD8^-$ and $CD4^-/CD8^+$ phenotypes and an increase in the levels of $CD4^+/CD8^-$ and $CD4^+/CD8^+$ were recorded. Elevated IgG/IgM levels were also observed in the MSN treated animals. The results indicate that MSNs showed a greater extent of damage than colloidal silica NPs [271]. However, a careful study of the toxicity is needed to establish the safety of MSNs.

6.4. Biocompatibility of MSNs in Humans

The biocompatibility of silica nanoparticles has long been a topic of controversy as studies conducted by researchers have yielded variable results. Nevertheless, the Food and Drug Administration (FDA) approval of hybrid silica nanoparticles for bioimaging marks an event of utmost importance. These particles were found to be ~7 nm in size within which fluorescent dye, Cy5 was incorporated. These particles were labelled with ^{124}I and surface functionalized with peptide cyclo-(Arg-Gly-Asp-Tyr) (cRGDY) to selectively target integrin-expressing tumours. C dots were synthesized in such a way that they had limited reticuloendothelial system (RES) uptake and promote renal excretion. Preliminary experiments on in vivo safety by Choi et al. (Cornell University) revealed that these fluorescent silica nanoparticles were safe and did not show any toxicity in mice. These particles were also found to be an effective bioimaging probe for cancer imaging [21,22]. Burns et al. carried out in vivo biodistribution studies of the developed C dots in nude mice wherein nanoparticles were injected intravenously. The particles were found to show rapid renal clearance within 45 min of injection and majority of these particles accumulated in the liver. To further modify the clearance, the particles were coated with methoxy-terminated poly(ethylene glycol) chains. By careful manipulation of the surface features of C dots, they can be used for wide variety of biomedical applications including imaging and therapy [22]. Based on the encouraging results of pre-clinical studies, these nanoparticles received approval from the FDA as an Investigational New Drug (IND) to conduct the human clinical trial, phase I. The first human clinical trials suggested its safety for human use. A pilot clinical trial was conducted in five metastatic melanoma patients to assess the pharmacokinetic (PK) profile of C dots following a single injection dose. The PK profiles, renal excretion, metabolic profile assessment in patients suggested that the particles were well tolerated, preferentially accumulated in the tumour site and were found to be safe for human use [272,273].

A study wherein the potential of ordered mesoporous silica nanoparticles (OMS) in enhancing the bioavailability of fenofibrate in man was conducted by Bukara and collaborators which can be considered as another breakthrough step acting as a trigger in evoking interest among the researchers for the use of MSNs for biomedical applications. Promising results obtained by them in their preclinical studies [274] prompted them to complement those results with clinical studies. Fenofibrate was loaded into OMS and these were subsequently enclosed within capsules. The study was carried out with 12 volunteers who were administered a single dose of fenofibrate OMS and the marketed formulation of fenofibrate, Lipanthyl®. Safety assessment was performed by periodic monitoring of the vital signs, 12-lead electrocardiogram (ECG) and blood biochemical parameters in the subjects. The PK profile revealed an increase in the rate and extent of absorption of fenofibrate when incorporated in OMS as compared to the marketed product. In addition, the formulation was found to be well tolerated in the volunteers ensuring the safety of the developed OMS formulation [235].

7. Recent Patents Filed in the Field of MSNs for Biomedical Applications

Ever since its first production, modifications in terms of synthesis aiming to control the particle size and pore volume has led to the filing of several patents on MSNs. Owing to its versatile nature of loading therapeutic agents, both hydrophilic and hydrophobic, patents filed on MSNs mainly include investigating them for biomedical applications, biosensors, imaging and as adsorbents. In the following section, we have laid emphasis on reviewing the recent patents related to the biomedical applications of MSNs.

A novel approach of coating the MSNs with lipids coined as 'protocells' has received significant attention in the fabrication of drug delivery systems. These combine the advantages of liposomes (low toxicity, long circulation times) with the advantages of MSNs (tunable size, shape and loading capacity) (Figure 6). Numerous studies have shown positive results, a few of which are touched upon here.

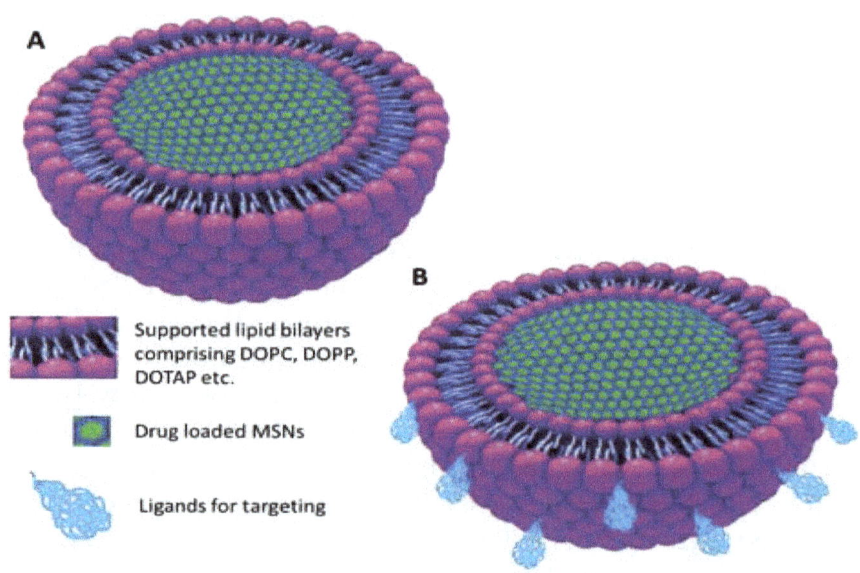

Figure 6. Representation of (**A**) Non-targeted protocell and (**B**) Targeted protocell.

A protocell of MSN encapsulated within lipid bilayer was designed by Ashley and collaborators wherein, MSNs were prepared by aerosol-assisted evaporation-induced self-assembly (EISA) procedure. The MSNs were encapsulated within supported lipid bilayers. The lipid bilayer components (cholesterol and phospholipids) were covalently attached to the glycidoxypropylsilane or APTES functionalized MSNs. Levofloxacin was loaded into the pores of the MSNs. The lipid bilayers were composed of either 1,2-dioleoyl-sn-glycero-3-phosphocholine (DOPC), 1,2-dioleoyl-sn-glycero-3-phosphoethanolamine (DOPE) or 1,2-distearoyl-sn-glycero-3-phosphocholine (DSPC). The protocells were rendered target specific by anchoring peptides (e.g., RGD peptide comprising of Arg-Gly-Asp) onto its surface. The protocells were PEGylated with polyethylene glycol to enhance its circulation time in the body. The pore size of the MSNs ranged from 1 nm to 75 nm. A high drug loading of about 20–55 wt % of the protocell was obtained for individual antibiotics. Fcy targeted protocells were found to show enhanced uptake by THP-1 cells resulting in the effective killing of intracellular organism *F. tularensis*. Only 2 wt % levofloxacin loaded protocell was also found to be cytotoxic as compared to that of free levofloxacin. Biodistribution studies in Balb/c mice showed that Fcy targeted protocells were distributed in various organs of potential *F. tularensis* infection such as lung, liver, spleen and lymph nodes. The results revealed that the biodistribution like many other nanoparticles depends on their size and size distribution. Based on literature reports and approximation of previous work on other antibiotics, the inventors also claimed that oral administration of protocells was far more effective than inhalation therapy for respiratory tularemia. However, these protocells have to be filled in capsules coated with a suitable polymer to prevent its degradation from the gastric environment. The application of protocells could also be extended to incorporate various other antibiotics, macromolecules such as DNA and histone packaged plasmid into the protocells to enhance its penetration into the nucleus of a cell and deposit its contents [275].

Jeffrey and collaborators fabricated MSNs which were functionalized with targeting ligands specific to white blood cells or arterial, venous or capillary vessels. These targeting ligands were either Fc gamma from IgG, human complement C3, ephrin B2 and SP94 peptide. These MSNs were further encapsulated within lipid bi- or multi-layers to form protocells. Polyethyleneglycol-polyethyleneimine (PEG-PEI) was tethered to the surface of MSNs to enhance the colloidal stability of the formulation. The MSNs were around 50 nm in size and positively charged. This helps to bind itself to endothelial cells, serum proteins and white blood cells. To elucidate the binding of these MSNs, they were injected into veins of ex vivo chick embryos. PEI-PEG-MSNs were found to be bound to endothelial cells as well as stationary and circulating white blood cells following injection [276].

Similar use of protocells was extended and reported for multicomponent delivery of drugs DOX, 5-fluorouracil and cisplatin to cancer cells. The protocells constituted MSNs which were surrounded by lipid bilayers also referred to as 'supported lipid bilayer' (SLB) and further functionalized with targeting ligand SP94 peptides which are overexpressed in liver cancer. These ligands were conjugated on the surface of amino-modified MSNs by a PEG spacer. The lipids chosen were *N*-[1-(2,3-Dioleoyloxy)propyl]-*N*,*N*,*N*-trimethylammonium methyl-sulfate (DOTAP), 1,2-dioleoyl-sn-glycero-3-phospho-L-serine (DOPS) which functions as a pore sealing agent and thereby restricts the release of the drug. Once internalized by the cells, the SLBs get destabilized by endosome acidification, thus releasing the drug. The protocells could also be tethered with nuclear localization sequence (NLS) to enhance the penetration of the drug into the nucleus of the cells. In vitro cellular uptake of the protocells by Hep3B cells (hepatocellular carcinoma) supported the hypothesis of active targeting by the developed protocells [277].

Toroidal MSNs were synthesized and their potential use as a carrier for the transport of different cargos ranging from small molecules to siRNA, mRNA and plasmids was explored by Brinker and Lin. Both ellipsoidal (eMSN) and toroidal shaped MSNs (tMSNs) were synthesized by varying the reaction procedure and the reactants. 'Torus' shaped MSNs refer to MSN with a central pore and two other pores into which macromolecules can be easily loaded. The internal surface area was found to be in the range of 1.1 to 0.5 cc/g with a payload of 50%. These were functionalized with amino groups and modified with PEG to improve the circulation time. Ligands, Fc gamma from IgG, human complement C3, ephrin B2 and SP94 peptide were tethered onto the MSNs for target specificity. DOPC and DOPP (dioctylphenylphosphonate) lipids can be coated onto the MSNs to seal the pores and also improve the biocompatibility. Cellular uptake studies were performed on a variety of cell lines such as human endothelial cells like EAhy 926, ATCC-CRL-2922 and mouse macrophages ATCC-TIB-71 and Raw 264-7. The successful internalization of the MSNs was proved by the in vivo studies. The developed MSNs can be a possible carrier to load large linear molecules due to its unique structure.

They can also be loaded with a variety of small molecules ranging from anti-cancer, anti-inflammatory, antiviral and so forth [278].

Protocells for the efficient delivery of chemotherapeutic agents for the treatment of hepatocellular carcinoma was formulated. The protocells contained nanoparticles protected by supported lipid bilayers comprising of DOTAP, DOPG (1,2-dioleoyl-sn-glycero-3-phosphoglycerol) or DOPE as lipids. The nanoparticles were loaded with DOX, cisplatin and 5-fluorouracil as model cargo. The surface of the protocells was tethered to a novel binding peptide c-MET. The pores can also be loaded with small interfering RNA, microRNA. The surface of the nanoparticles was modified with amino groups to sustain the drug release. These were coated with liposomes by electrostatically fusing them to nanoporous silica core. The surface was coated with a fusogenic peptide that promotes the endosomal escape of protocells. They can also be coated with nuclear localization sequence to enhance the uptake by the nucleus. The applicability of these protocells can also be extended for the transdermal delivery of the drugs wherein the supported lipid bilayers contained permeation enhancers to enhance the permeability via the stratum corneum [279].

Nel et al. developed phospholipid bilayer coated MSN loaded with gemcitabine (GEM) for the treatment of human pancreatic ductal adenocarcinoma (PDAC). The MSNs were synthesized and loaded with GEM. The lipid membrane was rehydrated with GEM-MSNs which led to the coating and capping of the pores of the MSNs. In addition to this, paclitaxel was dissolved in the organic solvent along with the lipids thus leading to MSNs with two drugs; one in the pores and other embedded in the lipid bilayer. The loading of GEM into the MSNs was found to be around 20% *w/w*. Transforming growth factor β (TGF-β) inhibitor, LY364947 was adsorbed onto MSNs. These TGF-β inhibitors help in enhancing the permeation of GEM laden MSNs to the tumour sites. This proof-of-concept was established in BxPC3 xenograft mouse models (pancreatic tumour model). The delivery system showed enhanced uptake in tumours showing a significant reduction in tumour volume. To prolong the circulation time, the MSNs were coated with PEI/PEG [280].

Silica nanoparticles loaded with antibiotics and their surface coated with a polymer to prevent premature release of the drug were developed by Avni and collaborators. The formulation was designed such that the cargo will be released only in response to stimuli. In this work, the drug within the nanoparticles will be released only if the substance released by the target cell has the property to degrade the gating molecules. Another application of this invention was in the diagnosis of diseases. Signaling molecule loaded silica nanoparticles were gated with nucleic acid molecules. Outside this particle, another molecule which produces a detectable signal was added. In the presence of a nucleic acid which is complementary to the gating molecule, they both hybridize resulting in the opening of the gates of the nanoparticles. In a similar way, the developed nanoparticles were used for various applications by coating the surface of the particles and making it responsive to stimuli [281].

Pore expanded MSNs with a pore diameter ranging from 1 nm to 100 nm for the loading of bioactive material and mainly protein was developed by Cheolhee. The pore expanding agent used was trimethylbenzene. Also, the surface of the MSNs was functionalized with ligands specific to the protein of interest to enhance the binding of the protein either to the inner or outer surface of the carrier. The ligand includes nickel, nickel-nitrilotriacetic acid (NTA), glutathione, dextrin, biotin or streptavidin. The protein of interest in this work was proteasome. Various other proteins such as bovine serum albumin (BSA), IgG proteins, β-galactosidase, horseradish peroxidase were introduced into the pores to study their effect. The surface of the MSNs was further functionalized with the ligand to enhance the intracellular drug delivery using peptides. The intracellular delivery efficiency of the MSNs was studied using fluorescent tagged MSNs. The MSNs were found to show an increased intracellular delivery of the agents as compared to the free proteins. The internalization mechanism of MSN-proteasome complex was studied in HeLa cell lines. It was observed that the complex exhibited energy-dependent caveolae-mediated and clathrin-mediated endocytosis. This drug delivery carrier could be further extended for the delivery of various other proteins and enzymes such as RNase, kinase, phosphatase, antibodies, miRNA or siRNA [282].

Weng et al. worked on improving the efficacy of a natural molecule, 16-hydroxy-cleroda-3,13-dine-15,16-olide (HCD) for the treatment of cancer. Even though HCD has shown great potential in inducing apoptosis, its use is limited by its poor solubility. HCD was incorporated into copper modified silica nanoparticles. To further prolong the release of the drug from the carrier, these nanoparticles were coated with Eudragit®S100 (Cu-MSN-HCD-S100). The loading of the drug was found to be around 18% of the weight of the carrier which was supported by the reduction in surface area with each coating. In vitro release profile of the drug showed a sustained release with Cu-MSN-HCD-S100 as compared to the uncoated MSNs. The cytotoxic potential of the developed formulation was observed in rat G6 glioma cell lines. These results were supported by in vivo studies in tumour xenograft C6 rat glioma bearing mouse models which showed a reduction in the tumour volume on oral administration of the formulation. The formulation was found to be safe without any major reported toxic effects [283].

Modified MSNs were fabricated by Lee and collaborators to monitor the redox-responsive drug release within the system. To validate this concept, doxorubicin-loaded MSN labeled with coumarin and tethered to cysteine was developed. The release of the drug was blocked by fluorescein isothiocyanate-β-cyclodextrin (FITC-β-CD) which was covalently bound to cysteine. These carriers are designated as redox-responsive fluorescent resonance energy transfer-based MSN drug delivery system (FRET-MSNs). These FRET systems have a unique feature of energy transfer between two fluorophores which is sensitive to changes in the donor (Coumarin-labeled cysteine) to acceptor (FITC-β-CD) separation distance. The change in the FRET signal was used to monitor the drug release. When the donor and acceptor are in proximity to MSN surface, a green emission peak at 520 nm was observed (FRET ON). In the presence of glutathione (GSH) which are overexpressed in cancer cells, the disulfide bonds get cleaved resulting in the opening of FITC-β-CD valve and release of drug which shows an increased blue fluorescence at 450 nm corresponding to coumarin (FRET OFF). The pore diameter of these carriers was found to be 2.3 nm with a particle size of around 100 nm. This theory was studied using HeLa cells treated with thioacetic acid (GSH synthesis scavenger) and *N*-ethylmaleimide (GSH scavenger). In the presence of thioacetic acid, a decrease in cell viability, as well as gradual decrease in FRET signal, was observed. The opposite was true in case of *N*-ethylmaleimide. Similarly, the same carrier can be used to monitor the release of a wide variety of drugs by suitably modifying the carrier system [284].

A comparatively new avenue of research for the use of MSNs is in the delivery of antibiotic drugs for the treatment of post-operative osteomyelitis and arthroplasty. Polyacrylate based bone cement materials for effective delivery of antibiotics was designed by Shou-Cang and collaborators. A sustained release of 70% of the active principle over a period of 80 days was observed when compared to only 5% release from the currently marketed antibiotic bone cement formulation, Smart-Set GHV.A co-delivery of antibiotics (gentamicin, vancomycin) and anti-inflammatory (indomethacin, ibuprofen) drug was achieved in the current invention. To formulate MSN based bone cement, the drug was loaded into the MSNs and polyacrylate was added to form a mixture to which monomer, methyl methacrylate was added and polymerized to form the bone cement. It was observed that as the content of MSN was increased from 6 wt % to above; an enhanced drug release was observed which was otherwise restricted to <7% as the majority of the drug would be embedded in the bone cement matrix. In the case of MSN, the drug could be released from the matrix via diffusion from the pores. The developed formulation also exhibited low cytotoxicity to mouse fibroblast cells ensuring the safety of the formulation. The compression strength and bending modulus of the bone cement were similar to that of the commercial product. Hence, the current invention can be used as an alternative to treat osteomyelitis, augmentation of the bone crew and bone-implant interface during joint replacement surgery, as bone filler and bone graft substitute [285].

Liu and Lay [286] reported the formulation of stimuli-responsive hollow silica vesicles coated with interpolymer complex for the delivery of bioactive agents. These carriers contained interpolymer complex where the first polymer PEG was immobilized on the surface and the second polymer, poly(methyl methacrylate) (PMMA) was complexed to the first one via hydrogen bond. The principle behind the release of active agent from the pore was related to a pH of the system. At around pH 5, the second polymer will remain complexed to the first one whereas, at pH 7 and above, the interpolymer complex dissociates releasing the drug. The dissociation of the PEG-PMMA complex was due to the deprotonation of PMMA leading to breaking of hydrogen bonds between methyl methacrylate (MMA) and ethylene glycol (EG). This leads to swelling of the complex and dissolving of anionic PMMA. The hollow silica particles were prepared using polystyrene as template and surface modified with amino groups. Calcein blue was loaded as the model cargo to study the behaviour of the delivery system. The ratio of methyl methacrylate: ethylene glycol was in the ratio of 1:3.4. PMMA of varying molecular weights was tried and 6.5 kDa formed a good complex with PEG as it could easily intercalate within the gaps of PEG chains thus providing flexible, smooth PEG-PMMA complex. The developed formulation was evaluated for the proof of concept by in vitro studies. These can be used for delivery of drugs susceptible to gastric pH and can be given via oral route by suitably formulating with additives.

Zink et al. formulated MSNs with its surface modified with mPEG and further coated with a polymer such as a polyethyleneimine (PEI) for the delivery of siRNA and plasmid DNA. Along with this, phosphonate modified MSNs were also synthesized and loaded with drugs. Also, doxorubicin, paclitaxel was loaded into the MSNs. The polymer chain length can effectively control the toxicity of the synthesized MSNs still maintaining the necessary function. To evaluate the toxicity of PEI as a polymer, MSNs were coated with different molecular weights of PEI polymer like 0.6, 1.2, 1.8, 10 and 25 KD. The cytotoxicity potential of the developed formulation was determined in HEPA-1 cells. The results revealed the absence of any toxicity in particles coated with 0.6, 1.2 and 1.8 KD polymers whereas 10 KD polymer showed toxicity at 50 μg/mL whereas 25 KD polymer showed a decline in MTS (3-(4,5-dimethylthiazol-2-yl)-5-(3-carboxymethoxyphenyl)-2-(4-sulfophenyl)-2H-tetrazolium) activity at more than 12.5 μg/mL. In addition to this, paclitaxel was also loaded into the pores to determine the activity of the carrier. The cellular uptake of the paclitaxel-loaded MSNs was determined in PANC-1 and BxPC3 cells (human pancreatic ductal carcinoma). The MSN-PEI-1.2 KD particles exhibited significant cytotoxicity and cellular uptake of paclitaxel whereas MSN-PEI-25 KD showed slight particle related toxicity at a concentration of 25 μg/mL as compared to that of paclitaxel suspension in aqueous media [287].

Liong and collaborators developed MSNs to carry water-insoluble drugs like camptothecin (CPT) and paclitaxel (PCL) for the treatment of pancreatic carcinoma. To render the nanoparticles magnetic in nature for MR imaging, iron oxide nanocrystals were incorporated into the MSNs. They further loaded hydrophobic chemotherapeutic agents into the pores of MSNs. They modified the synthesis of iron oxide nanocrystals by thermal decomposition of iron-oleate complexes which later were merged with cetyltrimethylammonium bromide (CTAB) by the interaction between the hydrophobic tail of CTAB and hydrophobic oleate ligand. The mesoporous silica was formed around the iron oxide nanocrystals at a temperature of 65–80 °C with vigorous stirring to obtain nanoparticles in the range of 100–200 nm. They also successfully utilized the same method with other inorganic nanoparticles like gold and silver in place of iron. The complete removal of surfactant template was brought about by ion exchange method using ammonium nitrate. To avoid agglomeration of the particles, the surface of MSNs was modified with phosphonate groups (that is, trihydroxy silyl propyl methylphosphonate). On loading the drugs into the pores of MSNs, it was observed that only 30 nmol of the drug was loaded onto 1 mg of nanoparticles. To enhance the cellular uptake by cancer cells, the MSNs were functionalized with folic acid moiety. This study was confirmed by cellular uptake studies in pancreatic cell lines (PANC-1, Capan-1 and AsPC-1), colon cancer cell line (SW480) and stomach cancer cell line (MKN-45). Fluorescent MSN clearly indicated the cytotoxic potential of CPT. They also studied the mechanism of cellular uptake in human pancreatic cell line PANC-1 and hepatoma cell line Hepa-1 cells. The results suggested that the uptake of FMSN takes place via temperature and energy dependent manner. This was confirmed by treating the cells with metabolic inhibitors such as sodium azide/sucrose/bafilomycin A, nocodazole/brefeldin A which inhibited the cellular uptake of FMSNs [288].

Sulfasalazine loaded charged MSNs were fabricated by Lee et al. for the effective therapy against diseases of the lower gastrointestinal tract (inflammatory bowel disease, ulcerative colitis, Crohn's disease). The surface of MSNs was functionalized with *N*-trimethoxysilylpropyl-*N*,*N*,*N*-trimethylammonium chloride via co-condensation method at varying concentration of 2%, 5%, 8% and 12% *v/v* designated as MSN-TA1, MSN-TA2, MSN-TA3 and MSN-TA4 respectively. Sulfasalazine and a dye named orange II were loaded into the pores of the MSNs. The loading percentage was found to be about 1.7 to 4% in water and DMSO as solvent respectively. The concentration of the dye played a significant role in the adsorption capacity. Higher the concentration of orange II, greater was the adsorption of the dye which suggested diffusion dependent adsorption. However, adsorption was found to be greater with the increased density of TA groups on the surface of MSNs. Similar results were observed with that of sulfasalazine as well. However, the loading efficiency was found to be lesser due to the hydrophobic nature of the drug. pH range of 2–5 was found to be optimum for the loading of the drug as at this pH strong electrostatic attraction was found to be present. The in vitro release profile revealed that MSN-TA4 showed a comparatively slower release of the drug compared to the rest of the modifications and unmodified MSN. Their work indicates that the release and adsorption of the drug onto MSNs could be tailored by tethering TA onto the surface of MSNs [289].

Lin et al. utilized room temperature ionic liquids (RTIL) as a template for the synthesis of MSNs. The organic cation used in this work includes alkylammonium and alkylphosphonium cations and heterocyclic cations like *N*-alkyl pyridinium and *N*,*N′*-dialkyl imidazolium. These organic cations were treated with suitable anions, such as tetrafluoroborate, hexafluorophosphate, halides such as fluoride, chloride, bromide and iodide to form RTIL. The pores of the MSNs were loaded with antimicrobial agents. These agents could also form part of the cationic group of the RTIL. They suggested that to obtain a delayed release of the drug either the antimicrobial ammonium species can be used as the template of MSN or the pores can be reloaded with the antimicrobial quaternary ammonium salts. To control the release of the drug from the template, the surface of the MSNs can be further coated with a polymer like poly (lactic acid) or any bioadhesive polymer to render the MSNs bioadhesive which can further prolong the drug release. In the present invention, MSNs with different shapes such as spheres, ellipsoids, rods and tubes were synthesized using different tetraalkoxysilanes namely 1-tetradecyl-3-methylimidazolium bromide (C_{14}MIMBr), 1-hexadecyl-3-methylimidazolium bromide (C_{16}MIMBr), 1-octadecyl-3-methylimidazolium bromide (C_{18}MIMBr), 1-tetradecyloxymethyl-3-methylimidazolium chloride (C_{14}OCMIMCl) and cetyl pyridinium bromide (CPBr) respectively. The pores of the MSNs were capped with certain amino acids to alter the drug release. The antibacterial activity of the developed MSNs was determined by disk diffusion assays, minimal inhibitory concentration (MIC), and minimal bactericidal concentration (MBC) against *Escherichia coli* K12. They were also claimed to be effective against fungi. The inventors also developed cetylpyridinium chloride (CPC) containing MSN formulation for the treatment of an oral volatile sulfur compounds (VSC)-prone condition leading to oral malodor problems. The pore surface was blocked with zinc-binding amino acids such as glutamic acid, histidine and aspartic acid groups. In neutral or weakly basic conditions, CPC molecules slowly diffuse out of the pores and suppress the anaerobic protein digestion activities of gram negative bacteria thus preventing VSC formation. The MSN formulation can be administered via oral, topical or parenteral routes depending on the final use. The MSNs can be further formulated using suitable diluents or carriers to convert it into tablets or topical ointments, gels [290].

8. Conclusions

In this review, we have touched upon some exciting research utilizing mesoporous silica nanocarriers as drug delivery systems. Their unique properties of tunable pore size, pore volume, high loading capacity makes them widely exploited nanocarriers. Varying the molar composition of the reactants, type of reactants and the reaction conditions, MSNs with different particle size, shape and pore volume can be obtained. Tailoring the surface properties and pore size of MSNs helps enhance the loading and modify the drug release profile. The major research on MSNs is focused on the use of these in the treatment of cancer wherein variety of ligands can be anchored onto the surface of MSNs due to the ease of functionalization. Moreover, these smart systems can be used to deliver drug at the site of interest by various external and internal stimuli such as pH, temperature, light, chemicals, enzymes, ultrasound and so forth. Review of the patents filed shows that majority of the research focuses on exploring the possible use of protocells (MSNs coated with supported lipid bilayers) for drug and macromolecule delivery. With this kind of systems, it is possible to protect the cargo from the external environment and also achieve 'zero' premature release. However, the pharmacokinetics and biodistribution of these carriers vary depending on its characteristics and the route of administration. Implications associated with long-term use of MSNs remain unanswered. This lacuna holds back the technology platform from stepping to the next level of clinical use.

9. Current and Future Perspectives

Although FDA has approved only a few nanomedicines for treatment and use in the clinics, these novel systems have been successful in laying a huge impact in the field of disease therapy and have the potential to change the conventional treatment or diagnosis. Ever since the first identification of the potential application of MSNs as carriers for drug delivery, exhaustive research is being carried out to prove the importance of this technology in the therapy of multiple diseases. Majority of the work focuses on the use of these carriers for site-specific delivery of chemotherapeutic agents. Nonetheless, regulatory and technical obstacles limit the safe and efficient translation and regulatory approval of these products. Unlike other nanocarriers, the fabrication of MSNs is a simple and cost-effective process. Moreover, these MSNs have an additional scope of being a multifunctional nanocarrier for spatial, temporal placement of drugs and also for theranostic purpose and imaging, and also supports multidrug loading. Remarkable outcomes have been achieved in this regard in both cellular and preclinical studies. However, certain challenges lay ahead in the successful translation of this platform to bedside. Synthesis of MSNs with consistent characteristics and quality can be a major challenge. The industrial transfer of technology mainly depends on scalability and hence the synthesis of MSNs at production scale may be a barrier to its commercialization. There is a need for a better understanding and control of the manufacturing process to ensure reproducibility in the product. In addition, all drugs cannot be loaded in the same concentration and hence the amount of MSN may vary from case to case which may play a role in determining the maximum tolerated dose of MSN. Certain process analytical tools such as custom-built fluorescence correlation spectroscopy (FCS) coupled with size exclusion/gel permeation chromatography (GPC) adopted by Chen et al. [291] would aid in monitoring the particle size and long term stability and thus reduce batch-to-batch variation. While the inherent toxicity issues of most of the inorganic nanoparticles remains a major issue, encouraging reports on the efficacy and biocompatibility of MSNs in animal models shows the tremendous potential of shifting this platform to clinical levels. However, the difference in the physiology of small animals and humans may lead to failure of these carriers in clinical trials. Lack of in-depth understanding of the interaction between MSNs and the biological system needs to be addressed. Comprehensive in vitro screening assays with varying ligands to ensure optimum uptake, stability, specificity and pharmacokinetic profile would be useful in developing a more reliable product for clinical trials especially for anticancer therapy and the same could be extended as a guide to develop more reliable MSN products for other biomedical purposes as well. Recently, a ray of light for the use of silica nanoparticles was seen in the form of FDA's approval to conduct stage I human clinical trial for Cornell dots (C dots). This marked an important step towards the acceptance of silica nanoparticles. Following this, first-in human studies by Bukara and group [235] demonstrated the safety of MSNs. Nevertheless, the potential challenge to the clinical translation of MSN-based drug delivery system lies in the lack of substantial evidence on its chronic toxicity studies, genotoxicity and teratogenic potential, long-term tissue compatibility. Thorough understanding of the degradation mechanism of mesoporous silica in vivo is yet to be established. Efforts are to be made by researchers like us to bridge the gap between the preclinical and clinical use of MSNs to achieve marked progress in this subject. We anticipate that if a careful assessment during the production and in vitro evaluation along with studies to ascertain the biosafety of MSNs is performed, these novel designs can be a vital breakthrough in the future for clinical applications in the diagnosis, imaging and treatment catering to the needs of patients.

Acknowledgments: The authors would like to acknowledge Manipal Academy of Higher Education (MAHE), Manipal, India for providing financial support and infra-structure to carry out the work.

References

1. Krukemeyer, M.G.; Krenn, V.; Huebner, F.; Wagner, W.; Resch, R. History and Possible Uses of Nanomedicine Based on Nanoparticles and Nanotechnological Progress. *J. Nanomed. Nanotechnol.* **2015**, *6*, 1–7. [CrossRef]
2. Mudshinge, S.R.; Deore, A.B.; Patil, S.; Bhalgat, C.M. Nanoparticles: Emerging carriers for drug delivery. *Saudi Pharm. J.* **2011**, *19*, 129–141. [CrossRef] [PubMed]
3. Kankala, R.K.; Zhang, Y.S.; Wang, S.-B.; Lee, C.-H.; Chen, A.-Z. Supercritical Fluid Technology: An Emphasis on Drug Delivery and Related Biomedical Applications. *Adv. Healthc. Mater.* **2017**, *6*, 1700433. [CrossRef] [PubMed]
4. Kankala, R.K.; Zhu, K.; Sun, X.-N.; Liu, C.-G.; Wang, S.-B.; Chen, A.-Z. Cardiac Tissue Engineering on the Nanoscale. *ACS Biomater. Sci. Eng.* **2018**, *4*, 800–818. [CrossRef]
5. Gong, T.; Xie, J.; Liao, J.; Zhang, T.; Lin, S.; Lin, Y. Nanomaterials and bone regeneration. *Bone Res.* **2015**, *3*, 15029. [CrossRef] [PubMed]
6. Alhariri, M.; Azghani, A.; Omri, A. Liposomal antibiotics for the treatment of infectious diseases. *Expert Opin. Drug Deliv.* **2013**, *10*, 1515–1532. [CrossRef] [PubMed]
7. Deshpande, P.P.; Biswas, S.; Torchilin, V.P. Current trends in the use of liposomes for tumor targeting. *Nanomedicine* **2013**, *8*, 1509–1528. [CrossRef] [PubMed]
8. Puri, A.; Loomis, K.; Smith, B.; Lee, J.-H.; Yavlovich, A.; Heldman, E.; Blumenthal, R. Lipid-based nanoparticles as pharmaceutical drug carriers: From concepts to clinic. *Crit. Rev. Ther. Drug Carr. Syst.* **2009**, *26*, 523–580. [CrossRef]
9. Gad, A.; Kydd, J.; Piel, B.; Rai, P. Targeting Cancer using Polymeric Nanoparticle mediated Combination Chemotherapy. *Int. J. Nanomed. Nanosurg.* **2016**, *2*. [CrossRef]
10. Cheng, C.J.; Tietjen, G.T.; Saucier-Sawyer, J.K.; Saltzman, W.M. A holistic approach to targeting disease with polymeric nanoparticles. *Nat. Rev. Drug Discov.* **2015**, *14*, 239–247. [CrossRef] [PubMed]
11. Han, Y.-H.; Kankala, R.; Wang, S.-B.; Chen, A.-Z. Leveraging Engineering of Indocyanine Green-Encapsulated Polymeric Nanocomposites for Biomedical Applications. *Nanomaterials* **2018**, *8*, 360. [CrossRef] [PubMed]
12. Pandita, D.; Poonia, N.; Kumar, S.; Lather, V.; Madaan, K. Dendrimers in drug delivery and targeting: Drug-dendrimer interactions and toxicity issues. *J. Pharm. Bioallied Sci.* **2014**, *6*, 139–150. [CrossRef] [PubMed]
13. Hiemenz, J.W.; Walsh, T.J. Lipid formulations of amphotericin B: Recent progress and future directions. *Clin. Infect. Dis.* **1996**, *22* (Suppl. 2), S133–S144. [CrossRef] [PubMed]
14. Kaposi's sarcoma: DaunoXome approved. *AIDS Treat. News* **1996**, 3–4.
15. Barenholz, Y. (Chezy) Doxil®—The first FDA-approved nano-drug: Lessons learned. *J. Control. Release* **2012**, *160*, 117–134. [CrossRef] [PubMed]
16. Batist, G.; Barton, J.; Chaikin, P.; Swenson, C.; Welles, L. Myocet (liposome-encapsulated doxorubicin citrate): A new approach in breast cancer therapy. *Expert Opin. Pharm.* **2002**, *3*, 1739–1751. [CrossRef] [PubMed]
17. Junghanns, J.-U.A.H.; Müller, R.H. Nanocrystal technology, drug delivery and clinical applications. *Int. J. Nanomed.* **2008**, *3*, 295–309. [PubMed]
18. Giner-Casares, J.J.; Henriksen-Lacey, M.; Coronado-Puchau, M.; Liz-Marzán, L.M. Inorganic nanoparticles for biomedicine: Where materials scientists meet medical research. *Mater. Today* **2016**, *19*, 19–28. [CrossRef]
19. Kankala, R.K.; Tsai, P.-Y.; Kuthati, Y.; Wei, P.-R.; Liu, C.-L.; Lee, C.-H. Overcoming multidrug resistance through co-delivery of ROS-generating nano-machinery in cancer therapeutics. *J. Mater. Chem. B* **2017**, *5*, 1507–1517. [CrossRef]

20. Kuthati, Y.; Kankala, R.K.; Lee, C.-H. Layered double hydroxide nanoparticles for biomedical applications: Current status and recent prospects. *Appl. Clay Sci.* **2015**, *112–113*, 100–116. [CrossRef]
21. Choi, J.; Burns, A.A.; Williams, R.M.; Zhou, Z.; Flesken-Nikitin, A.; Zipfel, W.R.; Wiesner, U.; Nikitin, A.Y. Core-shell silica nanoparticles as fluorescent labels for nanomedicine. *J. Biomed. Opt.* **2007**, *12*, 64007. [CrossRef] [PubMed]
22. Burns, A.A.; Vider, J.; Ow, H.; Herz, E.; Penate-Medina, O.; Baumgart, M.; Larson, S.M.; Wiesner, U.; Bradbury, M. Fluorescent Silica Nanoparticles with Efficient Urinary Excretion for Nanomedicine. *Nano Lett.* **2009**, *9*, 442–448. [CrossRef] [PubMed]
23. Slowing, I.I.; Trewyn, B.G.; Lin, V.S.-Y. Mesoporous Silica Nanoparticles for Intracellular Delivery of Membrane-Impermeable Proteins. *J. Am. Chem. Soc.* **2007**, *129*, 8845–8849. [CrossRef] [PubMed]
24. Deodhar, G.V.; Adams, M.L.; Trewyn, B.G. Controlled release and intracellular protein delivery from mesoporous silica nanoparticles. *Biotechnol. J.* **2017**, *12*, 1600408. [CrossRef] [PubMed]
25. Cha, W.; Fan, R.; Miao, Y.; Zhou, Y.; Qin, C.; Shan, X.; Wan, X.; Li, J. Mesoporous Silica Nanoparticles as Carriers for Intracellular Delivery of Nucleic Acids and Subsequent Therapeutic Applications. *Molecules* **2017**, *22*, 782. [CrossRef] [PubMed]
26. Tao, C.; Zhu, Y.; Xu, Y.; Zhu, M.; Morita, H.; Hanagata, N. Mesoporous silica nanoparticles for enhancing the delivery efficiency of immunostimulatory DNA drugs. *Dalton Trans.* **2014**, *43*, 5142–5150. [CrossRef] [PubMed]
27. Möller, K.; Müller, K.; Engelke, H.; Bräuchle, C.; Wagner, E.; Bein, T. Highly efficient siRNA delivery from core–shell mesoporous silica nanoparticles with multifunctional polymer caps. *Nanoscale* **2016**, *8*, 4007–4019. [CrossRef] [PubMed]
28. Hanafi-Bojd, M.Y.; Ansari, L.; Malaekeh-Nikouei, B. Codelivery of anticancer drugs and siRNA by mesoporous silica nanoparticles. *Ther. Deliv.* **2016**, *7*, 649–655. [CrossRef] [PubMed]
29. Riikonen, J.; Xu, W.; Lehto, V.-P. Mesoporous systems for poorly soluble drugs—Recent trends. *Int. J. Pharm.* **2018**, *536*, 178–186. [CrossRef] [PubMed]
30. Maleki, A.; Kettiger, H.; Schoubben, A.; Rosenholm, J.M.; Ambrogi, V.; Hamidi, M. Mesoporous silica materials: From physico-chemical properties to enhanced dissolution of poorly water-soluble drugs. *J. Control. Release* **2017**, *262*, 329–347. [CrossRef] [PubMed]
31. Wang, Y.; Zhao, Q.; Han, N.; Bai, L.; Li, J.; Liu, J.; Che, E.; Hu, L.; Zhang, Q.; Jiang, T.; et al. Mesoporous silica nanoparticles in drug delivery and biomedical applications. *Nanomed. Nanotechnol. Biol. Med.* **2015**, *11*, 313–327. [CrossRef] [PubMed]
32. Mamaeva, V.; Sahlgren, C.; Lindén, M. Mesoporous silica nanoparticles in medicine—Recent advances. *Adv. Drug Deliv. Rev.* **2013**, *65*, 689–702. [CrossRef] [PubMed]
33. Tao, Z. Mesoporous silica-based nanodevices for biological applications. *RSC Adv.* **2014**, *4*, 18961–18980. [CrossRef]
34. Huo, Q.; Margolese, D.I.; Stucky, G.D. Stucky Surfactant Control of Phases in the Synthesis of Mesoporous Silica-Based Materials. *Chem. Mater.* **1996**, *8*, 1147–1160. [CrossRef]
35. Beck, J.S.; Vartuli, J.C.; Roth, W.J.; Leonowicz, M.E.; Kresge, C.T.; Schmitt, K.D.; Chu, C.T.W.; Olson, D.H.; Sheppard, E.W.; McCullen, S.B.; et al. A new family of mesoporous molecular sieves prepared with liquid crystal templates. *J. Am. Chem. Soc.* **1992**, *114*, 10834–10843. [CrossRef]
36. Trewyn, B.G.; Slowing, I.I.; Giri, S.; Chen, H.-T.; Lin, V.S.-Y. Synthesis and Functionalization of a Mesoporous Silica Nanoparticle Based on the Sol–Gel Process and Applications in Controlled Release. *Acc. Chem. Res.* **2007**, *40*, 846–853. [CrossRef] [PubMed]
37. Oye, G.; Sjöblom, J.; Stöcker, M. Synthesis, characterization and potential applications of new materials in the mesoporous range. *Adv. Colloid Interface Sci.* **2001**, *89–90*, 439–466. [CrossRef]
38. Zhao, D.; Huo, Q.; Feng, J.; Chmelka, B.F.; Stucky, G.D. Nonionic Triblock and Star Diblock Copolymer and Oligomeric Surfactant Syntheses of Highly Ordered, Hydrothermally Stable, Mesoporous Silica Structures. *J. Am. Chem. Soc.* **1998**, *120*, 6024–6036. [CrossRef]
39. Tozuka, Y.; Wongmekiat, A.; Kimura, K.; Moribe, K.; Yamamura, S.; Yamamoto, K. Effect of Pore Size of FSM-16 on the Entrapment of Flurbiprofen in Mesoporous Structures. *Chem. Pharm. Bull.* **2005**, *53*, 974–977. [CrossRef] [PubMed]

40. Nandiyanto, A.B.D.; Kim, S.-G.; Iskandar, F.; Okuyama, K. Synthesis of spherical mesoporous silica nanoparticles with nanometer-size controllable pores and outer diameters. *Microporous Mesoporous Mater.* **2009**, *120*, 447–453. [CrossRef]
41. Heikkilä, T.; Salonen, J.; Tuura, J.; Hamdy, M.S.; Mul, G.; Kumar, N.; Salmi, T.; Murzin, D.Y.; Laitinen, L.; Kaukonen, A.M.; et al. Mesoporous silica material TUD-1 as a drug delivery system. *Int. J. Pharm.* **2007**, *331*, 133–138. [CrossRef] [PubMed]
42. Kumar, D.; Schumacher, K.; von Hohenesche, C.D.F.; Grun, M.; Unger, K.K. MCM-41, MCM-48 and related mesoporous adsorbents: Their synthesis and characterisation. *Colloids Surf. A Physicochem. Eng. Asp.* **2001**, *187–188*, 109–116. [CrossRef]
43. Wang, S. Ordered mesoporous materials for drug delivery. *Microporous Mesoporous Mater.* **2009**, *117*, 1–9. [CrossRef]
44. Wang, S.; Li, H. Structure directed reversible adsorption of organic dye on mesoporous silica in aqueous solution. *Microporous Mesoporous Mater.* **2006**, *97*, 21–26. [CrossRef]
45. Ukmar, T.; Planinsek, O. Ordered mesoporous silicates as matrices for controlled release of drugs. *Acta Pharm.* **2010**, *60*, 373–385. [CrossRef] [PubMed]
46. Zhao, D.; Zhou, W.; Wan, Y. *Ordered Mesoporous Materials*; Wiley-VCH Verlag GmbH & Co. KGaA: Weinheim, Germany, 2013; ISBN 3527647899.
47. Kim, K.S.; Park, M.; Kim, T.W.; Kim, J.-E.; Papoulis, D.; Komarneni, S.; Choi, J. Adsorbate-dependent uptake behavior of topographically bi-functionalized ordered mesoporous silica materials. *J. Porous Mater.* **2015**, *22*, 1297–1303. [CrossRef]
48. Lu, G.Q.; Zhao, X.S. *Nanoporous Materials: Science and Engineering*; Series on Chemical Engineering; Imperial College Press: London, UK; World Scientific Publishing Co.: Singapore, 2004; Volume 4, ISBN 978-1-86094-210-5.
49. Ge, S.; Geng, W.; He, X.; Zhao, J.; Zhou, B.; Duan, L.; Wu, Y.; Zhang, Q. Effect of framework structure, pore size and surface modification on the adsorption performance of methylene blue and Cu^{2+} in mesoporous silica. *Colloids Surf. A Physicochem. Eng. Asp.* **2018**, *539*, 154–162. [CrossRef]
50. Mayoral, A.; Blanco, R.M.; Diaz, I. Location of enzyme in lipase-SBA-12 hybrid biocatalyst. *J. Mol. Catal. B Enzym.* **2013**, *90*, 23–25. [CrossRef]
51. Galarneau, A.; Cambon, H.; Di Renzo, F.; Ryoo, R.; Choi, M.; Fajula, F. Microporosity and connections between pores in SBA-15 mesostructured silicas as a function of the temperature of synthesis. *New J. Chem.* **2003**, *27*, 73–79. [CrossRef]
52. Lercher, J.A.; Kaliaguine, S.; Gobin, O.C. *SBA-16 Materials Synthesis, Diffusion and Sorption Properties*; Technical University of Munich: Munich, Germany, 2006.
53. Kleitz, F.; Liu, D.; Gopinathan, M.A.; Park, I.-S.; Solovyov, L.A.; Shmakov, A.N.; Ryoo, R. Large Cage Face-Centered-Cubic Fm3m Mesoporous Silica: Synthesis and Structure. *J. Phys. Chem. B* **2003**, *107*, 14296–14300. [CrossRef]
54. Kalbasi, J.R.; Zirakbash, A. Synthesis, characterization and drug release studies of poly(2-hydroxyethyl methacrylate)/KIT-5 nanocomposite as an innovative organic–inorganic hybrid carrier system. *RSC Adv.* **2015**, *5*, 12463–12471. [CrossRef]
55. Jammaer, J.; Aerts, A.; D'Haen, J.; Seo, J.W.; Martens, J.A. Convenient synthesis of ordered mesoporous silica at room temperature and quasi-neutral pH. *J. Mater. Chem.* **2009**, *19*, 8290–8293. [CrossRef]
56. Vialpando, M.; Aerts, A.; Persoons, J.; Martens, J.; Van Den Mooter, G. Evaluation of ordered mesoporous silica as a carrier for poorly soluble drugs: Influence of pressure on the structure and drug release. *J. Pharm. Sci.* **2011**, *100*, 3411–3420. [CrossRef] [PubMed]
57. Stober, W.; Fink, A.; Bohn, E. Controlled growth of monodisperse silica spheres in the micron size range. *J. Colloid Interface Sci.* **1968**, *26*, 62–69. [CrossRef]
58. Grün, M.; Lauer, I.; Unger, K.K. The synthesis of micrometer- and submicrometer-size spheres of ordered mesoporous oxide MCM-41. *Adv. Mater.* **1997**, *9*, 254–257. [CrossRef]
59. Blin, J.L.; Impéror-Clerc, M. Mechanism of self-assembly in the synthesis of silica mesoporous materials: In situ studies by X-ray and neutron scattering. *Chem. Soc. Rev.* **2013**, *42*, 4071–4082. [CrossRef] [PubMed]
60. Gao, C.; Qiu, H.; Zeng, W.; Sakamoto, Y.; Terasaki, O.; Sakamoto, K.; Chen, Q.; Che, S. Formation Mechanism of Anionic Surfactant-Templated Mesoporous Silica. *Chem. Mater.* **2006**, *18*, 3904–3914. [CrossRef]

61. Flodström, K.; Wennerström, H.; Alfredsson, V. Mechanism of Mesoporous Silica Formation. A Time-Resolved NMR and TEM Study of Silica–Block Copolymer Aggregation. *Langmuir* **2004**, *20*, 680–688. [CrossRef] [PubMed]
62. Attard, G.S.; Glyde, J.C.; Göltner, C.G. Liquid-crystalline phases as templates for the synthesis of mesoporous silica. *Nature* **1995**, *378*, 366–368. [CrossRef]
63. Sundblom, A.; Oliveira, C.L.P.; Palmqvist, A.E.C.; Pedersen, J.S. Modeling In Situ Small-Angle X-ray Scattering Measurements Following the Formation of Mesostructured Silica. *J. Phys. Chem. C* **2009**, *113*, 7706–7713. [CrossRef]
64. Hollamby, M.J.; Borisova, D.; Brown, P.; Eastoe, J.; Grillo, I.; Shchukin, D. Growth of Mesoporous Silica Nanoparticles Monitored by Time-Resolved Small-Angle Neutron Scattering. *Langmuir* **2012**, *28*, 4425–4433. [CrossRef] [PubMed]
65. Edler, K.J. Current Understanding of Formation Mechanisms in Surfactant-Templated Materials. *Aust. J. Chem.* **2005**, *58*, 627–643. [CrossRef]
66. Yi, Z.; Dumée, L.F.; Garvey, C.J.; Feng, C.; She, F.; Rookes, J.E.; Mudie, S.; Cahill, D.M.; Kong, L. A New Insight into Growth Mechanism and Kinetics of Mesoporous Silica Nanoparticles by In Situ Small Angle X-ray Scattering. *Langmuir* **2015**, *31*, 8478–8487. [CrossRef] [PubMed]
67. Danks, A.E.; Hall, S.R.; Schnepp, Z. The evolution of "sol–gel" chemistry as a technique for materials synthesis. *Mater. Horiz.* **2016**, *3*, 91–112. [CrossRef]
68. Fowler, C.E.; Khushalani, D.; Lebeau, B.; Mann, S. Nanoscale Materials with Mesostructured Interiors. *Adv. Mater.* **2001**, *13*, 649–652. [CrossRef]
69. Sadasivan, S.; Fowler, C.E.; Khushalani, D.; Mann, S. Nucleation of MCM-41 Nanoparticles by Internal Reorganization of Disordered and Nematic-Like Silica–Surfactant Clusters. *Angew. Chem. Int. Ed.* **2002**, *41*, 2151–2153. [CrossRef]
70. Möller, K.; Kobler, J.; Bein, T. Colloidal suspensions of mercapto-functionalized nanosized mesoporous silica. *J. Mater. Chem.* **2007**, *17*, 624–631. [CrossRef]
71. Brinker, C.J.; Lu, Y.; Sellinger, A.; Fan, H. Evaporation-Induced Self-Assembly: Nanostructures Made Easy. *Adv. Mater.* **1999**, *11*, 579–585. [CrossRef]
72. Fontecave, T.; Boissiere, C.; Baccile, N.; Plou, F.J.; Sanchez, C. Using Evaporation-Induced Self-Assembly for the Direct Drug Templating of Therapeutic Vectors with High Loading Fractions, Tunable Drug Release, and Controlled Degradation. *Chem. Mater.* **2013**, *25*, 4671–4678. [CrossRef]
73. Shi, S.; Chen, F.; Cai, W. Biomedical applications of functionalized hollow mesoporous silica nanoparticles: Focusing on molecular imaging. *Nanomedicine* **2013**, *8*, 2027–2039. [CrossRef] [PubMed]
74. Chen, F.; Hong, H.; Shi, S.; Goel, S.; Valdovinos, H.F.; Hernandez, R.; Theuer, C.P.; Barnhart, T.E.; Cai, W. Engineering of Hollow Mesoporous Silica Nanoparticles for Remarkably Enhanced Tumor Active Targeting Efficacy. *Sci. Rep.* **2015**, *4*, 5080. [CrossRef] [PubMed]
75. Zhu, Y.; Shi, J.; Chen, H.; Shen, W.; Dong, X. A facile method to synthesize novel hollow mesoporous silica spheres and advanced storage property. *Microporous Mesoporous Mater.* **2005**, *84*, 218–222. [CrossRef]
76. Li, Y.; Shi, J.; Hua, Z.; Chen, H.; Ruan, M.; Yan, D. Hollow Spheres of Mesoporous Aluminosilicate with a Three-Dimensional Pore Network and Extraordinarily High Hydrothermal Stability. *Nano Lett.* **2003**, *3*, 609–612. [CrossRef]
77. Lou, X.W.; Archer, L.A.; Yang, Z. Hollow Micro-/Nanostructures: Synthesis and Applications. *Adv. Mater.* **2008**, *20*, 3987–4019. [CrossRef]
78. She, X.; Chen, L.; Li, C.; He, C.; He, L.; Kong, L. Functionalization of Hollow Mesoporous Silica Nanoparticles for Improved 5-FU Loading. *J. Nanomater.* **2015**, *2015*, 1–9. [CrossRef]
79. Liu, J.; Luo, Z.; Zhang, J.; Luo, T.; Zhou, J.; Zhao, X.; Cai, K. Hollow mesoporous silica nanoparticles facilitated drug delivery via cascade pH stimuli in tumor microenvironment for tumor therapy. *Biomaterials* **2016**, *83*, 51–65. [CrossRef] [PubMed]
80. Ghasemi, S.; Farsangi, Z.J.; Beitollahi, A.; Mirkazemi, M.; Rezayat, S.M.; Sarkar, S. Synthesis of hollow mesoporous silica (HMS) nanoparticles as a candidate for sulfasalazine drug loading. *Ceram. Int.* **2017**, *43*, 11225–11232. [CrossRef]
81. Sasidharan, M.; Zenibana, H.; Nandi, M.; Bhaumik, A.; Nakashima, K. Synthesis of mesoporous hollow silica nanospheres using polymeric micelles as template and their application as a drug-delivery carrier. *Dalton Trans.* **2013**, *42*, 13381–13389. [CrossRef] [PubMed]

82. Zhou, X.; Cheng, X.; Feng, W.; Qiu, K.; Chen, L.; Nie, W.; Yin, Z.; Mo, X.; Wang, H.; He, C. Synthesis of hollow mesoporous silica nanoparticles with tunable shell thickness and pore size using amphiphilic block copolymers as core templates. *Dalton Trans.* **2014**, *43*, 11834–11842. [CrossRef] [PubMed]
83. Li, Y.; Li, N.; Pan, W.; Yu, Z.; Yang, L.; Tang, B. Hollow Mesoporous Silica Nanoparticles with Tunable Structures for Controlled Drug Delivery. *ACS Appl. Mater. Interfaces* **2017**, *9*, 2123–2129. [CrossRef] [PubMed]
84. Wang, X.; Feng, J.; Bai, Y.; Zhang, Q.; Yin, Y. Synthesis, Properties, and Applications of Hollow Micro-/Nanostructures. *Chem. Rev.* **2016**, *116*, 10983–11060. [CrossRef] [PubMed]
85. Kong, M.; Tang, J.; Qiao, Q.; Wu, T.; Qi, Y.; Tan, S.; Gao, X.; Zhang, Z. Biodegradable Hollow Mesoporous Silica Nanoparticles for Regulating Tumor Microenvironment and Enhancing Antitumor Efficiency. *Theranostics* **2017**, *7*, 3276–3292. [CrossRef] [PubMed]
86. Lin, Y.-S.; Wu, S.-H.; Tseng, C.-T.; Hung, Y.; Chang, C.; Mou, C.-Y. Synthesis of hollow silica nanospheres with a microemulsion as the template. *Chem. Commun.* **2009**, *0*, 3542–3544. [CrossRef] [PubMed]
87. Ding, L.; Su, B. An electrochemistry assisted approach for fast, low-cost and gram-scale synthesis of mesoporous silica nanoparticles. *RSC Adv.* **2015**, *5*, 65922–65926. [CrossRef]
88. Bian, S.; Gao, K.; Shen, H.; Jiang, X.; Long, Y.; Chen, Y. Organic/inorganic hybrid mesoporous silica membrane rapidly synthesized by a microwave-assisted method and its application in enzyme adsorption and electrocatalysis. *J. Mater. Chem. B* **2013**, *1*, 3267–3276. [CrossRef]
89. Wu, C.-G.; Bein, T. Microwave synthesis of molecular sieve MCM-41. *Chem. Commun.* **1996**, 925–926. [CrossRef]
90. Vetrivel, S.; Chen, C.-T.; Kao, H.-M. The ultrafast sonochemical synthesis of mesoporous silica MCM-41. *New J. Chem.* **2010**, *34*, 2109–2112. [CrossRef]
91. Snoussi, Y.; Bastide, S.; Abderrabba, M.; Chehimi, M.M. Sonochemical synthesis of Fe_3O_4@NH_2-mesoporous silica@Polypyrrole/Pd: A core/double shell nanocomposite for catalytic applications. *Ultrason. Sonochem.* **2018**, *41*, 551–561. [CrossRef] [PubMed]
92. Mourhly, A.; Khachani, M.; Hamidi, A.E.; Kacimi, M.; Halim, M.; Arsalane, S. The Synthesis and Characterization of Low-cost Mesoporous Silica SiO_2 from Local Pumice Rock Regular Paper. *Nanomater. Nanotechnol.* **2015**, *5*. [CrossRef]
93. Akinjokun, A.I.; Ojumu, T.V.; Ogunfowokan, A.O. Biomass, Abundant Resources for Synthesis of Mesoporous Silica Material. In *Microporous and Mesoporous Materials*; InTech: Vienna, Austria, 2016; pp. 105–117.
94. Lin, Y.-S.; Haynes, C.L. Impacts of Mesoporous Silica Nanoparticle Size, Pore Ordering, and Pore Integrity on Hemolytic Activity. *J. Am. Chem. Soc.* **2010**, *132*, 4834–4842. [CrossRef] [PubMed]
95. Williams, S.; Neumann, A.; Bremer, I.; Su, Y.; Dräger, G.; Kasper, C.; Behrens, P. Nanoporous silica nanoparticles as biomaterials: Evaluation of different strategies for the functionalization with polysialic acid by step-by-step cytocompatibility testing. *J. Mater. Sci. Mater. Med.* **2015**, *26*, 125. [CrossRef] [PubMed]
96. Qiao, Z.-A.; Zhang, L.; Guo, M.; Liu, Y.; Huo, Q. Synthesis of Mesoporous Silica Nanoparticles via Controlled Hydrolysis and Condensation of Silicon Alkoxide. *Chem. Mater.* **2009**, *21*, 3823–3829. [CrossRef]
97. Möller, K.; Kobler, J.; Bein, T. Colloidal Suspensions of Nanometer-Sized Mesoporous Silica. *Adv. Funct. Mater.* **2007**, *17*, 605–612. [CrossRef]
98. Feng, P.; Bu, X.; Pine, D.J. Control of Pore Sizes in Mesoporous Silica Templated by Liquid Crystals in Block Copolymer—Cosurfactant—Water Systems. *Langmuir* **2000**, *16*, 5304–5310. [CrossRef]
99. El-Safty, S.A.; Evans, J. Formation of highly ordered mesoporous silica materials adopting lyotropic liquid crystal mesophases. *J. Mater. Chem.* **2002**, *12*, 117–123. [CrossRef]
100. Sayari, A.; Yang, Y. Nonionic oligomeric polymer directed synthesis of highly ordered large pore periodic mesoporous organosilica. *Chem. Commun.* **2002**, *0*, 2582–2583. [CrossRef]
101. Ganesh, M.; Lee, S.G. Synthesis, Characterization and Drug Release Capability of New Cost Effective Mesoporous Silica Nano Particle for Ibuprofen Drug Delivery. *Int. J. Control Autom.* **2013**, *6*, 207–216. [CrossRef]
102. Richer, R. Direct synthesis of functionalized mesoporous silica by non-ionic alkylpolyethyleneoxide surfactant assembly. *Chem. Commun.* **1998**, *0*, 1775–1777. [CrossRef]
103. Prouzet, E.; Cot, F.; Nabias, G.; Larbot, A.; Kooyman, P.; Pinnavaia, T.J. Assembly of Mesoporous Silica Molecular Sieves Based on Nonionic Ethoxylated Sorbitan Esters as Structure Directors. *Chem. Mater.* **1999**, *11*, 1498–1503. [CrossRef]

104. Blin, J.L.; Michaux, F.; Stébé, M.J. Nanostuctured mesoporous materials from different silica sources using fluorinated surfactants as templates. *Colloids Surf. A Physicochem. Eng. Asp.* **2016**, *510*, 104–112. [CrossRef]
105. Brevet, D.; Jouannin, C.; Tourné-Péteilh, C.; Devoisselle, J.-M.; Vioux, A.; Viau, L. Self-encapsulation of a drug-containing ionic liquid into mesoporous silica monoliths or nanoparticles by a sol–gel process. *RSC Adv.* **2016**, *6*, 82916–82923. [CrossRef]
106. Kwon, S.; Singh, R.K.; Perez, R.A.; Abou Neel, E.A.; Kim, H.-W.; Chrzanowski, W. Silica-based mesoporous nanoparticles for controlled drug delivery. *J. Tissue Eng.* **2013**, *4*, 2041731413503357. [CrossRef] [PubMed]
107. Zainal, N.A.; Rizal, S.; Shukor, A.; Azwana, H.; Wab, A.; Razak, K.A. Study on the Effect of Synthesis Parameters of Silica Nanoparticles Entrapped with Rifampicin. *Chem. Eng. Trans.* **2013**, *32*, 2245–2250. [CrossRef]
108. Wang, Y. Synthesis and formation of hierarchical mesoporous silica network in acidic aqueous solutions of sodium silicate and cationic surfactant. *Colloid J.* **2010**, *72*, 737–742. [CrossRef]
109. Das, D.; Yang, Y.; O'Brien, J.S.; Breznan, D.; Nimesh, S.; Bernatchez, S.; Hill, M.; Sayari, A.; Vincent, R.; Kumarathasan, P. Synthesis and Physicochemical Characterization of Mesoporous SiO_2 Nanoparticles. *J. Nanomater.* **2014**, *2014*, 1–12. [CrossRef]
110. Yi, J.; Kruk, M. Pluronic-P123-Templated Synthesis of Silica with Cubic *Ia3d* Structure in the Presence of Micelle Swelling Agent. *Langmuir* **2015**, *31*, 7623–7632. [CrossRef] [PubMed]
111. Yamamoto, E.; Mori, S.; Shimojima, A.; Wada, H.; Kuroda, K. Fabrication of colloidal crystals composed of pore-expanded mesoporous silica nanoparticles prepared by a controlled growth method. *Nanoscale* **2017**, *9*, 2464–2470. [CrossRef] [PubMed]
112. Dunphy, D.R.; Sheth, P.H.; Garcia, F.L.; Brinker, C.J. Enlarged Pore Size in Mesoporous Silica Films Templated by Pluronic F127: Use of Poloxamer Mixtures and Increased Template/SiO_2 Ratios in Materials Synthesized by Evaporation-Induced Self-Assembly. *Chem. Mater.* **2015**, *27*, 75–84. [CrossRef]
113. El-Toni, A.; Ibrahim, M.; Labis, J.; Khan, A.; Alhoshan, M. Optimization of Synthesis Parameters for Mesoporous Shell Formation on Magnetic Nanocores and Their Application as Nanocarriers for Docetaxel Cancer Drug. *Int. J. Mol. Sci.* **2013**, *14*, 11496–11509. [CrossRef] [PubMed]
114. Bouchoucha, M.; Côté, M.-F.; Caudreault, R.C.; Fortin, M.-A.; Kleitz, F. Size-Controlled Functionalized Mesoporous Silica Nanoparticles for Tunable Drug Release and Enhanced Anti-Tumoral Activity. *Chem. Mater.* **2016**, *28*, 4243–4258. [CrossRef]
115. Ma, K.; Werner-Zwanziger, U.; Zwanziger, J.; Wiesner, U. Controlling Growth of Ultrasmall Sub-10 nm Fluorescent Mesoporous Silica Nanoparticles. *Chem. Mater.* **2013**, *25*, 677–691. [CrossRef]
116. Kim, J.W.; Kim, L.U.; Kim, C.K. Size Control of Silica Nanoparticles and Their Surface Treatment for Fabrication of Dental Nanocomposites. *Biomacromolecules* **2007**, *8*, 215–222. [CrossRef] [PubMed]
117. Chiang, Y.-D.; Lian, H.-Y.; Leo, S.-Y.; Wang, S.-G.; Yamauchi, Y.; Wu, K.C.-W. Controlling Particle Size and Structural Properties of Mesoporous Silica Nanoparticles Using the Taguchi Method. *J. Phys. Chem. C* **2011**, *115*, 13158–13165. [CrossRef]
118. Yamada, H.; Urata, C.; Ujiie, H.; Yamauchi, Y.; Kuroda, K. Preparation of aqueous colloidal mesostructured and mesoporous silica nanoparticles with controlled particle size in a very wide range from 20 nm to 700 nm. *Nanoscale* **2013**, *5*, 6145–6153. [CrossRef] [PubMed]
119. Vazquez, N.I.; Gonzalez, Z.; Ferrari, B.; Castro, Y. Synthesis of mesoporous silica nanoparticles by sol–gel as nanocontainer for future drug delivery applications. *Bol. Soc. Esp. Cerám. Vidr.* **2017**, *56*, 139–145. [CrossRef]
120. Wanyika, H.; Gatebe, E.; Kioni, P.; Tang, Z.; Gao, Y. Synthesis and characterization of ordered mesoporous silica nanoparticles with tunable physical properties by varying molar composition of reagents. *Afr. J. Pharm. Pharmacol.* **2011**, *5*, 2402–2410. [CrossRef]
121. Yano, K.; Fukushima, Y. Synthesis of mono-dispersed mesoporous silica spheres with highly ordered hexagonal regularity using conventional alkyltrimethylammonium halide as a surfactant. *J. Mater. Chem.* **2004**, *14*, 1579–1584. [CrossRef]
122. Vallet-Regi, M.; Rámila, A.; del Real, R.P.; Pérez-Pariente, J. A New Property of MCM-41: Drug Delivery System. *Chem. Mater.* **2001**, *13*, 308–311. [CrossRef]
123. Egger, S.M.; Hurley, K.R.; Datt, A.; Swindlehurst, G.; Haynes, C.L. Ultraporous Mesostructured Silica Nanoparticles. *Chem. Mater.* **2015**, *27*, 3193–3196. [CrossRef]
124. Ganguly, A.; Ahmad, T.; Ganguli, A.K. Silica Mesostructures: Control of Pore Size and Surface Area Using a Surfactant-Templated Hydrothermal Process. *Langmuir* **2010**, *26*, 14901–14908. [CrossRef] [PubMed]

125. Palmqvist, A.E.C. Synthesis of ordered mesoporous materials using surfactant liquid crystals or micellar solutions. *Curr. Opin. Colloid Interface Sci.* **2003**, *8*, 145–155. [CrossRef]
126. Gu, J.; Huang, K.; Zhu, X.; Li, Y.; Wei, J.; Zhao, W.; Liu, C.; Shi, J. Sub-150 nm mesoporous silica nanoparticles with tunable pore sizes and well-ordered mesostructure for protein encapsulation. *J. Colloid Interface Sci.* **2013**, *407*, 236–242. [CrossRef] [PubMed]
127. Muñoz, B.; Rámila, A.; Pérez-Pariente, J.; Díaz, I.; Vallet-Regí, M. MCM-41 Organic Modification as Drug Delivery Rate Regulator. *Chem. Mater.* **2002**. [CrossRef]
128. Izquierdo-Barba, I.; Martinez, Á.; Doadrio, A.L.; Pérez-Pariente, J.; Vallet-Regí, M. Release evaluation of drugs from ordered three-dimensional silica structures. *Eur. J. Pharm. Sci.* **2005**, *26*, 365–373. [CrossRef] [PubMed]
129. Möller, K.; Bein, T. Talented Mesoporous Silica Nanoparticles. *Chem. Mater.* **2017**, *29*, 371–388. [CrossRef]
130. Huang, M.; Liu, L.; Wang, S.; Zhu, H.; Wu, D.; Yu, Z.; Zhou, S. Dendritic Mesoporous Silica Nanospheres Synthesized by a Novel Dual-Templating Micelle System for the Preparation of Functional Nanomaterials. *Langmuir* **2017**, *33*, 519–526. [CrossRef] [PubMed]
131. Yu, Y.-J.; Xing, J.-L.; Pang, J.-L.; Jiang, S.-H.; Lam, K.-F.; Yang, T.-Q.; Xue, Q.-S.; Zhang, K.; Wu, P. Facile Synthesis of Size Controllable Dendritic Mesoporous Silica Nanoparticles. *ACS Appl. Mater. Interfaces* **2014**, *6*, 22655–22665. [CrossRef] [PubMed]
132. Huang, X.; Li, L.; Liu, T.; Hao, N.; Liu, H.; Chen, D.; Tang, F. The Shape Effect of Mesoporous Silica Nanoparticles on Biodistribution, Clearance, and Biocompatibility In Vivo. *ACS Nano* **2011**, *5*, 5390–5399. [CrossRef] [PubMed]
133. Huang, X.; Teng, X.; Chen, D.; Tang, F.; He, J. The effect of the shape of mesoporous silica nanoparticles on cellular uptake and cell function. *Biomaterials* **2010**, *31*, 438–448. [CrossRef] [PubMed]
134. Cai, Q.; Luo, Z.-S.; Pang, W.-Q.; Fan, Y.-W.; Chen, X.-H.; Cui, F.-Z. Dilute Solution Routes to Various Controllable Morphologies of MCM-41 Silica with a Basic Medium. *Chem. Mater.* **2001**, *13*, 258–263. [CrossRef]
135. Han, L.; Zhou, Y.; He, T.; Song, G.; Wu, F.; Jiang, F.; Hu, J. One-pot morphology-controlled synthesis of various shaped mesoporous silica nanoparticles. *J. Mater. Sci.* **2013**, *48*, 5718–5726. [CrossRef]
136. Pang, X.; Gao, J.; Tang, F. Controlled preparation of rod- and top-like MCM-41 mesoporous silica through one-step route. *J. Non-Cryst. Solids* **2005**, *351*, 1705–1709. [CrossRef]
137. Björk, E.M.; Söderlind, F.; Odén, M. Tuning the Shape of Mesoporous Silica Particles by Alterations in Parameter Space: From Rods to Platelets. *Langmuir* **2013**, *29*, 13551–13561. [CrossRef] [PubMed]
138. Hao, N.; Li, L.; Tang, F. Facile preparation of ellipsoid-like MCM-41 with parallel channels along the short axis for drug delivery and assembly of Ag nanoparticles for catalysis. *J. Mater. Chem. A* **2014**, *2*, 11565–11568. [CrossRef]
139. Shen, S.; Gu, T.; Mao, D.; Xiao, X.; Yuan, P.; Yu, M.; Xia, L.; Ji, Q.; Meng, L.; Song, W.; et al. Synthesis of Nonspherical Mesoporous Silica Ellipsoids with Tunable Aspect Ratios for Magnetic Assisted Assembly and Gene Delivery. *Chem. Mater.* **2012**, *24*, 230–235. [CrossRef]
140. Cui, X.; Moon, S.-W.; Zin, W.-C. High-yield synthesis of monodispersed SBA-15 equilateral hexagonal platelet with thick wall. *Mater. Lett.* **2006**, *60*, 3857–3860. [CrossRef]
141. Chen, B.-C.; Lin, H.-P.; Chao, M.-C.; Mou, C.-Y.; Tang, C.-Y. Mesoporous Silica Platelets with Perpendicular Nanochannels via a Ternary Surfactant System. *Adv. Mater.* **2004**, *16*, 1657–1661. [CrossRef]
142. Huh, S.; Wiench, J.W.; Yoo, J.-C.; Pruski, M.; Lin, V.S.-Y. Organic Functionalization and Morphology Control of Mesoporous Silicas via a Co-Condensation Synthesis Method. *Chem. Mater.* **2003**, *15*, 4247–4256. [CrossRef]
143. Wang, Y.; Sun, Y.; Wang, J.; Yang, Y.; Li, Y.; Yuan, Y.; Liu, C. Charge-Reversal APTES-Modified Mesoporous Silica Nanoparticles with High Drug Loading and Release Controllability. *ACS Appl. Mater. Interfaces* **2016**, *8*, 17166–17175. [CrossRef] [PubMed]
144. Bouchoucha, M.; Gaudreault, R.C.; Fortin, M.-A.; Kleitz, F. Mesoporous Silica Nanoparticles: Selective Surface Functionalization for Optimal Relaxometric and Drug Loading Performances. *Adv. Funct. Mater.* **2014**, *24*, 5911–5923. [CrossRef]
145. Zhu, Y.; Shi, J.; Shen, W.; Chen, H.; Dong, X.; Ruan, M. Preparation of novel hollow mesoporous silica spheres and their sustained-release property. *Nanotechnology* **2005**, *16*, 2633–2638. [CrossRef]
146. Palanikumar, L.; Kim, H.Y.; Oh, J.Y.; Thomas, A.P.; Choi, E.S.; Jeena, M.T.; Joo, S.H.; Ryu, J.-H. Noncovalent Surface Locking of Mesoporous Silica Nanoparticles for Exceptionally High Hydrophobic Drug Loading and Enhanced Colloidal Stability. *Biomacromolecules* **2015**, *16*, 2701–2714. [CrossRef] [PubMed]

147. Vallet-Regí, M.; Balas, F.; Arcos, D. Mesoporous Materials for Drug Delivery. *Angew. Chem. Int. Ed.* **2007**, *46*, 7548–7558. [CrossRef] [PubMed]
148. Palanikumar, L.; Jeena, M.T.; Kim, K.; Yong Oh, J.; Kim, C.; Park, M.-H.; Ryu, J.-H. Spatiotemporally and Sequentially-Controlled Drug Release from Polymer Gatekeeper–Hollow Silica Nanoparticles. *Sci. Rep.* **2017**, *7*, 46540. [CrossRef] [PubMed]
149. Kao, K.-C.; Mou, C.-Y. Pore-expanded mesoporous silica nanoparticles with alkanes/ethanol as pore expanding agent. *Microporous Mesoporous Mater.* **2013**, *169*, 7–15. [CrossRef]
150. Kim, M.-H.; Na, H.-K.; Kim, Y.-K.; Ryoo, S.-R.; Cho, H.S.; Lee, K.E.; Jeon, H.; Ryoo, R.; Min, D.-H. Facile Synthesis of Monodispersed Mesoporous Silica Nanoparticles with Ultralarge Pores and Their Application in Gene Delivery. *ACS Nano* **2011**, *5*, 3568–3576. [CrossRef] [PubMed]
151. Qu, F.; Zhu, G.; Huang, S.; Li, S.; Sun, J.; Zhang, D.; Qiu, S. Controlled release of Captopril by regulating the pore size and morphology of ordered mesoporous silica. *Microporous Mesoporous Mater.* **2006**, *92*, 1–9. [CrossRef]
152. Doadrio, J.C.; Sousa, E.M.B.; Izquierdo-Barba, I.; Doadrio, A.L.; Perez-Pariente, J.; Vallet-Regí, M. Functionalization of mesoporous materials with long alkyl chains as a strategy for controlling drug delivery pattern. *J. Mater. Chem.* **2006**, *16*, 462–466. [CrossRef]
153. Balas, F.; Manzano, M.; Horcajada, P.; Vallet-Regí, M. Confinement and Controlled Release of Bisphosphonates on Ordered Mesoporous Silica-Based Materials. *J. Am. Chem. Soc.* **2006**, *128*, 8116–8117. [CrossRef] [PubMed]
154. Nieto, A.; Colilla, M.; Balas, F.; Vallet-Regí, M. Surface Electrochemistry of Mesoporous Silicas as a Key Factor in the Design of Tailored Delivery Devices. *Langmuir* **2010**, *26*, 5038–5049. [CrossRef] [PubMed]
155. Datt, A.; El-Maazawi, I.; Larsen, S.C. Aspirin Loading and Release from MCM-41 Functionalized with Aminopropyl Groups via Co-condensation or Postsynthesis Modification Methods. *J. Phys. Chem. C* **2012**, *116*, 18358–18366. [CrossRef]
156. Song, S.-W.; Hidajat, K.; Kawi, S. Functionalized SBA-15 Materials as Carriers for Controlled Drug Delivery: Influence of Surface Properties on Matrix−Drug Interactions. *Langmuir* **2005**, *21*, 9568–9575. [CrossRef] [PubMed]
157. Mishra, A.K.; Pandey, H.; Agarwal, V.; Ramteke, P.W.; Pandey, A.C. Nanoengineered mesoporous silica nanoparticles for smart delivery of doxorubicin. *J. Nanopart. Res.* **2014**, *16*, 2515. [CrossRef]
158. Han, N.; Wang, Y.; Bai, J.; Liu, J.; Wang, Y.; Gao, Y.; Jiang, T.; Kang, W.; Wang, S. Facile synthesis of the lipid bilayer coated mesoporous silica nanocomposites and their application in drug delivery. *Microporous Mesoporous Mater.* **2016**, *219*, 209–218. [CrossRef]
159. Murugan, C.; Rayappan, K.; Thangam, R.; Bhanumathi, R.; Shanthi, K.; Vivek, R.; Thirumurugan, R.; Bhattacharyya, A.; Sivasubramanian, S.; Gunasekaran, P.; et al. Combinatorial nanocarrier based drug delivery approach for amalgamation of anti-tumor agents in breast cancer cells: An improved nanomedicine strategy. *Sci. Rep.* **2016**, *6*, 34053. [CrossRef] [PubMed]
160. Kim, S.; Diab, R.; Joubert, O.; Canilho, N.; Pasc, A. Core–shell microcapsules of solid lipid nanoparticles and mesoporous silica for enhanced oral delivery of curcumin. *Colloids Surf. B Biointerfaces* **2016**, *140*, 161–168. [CrossRef] [PubMed]
161. Fu, Q.; Hargrove, D.; Lu, X. Improving paclitaxel pharmacokinetics by using tumor-specific mesoporous silica nanoparticles with intraperitoneal delivery. *Nanomed. Nanotechnol. Biol. Med.* **2016**, *12*, 1951–1959. [CrossRef] [PubMed]
162. Kumar, B.; Kulanthaivel, S.; Mondal, A.; Mishra, S.; Banerjee, B.; Bhaumik, A.; Banerjee, I.; Giri, S. Mesoporous silica nanoparticle based enzyme responsive system for colon specific drug delivery through guar gum capping. *Colloids Surf. B Biointerfaces* **2017**, *150*, 352–361. [CrossRef] [PubMed]
163. Saroj, S.; Rajput, S.J. Tailor-made pH-sensitive polyacrylic acid functionalized mesoporous silica nanoparticles for efficient and controlled delivery of anti-cancer drug Etoposide. *Drug Dev. Ind. Pharm.* **2018**, *44*, 1198–1211. [CrossRef] [PubMed]
164. Thiyagarajan, V.; Lin, S.-X.; Lee, C.-H.; Weng, C.-F. A focal adhesion kinase inhibitor 16-hydroxy-cleroda-3,13-dien-16,15-olide incorporated into enteric-coated nanoparticles for controlled anti-glioma drug delivery. *Colloids Surf. B Biointerfaces* **2016**, *141*, 120–131. [CrossRef] [PubMed]

165. Ganesh, M.; Ubaidulla, U.; Hemalatha, P.; Peng, M.M.; Jang, H.T. Development of Duloxetine Hydrochloride Loaded Mesoporous Silica Nanoparticles: Characterizations and In Vitro Evaluation. *AAPS PharmSciTech* **2015**, *16*, 944–951. [CrossRef] [PubMed]
166. Mohseni, M.; Gilani, K.; Mortazavi, S.A. Preparation and characterization of rifampin loaded mesoporous silica nanoparticles as a potential system for pulmonary drug delivery. *Iran. J. Pharm. Res.* **2015**, *14*, 27–34. [PubMed]
167. El Nabarawi, M.A.; Hassen, D.H.; Taha, A.A. Inclusion and characterization of ketoprofen into different mesoporous silica nanoparticles using three loading methods. *Int. J. Pharm. Pharm. Sci.* **2014**, *6*, 183–191.
168. Yoncheva, K.; Popova, M.; Szegedi, A.; Mihaly, J.; Tzankov, B.; Lambov, N.; Konstantinov, S.; Tzankova, V.; Pessina, F.; Valoti, M. Functionalized mesoporous silica nanoparticles for oral delivery of budesonide. *J. Solid State Chem.* **2014**, *211*, 154–161. [CrossRef]
169. Mudakavi, R.J.; Raichur, A.M.; Chakravortty, D. Lipid coated mesoporous silica nanoparticles as an oral delivery system for targeting and treatment of intravacuolar Salmonella infections. *RSC Adv.* **2014**, *4*, 61160–61166. [CrossRef]
170. Mudakavi, R.J.; Vanamali, S.; Chakravortty, D.; Raichur, A.M. Development of arginine based nanocarriers for targeting and treatment of intracellular *Salmonella*. *RSC Adv.* **2017**, *7*, 7022–7032. [CrossRef]
171. Koneru, B.; Shi, Y.; Wang, Y.-C.; Chavala, S.; Miller, M.; Holbert, B.; Conson, M.; Ni, A.; Di Pasqua, A. Tetracycline-Containing MCM-41 Mesoporous Silica Nanoparticles for the Treatment of *Escherichia coli*. *Molecules* **2015**, *20*, 19690–19698. [CrossRef] [PubMed]
172. Alexa, I.F.; Ignat, M.; Popovici, R.F.; Timpu, D.; Popovici, E. In vitro controlled release of antihypertensive drugs intercalated into unmodified SBA-15 and MgO modified SBA-15 matrices. *Int. J. Pharm.* **2012**, *436*, 111–119. [CrossRef] [PubMed]
173. Doadrio, A.L.; Sánchez-Montero, J.M.; Doadrio, J.C.; Salinas, A.J.; Vallet-Regí, M. Mesoporous silica nanoparticles as a new carrier methodology in the controlled release of the active components in a polypill. *Eur. J. Pharm. Sci.* **2017**, *97*, 1–8. [CrossRef] [PubMed]
174. Zou, Z.; He, D.; Cai, L.; He, X.; Wang, K.; Yang, X.; Li, L.; Li, S.; Su, X. Alizarin Complexone Functionalized Mesoporous Silica Nanoparticles: A Smart System Integrating Glucose-Responsive Double-Drugs Release and Real-Time Monitoring Capabilities. *ACS Appl. Mater. Interfaces* **2016**, *8*, 8358–8366. [CrossRef] [PubMed]
175. Huang, P.-K.; Lin, S.-X.; Tsai, M.-J.; Leong, M.; Lin, S.-R.; Kankala, R.; Lee, C.-H.; Weng, C.-F. Encapsulation of 16-Hydroxycleroda-3,13-Dine-16,15-Olide in Mesoporous Silica Nanoparticles as a Natural Dipeptidyl Peptidase-4 Inhibitor Potentiated Hypoglycemia in Diabetic Mice. *Nanomaterials* **2017**, *7*, 112. [CrossRef] [PubMed]
176. Shi, X.; Wang, Y.; Varshney, R.R.; Ren, L.; Zhang, F.; Wang, D.-A. In-vitro osteogenesis of synovium stem cells induced by controlled release of bisphosphate additives from microspherical mesoporous silica composite. *Biomaterials* **2009**, *30*, 3996–4005. [CrossRef] [PubMed]
177. Zhou, X.; Feng, W.; Qiu, K.; Chen, L.; Wang, W.; Nie, W.; Mo, X.; He, C. BMP-2 Derived Peptide and Dexamethasone Incorporated Mesoporous Silica Nanoparticles for Enhanced Osteogenic Differentiation of Bone Mesenchymal Stem Cells. *ACS Appl. Mater. Interfaces* **2015**, *7*, 15777–15789. [CrossRef] [PubMed]
178. Arriagada, F.; Correa, O.; Günther, G.; Nonell, S.; Mura, F.; Olea-Azar, C.; Morales, J. Morin Flavonoid Adsorbed on Mesoporous Silica, a Novel Antioxidant Nanomaterial. *PLoS ONE* **2016**, *11*, e0164507. [CrossRef] [PubMed]
179. Meng, H.; Xue, M.; Xia, T.; Ji, Z.; Tarn, D.Y.; Zink, J.I.; Nel, A.E. Use of Size and a Copolymer Design Feature To Improve the Biodistribution and the Enhanced Permeability and Retention Effect of Doxorubicin-Loaded Mesoporous Silica Nanoparticles in a Murine Xenograft Tumor Model. *ACS Nano* **2011**, *5*, 4131–4144. [CrossRef] [PubMed]
180. Ma, X.; Qu, Q.; Zhao, Y. Targeted Delivery of 5-Aminolevulinic Acid by Multifunctional Hollow Mesoporous Silica Nanoparticles for Photodynamic Skin Cancer Therapy. *ACS Appl. Mater. Interfaces* **2015**, *7*, 10671–10676. [CrossRef] [PubMed]
181. Khosravian, P.; Shafiee Ardestani, M.; Khoobi, M.; Ostad, S.N.; Dorkoosh, F.A.; Akbari Javar, H.; Amanlou, M. Mesoporous silica nanoparticles functionalized with folic acid/methionine for active targeted delivery of docetaxel. *OncoTargets Ther.* **2016**′ *9*, 7315–7330. [CrossRef] [PubMed]

182. Zhang, M.; Xu, C.; Wen, L.; Han, M.K.; Xiao, B.; Zhou, J.; Zhang, Y.; Zhang, Z.; Viennois, E.; Merlin, D. A Hyaluronidase-Responsive Nanoparticle-Based Drug Delivery System for Targeting Colon Cancer Cells. *Cancer Res.* **2016**, *76*, 7208–7218. [CrossRef] [PubMed]
183. Gary-Bobo, M.; Brevet, D.; Benkirane-Jessel, N.; Raehm, L.; Maillard, P.; Garcia, M.; Durand, J.-O. Hyaluronic acid-functionalized mesoporous silica nanoparticles for efficient photodynamic therapy of cancer cells. *Photodiagn. Photodyn. Ther.* **2012**, *9*, 256–260. [CrossRef] [PubMed]
184. Quan, G.; Pan, X.; Wang, Z.; Wu, Q.; Li, G.; Dian, L.; Chen, B.; Wu, C. Lactosaminated mesoporous silica nanoparticles for asialoglycoprotein receptor targeted anticancer drug delivery. *J. Nanobiotechnol.* **2015**, *13*, 7. [CrossRef] [PubMed]
185. Vaillant, O.; El Cheikh, K.; Warther, D.; Brevet, D.; Maynadier, M.; Bouffard, E.; Salgues, F.; Jeanjean, A.; Puche, P.; Mazerolles, C.; et al. Mannose-6-Phosphate Receptor: A Target for Theranostics of Prostate Cancer. *Angew. Chem. Int. Ed.* **2015**, *54*, 5952–5956. [CrossRef] [PubMed]
186. Gary-Bobo, M.; Mir, Y.; Rouxel, C.; Brevet, D.; Basile, I.; Maynadier, M.; Vaillant, O.; Mongin, O.; Blanchard-Desce, M.; Morère, A.; et al. Mannose-Functionalized Mesoporous Silica Nanoparticles for Efficient Two-Photon Photodynamic Therapy of Solid Tumors. *Angew. Chem. Int. Ed.* **2011**, *50*, 11425–11429. [CrossRef] [PubMed]
187. Wu, K.; Liao, Y.-T.; Liu, C.-H.; Yu, J. Liver cancer cells: Targeting and prolonged-release drug carriers consisting of mesoporous silica nanoparticles and alginate microspheres. *Int. J. Nanomed.* **2014**, *9*, 2767–2778. [CrossRef] [PubMed]
188. Chakravarty, R.; Goel, S.; Hong, H.; Chen, F.; Valdovinos, H.F.; Hernandez, R.; Barnhart, T.E.; Cai, W. Hollow mesoporous silica nanoparticles for tumor vasculature targeting and PET image-guided drug delivery. *Nanomedicine* **2015**, *10*, 1233–1246. [CrossRef] [PubMed]
189. Liu, K.; Wang, Z.; Wang, S.; Liu, P.; Qin, Y.; Ma, Y.; Li, X.-C.; Huo, Z.-J. Hyaluronic acid-tagged silica nanoparticles in colon cancer therapy: Therapeutic efficacy evaluation. *Int. J. Nanomed.* **2015**, *10*, 6445–6454. [CrossRef]
190. Chen, L.; She, X.; Wang, T.; He, L.; Shigdar, S.; Duan, W.; Kong, L. Overcoming acquired drug resistance in colorectal cancer cells by targeted delivery of 5-FU with EGF grafted hollow mesoporous silica nanoparticles. *Nanoscale* **2015**, *7*, 14080–14092. [CrossRef] [PubMed]
191. Radhakrishnan, K.; Tripathy, J.; Datey, A.; Chakravortty, D.; Raichur, A.M. Mesoporous silica–chondroitin sulphate hybrid nanoparticles for targeted and bio-responsive drug delivery. *New J. Chem.* **2015**, *39*, 1754–1760. [CrossRef]
192. Chen, X.; Sun, H.; Hu, J.; Han, X.; Liu, H.; Hu, Y. Transferrin gated mesoporous silica nanoparticles for redox-responsive and targeted drug delivery. *Colloids Surf. B Biointerfaces* **2017**, *152*, 77–84. [CrossRef] [PubMed]
193. Xie, X.; Li, F.; Zhang, H.; Lu, Y.; Lian, S.; Lin, H.; Gao, Y.; Jia, L. EpCAM aptamer-functionalized mesoporous silica nanoparticles for efficient colon cancer cell-targeted drug delivery. *Eur. J. Pharm. Sci.* **2016**, *83*, 28–35. [CrossRef] [PubMed]
194. Brevet, D.; Gary-Bobo, M.; Raehm, L.; Richeter, S.; Hocine, O.; Amro, K.; Loock, B.; Couleaud, P.; Frochot, C.; Morère, A.; et al. Mannose-targeted mesoporous silica nanoparticles for photodynamic therapy. *Chem. Commun.* **2009**, 1475–1477. [CrossRef] [PubMed]
195. Sarkar, A.; Ghosh, S.; Chowdhury, S.; Pandey, B.; Sil, P.C. Targeted delivery of quercetin loaded mesoporous silica nanoparticles to the breast cancer cells. *Biochim. Biophys. Acta Gen. Subj.* **2016**, *1860*, 2065–2075. [CrossRef] [PubMed]
196. Goel, S.; Chen, F.; Hong, H.; Valdovinos, H.F.; Hernandez, R.; Shi, S.; Barnhart, T.E.; Cai, W. $VEGF_{121}$-Conjugated Mesoporous Silica Nanoparticle: A Tumor Targeted Drug Delivery System. *ACS Appl. Mater. Interfaces* **2014**, *6*, 21677–21685. [CrossRef] [PubMed]
197. Xu, H.; Wang, Z.; Li, Y.; Guo, Y.; Zhou, H.; Li, Y.; Wu, F.; Zhang, L.; Yang, X.; Lu, B.; et al. Preparation and characterization of a dual-receptor mesoporous silica nanoparticle–hyaluronic acid–RGD peptide targeting drug delivery system. *RSC Adv.* **2016**, *6*, 40427–40435. [CrossRef]
198. Kankala, R.K.; Kuthati, Y.; Liu, C.-L.; Mou, C.-Y.; Lee, C.-H. Killing cancer cells by delivering a nanoreactor for inhibition of catalase and catalytically enhancing intracellular levels of ROS. *RSC Adv.* **2015**, *5*, 86072–86081. [CrossRef]

199. Kankala, R.K.; Liu, C.-G.; Chen, A.-Z.; Wang, S.-B.; Xu, P.-Y.; Mende, L.K.; Liu, C.-L.; Lee, C.-H.; Hu, Y.-F. Overcoming Multidrug Resistance through the Synergistic Effects of Hierarchical pH-Sensitive, ROS-Generating Nanoreactors. *ACS Biomater. Sci. Eng.* **2017**, *3*, 2431–2442. [CrossRef]
200. Jadhav, S.A.; Brunella, V.; Berlier, G.; Ugazio, E.; Scalarone, D. Effect of Multimodal Pore Channels on Cargo Release from Mesoporous Silica Nanoparticles. *J. Nanomater.* **2016**, *2016*, 1–7. [CrossRef]
201. Kamarudin, N.H.N.; Jalil, A.A.; Triwahyono, S.; Salleh, N.F.M.; Karim, A.H.; Mukti, R.R.; Hameed, B.H.; Ahmad, A. Role of 3-aminopropyltriethoxysilane in the preparation of mesoporous silica nanoparticles for ibuprofen delivery: Effect on physicochemical properties. *Microporous Mesoporous Mater.* **2013**, *180*, 235–241. [CrossRef]
202. Ahmadi, E.; Dehghannejad, N.; Hashemikia, S.; Ghasemnejad, M.; Tabebordbar, H. Synthesis and surface modification of mesoporous silica nanoparticles and its application as carriers for sustained drug delivery. *Drug Deliv.* **2014**, *21*, 164–172. [CrossRef] [PubMed]
203. Braz, W.R.; Rocha, N.L.; de Faria, E.H.; Silva, M.L.; Ciuffi, K.J.; Tavares, D.C.; Furtado, R.A.; Rocha, L.A.; Nassar, E.J. Incorporation of anti-inflammatory agent into mesoporous silica. *Nanotechnology* **2016**, *27*, 385103. [CrossRef] [PubMed]
204. Song, Y.; Li, Y.; Xu, Q.; Liu, Z. Mesoporous silica nanoparticles for stimuli-responsive controlled drug delivery: Advances, challenges, and outlook. *Int. J. Nanomed.* **2017**, *12*, 87–110. [CrossRef] [PubMed]
205. Nguyen, C.T.H.; Webb, R.I.; Lambert, L.K.; Strounina, E.; Lee, E.C.; Parat, M.-O.; McGuckin, M.A.; Popat, A.; Cabot, P.J.; Ross, B.P. Bifunctional Succinylated ε-Polylysine-Coated Mesoporous Silica Nanoparticles for pH-Responsive and Intracellular Drug Delivery Targeting the Colon. *ACS Appl. Mater. Interfaces* **2017**, *9*, 9470–9483. [CrossRef] [PubMed]
206. Ahmadi Nasab, N.; Hassani Kumleh, H.; Beygzadeh, M.; Teimourian, S.; Kazemzad, M. Delivery of curcumin by a pH-responsive chitosan mesoporous silica nanoparticles for cancer treatment. *Artif. Cells Nanomed. Biotechnol.* **2017**, 1–7. [CrossRef] [PubMed]
207. Hu, X.; Wang, Y.; Peng, B. Chitosan-Capped Mesoporous Silica Nanoparticles as pH-Responsive Nanocarriers for Controlled Drug Release. *Chem. Asian J.* **2014**, *9*, 319–327. [CrossRef] [PubMed]
208. Yuan, L.; Tang, Q.; Yang, D.; Zhang, J.Z.; Zhang, F.; Hu, J. Preparation of pH-Responsive Mesoporous Silica Nanoparticles and Their Application in Controlled Drug Delivery. *J. Phys. Chem. C* **2011**, *115*, 9926–9932. [CrossRef]
209. Cheng, W.; Nie, J.; Xu, L.; Liang, C.; Peng, Y.; Liu, G.; Wang, T.; Mei, L.; Huang, L.; Zeng, X. pH-Sensitive Delivery Vehicle Based on Folic Acid-Conjugated Polydopamine-Modified Mesoporous Silica Nanoparticles for Targeted Cancer Therapy. *ACS Appl. Mater. Interfaces* **2017**, *9*, 18462–18473. [CrossRef] [PubMed]
210. Zheng, J.; Tian, X.; Sun, Y.; Lu, D.; Yang, W. pH-sensitive poly(glutamic acid) grafted mesoporous silica nanoparticles for drug delivery. *Int. J. Pharm.* **2013**, *450*, 296–303. [CrossRef] [PubMed]
211. Hu, C.; Yu, L.; Zheng, Z.; Wang, J.; Liu, Y.; Jiang, Y.; Tong, G.; Zhou, Y.; Wang, X. Tannin as a gatekeeper of pH-responsive mesoporous silica nanoparticles for drug delivery. *RSC Adv.* **2015**, *5*, 85436–85441. [CrossRef]
212. Park, C.; Oh, K.; Lee, S.C.; Kim, C. Controlled Release of Guest Molecules from Mesoporous Silica Particles Based on a pH-Responsive Polypseudorotaxane Motif. *Angew. Chem. Int. Ed.* **2007**, *46*, 1455–1457. [CrossRef] [PubMed]
213. Bai, L.; Zhao, Q.; Wang, J.; Gao, Y.; Sha, Z.; Di, D.; Han, N.; Wang, Y.; Zhang, J.; Wang, S. Mechanism study on pH-responsive cyclodextrin capped mesoporous silica: Effect of different stalk densities and the type of cyclodextrin. *Nanotechnology* **2015**, *26*, 165704. [CrossRef] [PubMed]
214. Kuthati, Y.; Kankala, R.K.; Lin, S.-X.; Weng, C.-F.; Lee, C.-H. pH-Triggered Controllable Release of Silver–Indole-3 Acetic Acid Complexes from Mesoporous Silica Nanoparticles (IBN-4) for Effectively Killing Malignant Bacteria. *Mol. Pharm.* **2015**, *12*, 2289–2304. [CrossRef] [PubMed]
215. Wang, Y.; Han, N.; Zhao, Q.; Bai, L.; Li, J.; Jiang, T.; Wang, S. Redox-responsive mesoporous silica as carriers for controlled drug delivery: A comparative study based on silica and PEG gatekeepers. *Eur. J. Pharm. Sci.* **2015**, *72*, 12–20. [CrossRef] [PubMed]
216. Zhu, X.; Wang, C.-Q. pH and redox-operated nanovalve for size-selective cargo delivery on hollow mesoporous silica spheres. *J. Colloid Interface Sci.* **2016**, *480*, 39–48. [CrossRef] [PubMed]
217. Bathfield, M.; Reboul, J.; Cacciaguerra, T.; Lacroix-Desmazes, P.; Gérardin, C. Thermosensitive and Drug-Loaded Ordered Mesoporous Silica: A Direct and Effective Synthesis Using PEO-*b*-PNIPAM Block Copolymers. *Chem. Mater.* **2016**, *28*, 3374–3384. [CrossRef]

218. Zhao, Y.; Trewyn, B.G.; Slowing, I.I.; Lin, V.S.-Y. Mesoporous Silica Nanoparticle-Based Double Drug Delivery System for Glucose-Responsive Controlled Release of Insulin and Cyclic AMP. *J. Am. Chem. Soc.* **2009**, *131*, 8398–8400. [CrossRef] [PubMed]
219. Tan, L.; Yang, M.-Y.; Wu, H.-X.; Tang, Z.-W.; Xiao, J.-Y.; Liu, C.-J.; Zhuo, R.-X. Glucose- and pH-Responsive Nanogated Ensemble Based on Polymeric Network Capped Mesoporous Silica. *ACS Appl. Mater. Interfaces* **2015**, *7*, 6310–6316. [CrossRef] [PubMed]
220. Bhat, R.; Ribes, À.; Mas, N.; Aznar, E.; Sancenón, F.; Marcos, M.D.; Murguía, J.R.; Venkataraman, A.; Martínez-Máñez, R. Thrombin-Responsive Gated Silica Mesoporous Nanoparticles as Coagulation Regulators. *Langmuir* **2016**, *32*, 1195–1200. [CrossRef] [PubMed]
221. Gayam, S.R.; Venkatesan, P.; Sung, Y.-M.; Sung, S.-Y.; Hu, S.-H.; Hsu, H.-Y.; Wu, S.-P. An NAD(P)H:quinone oxidoreductase 1 (NQO1) enzyme responsive nanocarrier based on mesoporous silica nanoparticles for tumor targeted drug delivery in vitro and in vivo. *Nanoscale* **2016**, *8*, 12307–12317. [CrossRef] [PubMed]
222. Liu, J.; Zhang, B.; Luo, Z.; Ding, X.; Li, J.; Dai, L.; Zhou, J.; Zhao, X.; Ye, J.; Cai, K. Enzyme responsive mesoporous silica nanoparticles for targeted tumor therapy in vitro and in vivo. *Nanoscale* **2015**, *7*, 3614–3626. [CrossRef] [PubMed]
223. Radhakrishnan, K.; Gupta, S.; Gnanadhas, D.P.; Ramamurthy, P.C.; Chakravortty, D.; Raichur, A.M. Protamine-Capped Mesoporous Silica Nanoparticles for Biologically Triggered Drug Release. *Part. Part. Syst. Charact.* **2014**, *31*, 449–458. [CrossRef]
224. Xiao, Y.; Wang, T.; Cao, Y.; Wang, X.; Zhang, Y.; Liu, Y.; Huo, Q. Enzyme and voltage stimuli-responsive controlled release system based on β-cyclodextrin-capped mesoporous silica nanoparticles. *Dalton Trans.* **2015**, *44*, 4355–4361. [CrossRef] [PubMed]
225. Febvay, S.; Marini, D.M.; Belcher, A.M.; Clapham, D.E. Targeted Cytosolic Delivery of Cell-Impermeable Compounds by Nanoparticle-Mediated, Light-Triggered Endosome Disruption. *Nano Lett.* **2010**, *10*, 2211–2219. [CrossRef] [PubMed]
226. Liu, J.; Detrembleur, C.; De Pauw-Gillet, M.-C.; Mornet, S.; Jérôme, C.; Duguet, E. Gold Nanorods Coated with Mesoporous Silica Shell as Drug Delivery System for Remote Near Infrared Light-Activated Release and Potential Phototherapy. *Small* **2015**, *11*, 2323–2332. [CrossRef] [PubMed]
227. Li, W.-P.; Liao, P.-Y.; Su, C.-H.; Yeh, C.-S. Formation of Oligonucleotide-Gated Silica Shell-Coated Fe_3O_4-Au Core–Shell Nanotrisoctahedra for Magnetically Targeted and Near-Infrared Light-Responsive Theranostic Platform. *J. Am. Chem. Soc.* **2014**, *136*, 10062–10075. [CrossRef] [PubMed]
228. Baeza, A.; Guisasola, E.; Ruiz-Hernández, E.; Vallet-Regí, M. Magnetically Triggered Multidrug Release by Hybrid Mesoporous Silica Nanoparticles. *Chem. Mater.* **2012**, *24*, 517–524. [CrossRef]
229. Paris, J.L.; Cabañas, M.V.; Manzano, M.; Vallet-Regí, M. Polymer-Grafted Mesoporous Silica Nanoparticles as Ultrasound-Responsive Drug Carriers. *ACS Nano* **2015**, *9*, 11023–11033. [CrossRef] [PubMed]
230. Kim, H.-J.; Matsuda, H.; Zhou, H.; Honma, I. Ultrasound-Triggered Smart Drug Release from a Poly(dimethylsiloxane)– Mesoporous Silica Composite. *Adv. Mater.* **2006**, *18*, 3083–3088. [CrossRef]
231. Paris, J.L.; Villaverde, G.; Cabañas, M.V.; Manzano, M.; Vallet-Regí, M. From proof-of-concept material to PEGylated and modularly targeted ultrasound-responsive mesoporous silica nanoparticles. *J. Mater. Chem. B* **2018**, *6*, 2785–2794. [CrossRef]
232. Wang, T.; Sun, G.; Wang, M.; Zhou, B.; Fu, J. Voltage/pH-Driven Mechanized Silica Nanoparticles for the Multimodal Controlled Release of Drugs. *ACS Appl. Mater. Interfaces* **2015**, *7*, 21295–21304. [CrossRef] [PubMed]
233. Kuthati, Y.; Kankala, R.K.; Busa, P.; Lin, S.-X.; Deng, J.-P.; Mou, C.-Y.; Lee, C.-H. Phototherapeutic spectrum expansion through synergistic effect of mesoporous silica trio-nanohybrids against antibiotic-resistant gram-negative bacterium. *J. Photochem. Photobiol. B Biol.* **2017**, *169*, 124–133. [CrossRef] [PubMed]
234. McCarthy, C.A.; Ahern, R.J.; Dontireddy, R.; Ryan, K.B.; Crean, A.M. Mesoporous silica formulation strategies for drug dissolution enhancement: A review. *Expert Opin. Drug Deliv.* **2016**, *13*, 93–108. [CrossRef] [PubMed]
235. Bukara, K.; Schueller, L.; Rosier, J.; Martens, M.A.; Daems, T.; Verheyden, L.; Eelen, S.; Speybroeck, M.V.; Libanati, C.; Martens, J.A.; et al. Ordered mesoporous silica to enhance the bioavailability of poorly water-soluble drugs: Proof of concept in man. *Eur. J. Pharm. Biopharm.* **2016**, *108*, 220–225. [CrossRef] [PubMed]
236. Zhang, Y.; Wang, J.; Bai, X.; Jiang, T.; Zhang, Q.; Wang, S. Mesoporous Silica Nanoparticles for Increasing the Oral Bioavailability and Permeation of Poorly Water Soluble Drugs. *Mol. Pharm.* **2012**, *9*, 505–513. [CrossRef] [PubMed]

237. Thomas, M.J.K.; Slipper, I.; Walunj, A.; Jain, A.; Favretto, M.E.; Kallinteri, P.; Douroumis, D. Inclusion of poorly soluble drugs in highly ordered mesoporous silica nanoparticles. *Int. J. Pharm.* **2010**, *387*, 272–277. [CrossRef] [PubMed]
238. Sreejith, S.; Ma, X.; Zhao, Y. Graphene Oxide Wrapping on Squaraine-Loaded Mesoporous Silica Nanoparticles for Bioimaging. *J. Am. Chem. Soc.* **2012**, *134*, 17346–17349. [CrossRef] [PubMed]
239. Nakamura, T.; Sugihara, F.; Matsushita, H.; Yoshioka, Y.; Mizukami, S.; Kikuchi, K. Mesoporous silica nanoparticles for ^{19}F magnetic resonance imaging, fluorescence imaging, and drug delivery. *Chem. Sci.* **2015**, *6*, 1986–1990. [CrossRef] [PubMed]
240. Jun, B.-H.; Hwang, D.W.; Jung, H.S.; Jang, J.; Kim, H.; Kang, H.; Kang, T.; Kyeong, S.; Lee, H.; Jeong, D.H.; et al. Ultrasensitive, Biocompatible, Quantum-Dot-Embedded Silica Nanoparticles for Bioimaging. *Adv. Funct. Mater.* **2012**, *22*, 1843–1849. [CrossRef]
241. Helle, M.; Rampazzo, E.; Monchanin, M.; Marchal, F.; Guillemin, F.; Bonacchi, S.; Salis, F.; Prodi, L.; Bezdetnaya, L. Surface Chemistry Architecture of Silica Nanoparticles Determine the Efficiency of in Vivo Fluorescence Lymph Node Mapping. *ACS Nano* **2013**, *7*, 8645–8657. [CrossRef] [PubMed]
242. Vallet-Regí, M. Ordered Mesoporous Materials in the Context of Drug Delivery Systems and Bone Tissue Engineering. *Chem. Eur. J.* **2006**, *12*, 5934–5943. [CrossRef] [PubMed]
243. Izquierdo-Barba, I.; Ruiz-González, L.; Doadrio, J.C.; González-Calbet, J.M.; Vallet-Regí, M. Tissue regeneration: A new property of mesoporous materials. *Solid State Sci.* **2005**, *7*, 983–989. [CrossRef]
244. Luo, Z.; Deng, Y.; Zhang, R.; Wang, M.; Bai, Y.; Zhao, Q.; Lyu, Y.; Wei, J.; Wei, S. Peptide-laden mesoporous silica nanoparticles with promoted bioactivity and osteo-differentiation ability for bone tissue engineering. *Colloids Surf. B Biointerfaces* **2015**, *131*, 73–82. [CrossRef] [PubMed]
245. Wu, C.; Chang, J. Mesoporous bioactive glasses: Structure characteristics, drug/growth factor delivery and bone regeneration application. *Interface Focus* **2012**, *2*, 292–306. [CrossRef] [PubMed]
246. López-Noriega, A.; Arcos, D.; Izquierdo-Barba, I.; Sakamoto, Y.; Terasaki, O.; Vallet-Regí, M. Ordered Mesoporous Bioactive Glasses for Bone Tissue Regeneration. *Chem. Mater* **2006**, *18*, 3137–3144. [CrossRef]
247. Bozzuto, G.; Molinari, A. Liposomes as nanomedical devices. *Int. J. Nanomed.* **2015**, *10*, 975–999. [CrossRef] [PubMed]
248. Davis, M.E.; Chen, Z.; Shin, D.M. Nanoparticle therapeutics: An emerging treatment modality for cancer. *Nat. Rev. Drug Discov.* **2008**, *7*, 771–782. [CrossRef] [PubMed]
249. Palazzolo, S.; Bayda, S.; Hadla, M.; Caligiuri, I.; Corona, G.; Toffoli, G.; Rizzolio, F. The Clinical translation of Organic Nanomaterials for Cancer Therapy: A Focus on Polymeric Nanoparticles, Micelles, Liposomes and Exosomes. *Curr. Med. Chem.* **2017**, *24*. [CrossRef] [PubMed]
250. Kamaly, N.; Xiao, Z.; Valencia, P.M.; Radovic-Moreno, A.F.; Farokhzad, O.C. Targeted polymeric therapeutic nanoparticles: Design, development and clinical translation. *Chem. Soc. Rev.* **2012**, *41*, 2971–3010. [CrossRef] [PubMed]
251. Slowing, I.I.; Wu, C.-W.; Vivero-Escoto, J.L.; Lin, V.S.-Y. Mesoporous Silica Nanoparticles for Reducing Hemolytic Activity towards Mammalian Red Blood Cells. *Small* **2009**, *5*, 57–62. [CrossRef] [PubMed]
252. Nash, T.; Allison, A.C.; Harington, J.S. Physico-Chemical Properties of Silica in Relation to its Toxicity. *Nature* **1966**, *210*, 259–261. [CrossRef] [PubMed]
253. He, Q.; Zhang, Z.; Gao, F.; Li, Y.; Shi, J. In vivo Biodistribution and Urinary Excretion of Mesoporous Silica Nanoparticles: Effects of Particle Size and PEGylation. *Small* **2011**, *7*, 271–280. [CrossRef] [PubMed]
254. Yu, T.; Malugin, A.; Ghandehari, H. Impact of Silica Nanoparticle Design on Cellular Toxicity and Hemolytic Activity. *ACS Nano* **2011**, *5*, 5717–5728. [CrossRef] [PubMed]
255. Townson, J.L.; Lin, Y.-S.; Agola, J.O.; Carnes, E.C.; Leong, H.S.; Lewis, J.D.; Haynes, C.L.; Brinker, C.J. Re-examining the Size/Charge Paradigm: Differing in Vivo Characteristics of Size- and Charge-Matched Mesoporous Silica Nanoparticles. *J. Am. Chem. Soc.* **2013**, *135*, 16030–16033. [CrossRef] [PubMed]
256. Li, L.; Liu, T.; Fu, C.; Tan, L.; Meng, X.; Liu, H. Biodistribution, excretion, and toxicity of mesoporous silica nanoparticles after oral administration depend on their shape. *Nanomed. Nanotechnol. Biol. Med.* **2015**, *11*, 1915–1924. [CrossRef] [PubMed]
257. Zhao, Y.; Wang, Y.; Ran, F.; Cui, Y.; Liu, C.; Zhao, Q.; Gao, Y.; Wang, D.; Wang, S. A comparison between sphere and rod nanoparticles regarding their in vivo biological behavior and pharmacokinetics. *Sci. Rep.* **2017**, *7*, 4131. [CrossRef] [PubMed]

258. Hudson, S.P.; Padera, R.F.; Langer, R.; Kohane, D.S. The biocompatibility of mesoporous silicates. *Biomaterials* **2008**, *29*, 4045–4055. [CrossRef] [PubMed]
259. Lu, J.; Liong, M.; Li, Z.; Zink, J.I.; Tamanoi, F. Biocompatibility, biodistribution, and drug-delivery efficiency of mesoporous silica nanoparticles for cancer therapy in animals. *Small* **2010**, *6*, 1794–1805. [CrossRef] [PubMed]
260. Tang, F.; Li, L.; Chen, D. Mesoporous Silica Nanoparticles: Synthesis, Biocompatibility and Drug Delivery. *Adv. Mater.* **2012**, *24*, 1504–1534. [CrossRef] [PubMed]
261. Zhang, Q.; Wang, X.; Li, P.-Z.; Nguyen, K.T.; Wang, X.-J.; Luo, Z.; Zhang, H.; Tan, N.S.; Zhao, Y. Biocompatible, Uniform, and Redispersible Mesoporous Silica Nanoparticles for Cancer-Targeted Drug Delivery In Vivo. *Adv. Funct. Mater.* **2014**, *24*, 2450–2461. [CrossRef]
262. Shen, D.; Yang, J.; Li, X.; Zhou, L.; Zhang, R.; Li, W.; Chen, L.; Wang, R.; Zhang, F.; Zhao, D. Biphase Stratification Approach to Three-Dimensional Dendritic Biodegradable Mesoporous Silica Nanospheres. *Nano Lett.* **2014**, *14*, 923–932. [CrossRef] [PubMed]
263. He, Y.; Zeng, B.; Liang, S.; Long, M.; Xu, H. Synthesis of pH-Responsive Biodegradable Mesoporous Silica–Calcium Phosphate Hybrid Nanoparticles as a High Potential Drug Carrier. *ACS Appl. Mater. Interfaces* **2017**, *9*, 44402–44409. [CrossRef] [PubMed]
264. Liu, T.; Li, L.; Teng, X.; Huang, X.; Liu, H.; Chen, D.; Ren, J.; He, J.; Tang, F. Single and repeated dose toxicity of mesoporous hollow silica nanoparticles in intravenously exposed mice. *Biomaterials* **2011**, *32*, 1657–1668. [CrossRef] [PubMed]
265. Fu, C.; Liu, T.; Li, L.; Liu, H.; Chen, D.; Tang, F. The absorption, distribution, excretion and toxicity of mesoporous silica nanoparticles in mice following different exposure routes. *Biomaterials* **2013**, *34*, 2565–2575. [CrossRef] [PubMed]
266. Chen, Y.; Chen, H.; Shi, J. In Vivo Bio-Safety Evaluations and Diagnostic/Therapeutic Applications of Chemically Designed Mesoporous Silica Nanoparticles. *Adv. Mater.* **2013**, *25*, 3144–3176. [CrossRef] [PubMed]
267. Asefa, T.; Tao, Z. Biocompatibility of Mesoporous Silica Nanoparticles. *Chem. Res. Toxicol.* **2012**, *25*, 2265–2284. [CrossRef] [PubMed]
268. Napierska, D.; Thomassen, L.C.; Lison, D.; Martens, J.A.; Hoet, P.H. The nanosilica hazard: Another variable entity. *Part. Fibre Toxicol.* **2010**, *7*, 39. [CrossRef] [PubMed]
269. Martin, K.R. The chemistry of silica and its potential health benefits. *J. Nutr. Health Aging* **2007**, *11*, 94–97. [PubMed]
270. Croissant, J.G.; Fatieiev, Y.; Khashab, N.M. Degradability and Clearance of Silicon, Organosilica, Silsesquioxane, Silica Mixed Oxide, and Mesoporous Silica Nanoparticles. *Adv. Mater.* **2017**, *29*, 1604634. [CrossRef] [PubMed]
271. Kim, S.-H.; Lee, M.-S.; Kim, D.; Lee, T.K.; Kwon, T.K.; Yun, H.; Khang, S.-H. The comparative immunotoxicity of mesoporous silica nanoparticles and colloidal silica nanoparticles in mice. *Int. J. Nanomed.* **2013**, *8*, 147–158. [CrossRef] [PubMed]
272. Phillips, E.; Penate-Medina, O.; Zanzonico, P.B.; Carvajal, R.D.; Mohan, P.; Ye, Y.; Humm, J.; Gonen, M.; Kalaigian, H.; Schoder, H.; et al. Clinical translation of an ultrasmall inorganic optical-PET imaging nanoparticle probe. *Sci. Transl. Med.* **2014**, *6*, 260ra149. [CrossRef] [PubMed]
273. Benezra, M.; Penate-Medina, O.; Zanzonico, P.B.; Schaer, D.; Ow, H.; Burns, A.; DeStanchina, E.; Longo, V.; Herz, E.; Iyer, S.; et al. Multimodal silica nanoparticles are effective cancer-targeted probes in a model of human melanoma. *J. Clin. Investig.* **2011**, *121*, 2768–2780. [CrossRef] [PubMed]
274. Bukara, K.; Schueller, L.; Rosier, J.; Daems, T.; Verheyden, L.; Eelen, S.; Martens, J.A.; Van den Mooter, G.; Bugarski, B.; Kiekens, F. In Vivo Performance of Fenofibrate Formulated With Ordered Mesoporous Silica Versus 2-Marketed Formulations: A Comparative Bioavailability Study in Beagle Dogs. *J. Pharm. Sci.* **2016**, *105*, 2381–2385. [CrossRef] [PubMed]
275. Ashley, C.E.; Carnes, E.C.; Wu, T.; Felton, L.A.; Sasaki, D.Y. Antibiotic Protocells and Related Pharmaceutical Formulations and Methods of Treatment. U.S. Patent 20170165375A1, 15 June 2017. Available online: https://www.google.com/patents/US20170165375 (accessed on 7 November 2017).
276. Brinker, C.J.; Townson, J.; Lin, Y.-S.; Durfee, P.N. Core and Surface Modification of Mesoporous Silica Nanoparticles to Achieve Cell Specific Targeting In Vivo. U.S. Patent 20160287717A1, 6 October 2016. Available online: https://www.google.com/patents/US20160287717 (accessed on 7 November 2017).

277. Brinker, C.J.; Ashley, C.E.; Jiang, X.; Liu, J.; Peabody, D.S.; Wharton, W.R.; Carnes, E.; Chackerian, B.; Willman, C.L. Protocells and Their Use for Targeted Delivery of Multicomponent Cargos to Cancer Cells. U.S. Patent 8992984B1, 31 March 2015. Available online: https://www.google.com/patents/US8992984 (accessed on 7 November 2017).
278. Brinker, J.C.; Lin, Y. Torroidal Mesoporous Silica Nanoparticles (TMSNPS) and Related Protocells. U.S. Patent 20160338954A1, 24 November 2016. Available online: http://www.freepatentsonline.com/y2016/0338954.html (accessed on 7 November 2017).
279. Ashley, C.E.; Brinker, C.J.; Carnes, E.C.; Fekrazad, M.H.; Felton, L.A.; Negrete, O.; Padilla, D.P.; Wilkinson, B.S.; Wilkinson, D.C.; Willman, C.L. Porous Nanoparticle-Supported Lipid Bilayers (Protocells) for Targeted Delivery Including Transdermal Delivery of Cargo and Methods Thereof. U.S. Patent EP2765997A4, 24 June 2015. Available online: https://www.google.co.in/patents/EP2765997A4?cl=esCached (accessed on 7 November 2017).
280. Nel, A.E.; Zink, J.I.; Meng, H. Lipid Bilayer Coated Mesoporous Silica Nanoparticles with a High Loading Capacity for One or More Anticancer Agents. U.S. Patent 20160008283A1, 14 January 2016. Available online: https://www.google.com/patents/US20160008283?cl=en (accessed on 7 November 2017).
281. Oktem, H.A.; Ozalp, V.C.; Hernandez, F.J.; Hernandez, L.I. Applications and Tools Based on Silica Particles Coated with Biological or Synthetic Molecules. U.S. Patent 20170172935A1, 22 June 2017. Available online: https://www.google.com/patents/US20170172935 (accessed on 7 November 2017).
282. Won, C. Composition for Delivering Bioactive Material or Protein, and Use Thereof. U.S. Patent 20170172923A1, 22 June 2017. Available online: https://www.google.com/patents/US20170172923 (accessed on 7 November 2017).
283. Weng, C.-F.; Chia, Y.-C.; Lee, C.-H.; Varadharajan, T. HCD Formulation for Cancer Treatment. U.S. Patent 20160243236A1, 25 August 2016. Available online: https://www.google.com/patents/US20160243236 (accessed on 7 November 2017).
284. Lee, K.; Lai, J.; Shah, B. FRET-Based Mesoporous Silica Nanoparticles for Real-Time Monitoring of Drug Release. U.S. Patent 9408918B1, 9 August 2016. Available online: http://www.freepatentsonline.com/9408918.html (accessed on 7 November 2017).
285. Shou-Cang, S.; Kiong, N.W.; Chia, L.; Tan, R. Nanostructured Material Formulated with Bone Cement for Effective Antibiotic Delivery. U.S. Patent 9155814B2, 13 October 2015. Available online: https://www.google.com/patents/US9155814 (accessed on 7 November 2017).
286. Liu, Y.; Lay, C.L. Stimuli-Responsive Interpolymer Complex Coated Hollow Silica Vesicles. U.S. Patent 20150182468A1, 2 July 2015. Available online: https://www.google.com/patents/US20150182468 (accessed on 7 November 2017).
287. Zink, J.I.; Nel, A.E.; Xia, T.; Ji, Z.; Meng, H.; Li, Z.; Liong, M.; Xue, M.; Tarn, D.Y. Cationic Polymer Coated Mesoporous Silica Nanoparticles and Uses Thereof. U.S. Patent 20120207795A1, 16 August 2012.
288. Liong, M.; Lu, J.; Tamanoi, F.; Zink, J.I.; Nel, A. Mesoporous Silica Nanoparticles for Biomedical Applications. U.S. Patent 20100255103A1, 7 October 2010. Available online: https://www.google.ch/patents/US20100255103 (accessed on 7 November 2017).
289. Lee, C.-H.; Lo, L.-W.; Yang, C.-S.; Mou, C.-Y. Charged Mesoporous Silica Nanoparticle-Based Drug Delivery System for Controlled Release and Enhanced Bioavailability. U.S. Patent 20100104650A1, 29 April 2010. Available online: https://www.google.com/patents/US20100104650 (accessed on 7 November 2017).
290. Lin, V.; Trewyn, B.; Huh, S.; Whitman, C. Antimicrobial Mesoporous Silica Nanoparticles. U.S. Patent 20060018966A1, 26 January 2006. Available online: https://www.google.com/patents/US20060018966 (accessed on 7 November 2017).
291. Chen, F.; Ma, K.; Benezra, M.; Zhang, L.; Cheal, S.M.; Phillips, E.; Yoo, B.; Pauliah, M.; Overholtzer, M.; Zanzonico, P.; et al. Cancer-Targeting Ultrasmall Silica Nanoparticles for Clinical Translation: Physicochemical Structure and Biological Property Correlations. *Chem. Mater.* **2017**, *29*, 8766–8779. [CrossRef] [PubMed]

3

Exploring Light-Sensitive Nanocarriers for Simultaneous Triggered Antibiotic Release and Disruption of Biofilms Upon Generation of Laser-Induced Vapor Nanobubbles

Eline Teirlinck [1,2], Alexandre Barras [3], Jing Liu [1,2], Juan C. Fraire [1,2], Tatu Lajunen [4], Ranhua Xiong [1,2], Katrien Forier [1,2], Chengnan Li [3], Arto Urtti [4,5,6], Rabah Boukherroub [3], Sabine Szunerits [3], Stefaan C. De Smedt [1,2], Tom Coenye [7] and Kevin Braeckmans [1,2,3,*]

1 Laboratory of General Biochemistry and Physical Pharmacy, University of Ghent, 9000 Ghent, Belgium; Eline.Teirlinck@UGent.be (E.T.); jingli.Liu@UGent.be (J.L.); Juan.Fraire@UGent.be (J.C.F.); Ranhua.Xiong@UGent.be (R.X.); Katrien.Forier@UGent.be (K.F.); Stefaan.Desmedt@UGent.be (S.C.D.S.)
2 Centre for Nano- and Biophotonics, 9000 Ghent, Belgium
3 Univ. Lille, CNRS, Centrale Lille, ISEN, Univ. Valenciennes, UMR 8520—IEMN, 59000 Lille, France; alexandre.barras@univ-lille.fr (A.B.); neu_lcn@163.com (C.L.); rabah.boukherroub@univ-lille.fr (R.B.); Sabine.Szunerits@univ-lille1.fr (S.S.)
4 Drug Research Program, Faculty of Pharmacy, University of Helsinki, Viikinkaari 5 E, 00790 Helsinki, Finland; tatu.lajunen@helsinki.fi (T.L.); arto.urtti@helsinki.fi (A.U.)
5 School of Pharmacy, University of Eastern Finland, Yliopistonranta 1, 70211 Kuopio, Finland
6 Laboratory of Biohybrid Technologies, Institute of Chemistry, St. Petersburg State University, Universitetskii pr. 26, Peterhoff, St. 198504 Petersburg, Russia
7 Laboratory of Pharmaceutical Microbiology, University of Ghent, 9000 Ghent, Belgium; Tom.Coenye@UGent.be
* Correspondence: Kevin.Braeckmans@UGent.be;

Abstract: Impaired penetration of antibiotics through bacterial biofilms is one of the reasons for failure of antimicrobial therapy. Hindered drug diffusion is caused on the one hand by interactions with the sticky biofilm matrix and on the other hand by the fact that bacterial cells are organized in densely packed clusters of cells. Binding interactions with the biofilm matrix can be avoided by encapsulating the antibiotics into nanocarriers, while interfering with the integrity of the dense cell clusters can enhance drug transport deep into the biofilm. Vapor nanobubbles (VNB), generated from laser irradiated nanoparticles, are a recently reported effective way to loosen up the biofilm structure in order to enhance drug transport and efficacy. In the present study, we explored if the disruptive force of VNB can be used simultaneously to interfere with the biofilm structure and trigger antibiotic release from light-responsive nanocarriers. The antibiotic tobramycin was incorporated in two types of light-responsive nanocarriers—liposomes functionalized with gold nanoparticles (Lip-AuNP) and graphene quantum dots (GQD)—and their efficacy was evaluated on *Pseudomonas aeruginosa* biofilms. Even though the anti-biofilm efficacy of tobramycin was improved by liposomal encapsulation, electrostatic functionalization with 70 nm AuNP unfortunately resulted in premature leakage of tobramycin in a matter of hours. Laser-irradiation consequently did not further improve *P. aeruginosa* biofilm eradication. Adsorption of tobramycin to GQD, on the other hand, did result in a stable formulation with high encapsulation efficiency, without burst release of tobramycin from the nanocarriers. However, even though laser-induced VNB formation from GQD resulted in biofilm disruption, an enhanced anti-biofilm effect was not achieved due to tobramycin not being efficiently released from GQD. Even though this study was unsuccessful in designing suitable nanocarriers for simultaneous biofilm disruption and light-triggered release of tobramycin, it provides insights into the difficulties and challenges that need to be considered for future developments in this regard.

Keywords: vapor nanobubbles; laser treatment; triggered release; liposomes; gold nanoparticles; graphene quantum dots; biofilms; diffusion barrier

---

1. Introduction

Difficult to treat infectious diseases pose a significant threat to healthcare globally. An important reason why antibiotics are not effective is the formation of microbial biofilms. Biofilms offer protection to their inhabiting sessile cells by a plethora of mechanisms such as reduced metabolic activity, avoidance of oxidative stress and reduced penetration of antimicrobials [1]. The latter is referred to as the biofilm diffusion barrier and is essentially due to two reasons (Figure 1). First, sessile cells in biofilms produce a complex matrix of polysaccharides, extracellular DNA and enzymes, all of which can block or even inactivate antimicrobial agents [2–6]. A promising strategy in this regard is the encapsulation of antimicrobials into nanocarriers to shield them from physicochemical interactions with biofilm matrix constituents [7]. Nanocarriers ideally should combine efficient and stable drug encapsulation, while at the same time having the ability to release the drug when reaching the target cells. Triggered drug release can be achieved by relying on specific properties of the biofilm microenvironment. One example are rhamnolipids in biofilms related to cystic fibrosis lung infections which were shown to release amikacin from liposomes locally [8]. Another pertinent example is a change of local pH which can be exploited to achieve local release, for instance with pH-sensitive polymeric nanoparticles which released farnesol when present in acidic biofilm habitats [9]. A practical limitation of relying on endogenous triggers is that they are quite specific for particular types of biofilms whose composition might vary over time and disease state [7]. Externally controlled triggers, on the other hand, ensure a broader applicability as they are independent on the biofilm composition.

The second important contribution to the biofilm diffusion barrier is related to the specific biofilm architecture. Sessile cells in biofilms are packed together into dense clusters of tens to hundreds of micrometres in size [2]. Consequently, while the outer layer of cells in those clusters can be relatively easily reached, cells in deeper layers of the biofilm will experience delayed exposure to the antimicrobials, leading to an effective dose below the therapeutic window or giving them the chance to mount defence mechanisms. Therefore, to improve drug penetration into biofilms, strategies are required that interfere with the biofilm structure so that antimicrobials can more easily and rapidly reach all cells. A recently reported effective way to achieve this goal is the use of laser-induced vapor nanobubbles [10]. It relies on gold nanoparticles (AuNP) which can efficiently absorb laser energy of specific wavelengths. When AuNP are irradiated with short laser pulses, their temperature can increase by several hundreds of degrees, leading to a quick evaporation of the surrounding water and the formation of vapor nanobubbles (VNB) [11,12]. It has been shown that the mechanical impact of these expanding and subsequently imploding nanobubbles can cause a highly local but effective deformation of dense cell clusters in both Gram-positive and Gram-negative biofilms. This led to markedly enhanced penetration of the antibiotic tobramycin, increasing its effectiveness by 1–3 orders of magnitude depending on the micro-organism.

In the present study, we aimed to combine light-triggered nanocarriers and VNB-based biofilm disruption to come to a complete solution to the biofilm diffusion barrier problem (Figure 1). We developed two types of nanocarriers suited for encapsulation of tobramycin and having the possibility to generate laser-induced VNB to simultaneously release tobramycin and at the same time interfere with the biofilm structural integrity. For the first type of nanocarriers we combined AuNP with DOPC/DPPG liposomes because of their outstanding advantages as antibiotic drug carriers, such as biocompatibility, versatility and ability to penetrate biofilms [13,14]. While the liposomes themselves could enhance the effectiveness of tobramycin in *P. aeruginosa* biofilms, no beneficial effect was observed of applying laser irradiation and VNB formation. As this was due to spontaneous leaking of tobramycin from the liposomes upon functionalization with AuNP, we switched to graphene quantum dots (GQD) as an alternative nanocarrier. Thanks to their large surface area and various functional groups, they can be efficiently loaded with drugs on their surface [15] which can be released upon irradiation with light [16,17]. We showed that indeed tobramycin could be efficiently loaded onto GQD without premature release. In addition, pulsed laser irradiation of GQD resulted in VNB formation and enhanced diffusion of co-administered tobramycin, similar to what we have previously shown for AuNP. However, tobramycin loaded GQD did not have an enhanced anti-biofilm efficacy upon laser irradiation and VNB formation. Further experiments showed that this was surprisingly due to tobramycin not being released from the GQD upon laser irradiation. We conclude that the concept of VNB-triggered antibiotic release should be re-evaluated with other types of nanocarriers that can stably incorporate antibiotics (without leaking), while at the same time being able to release their cargo in response to light.

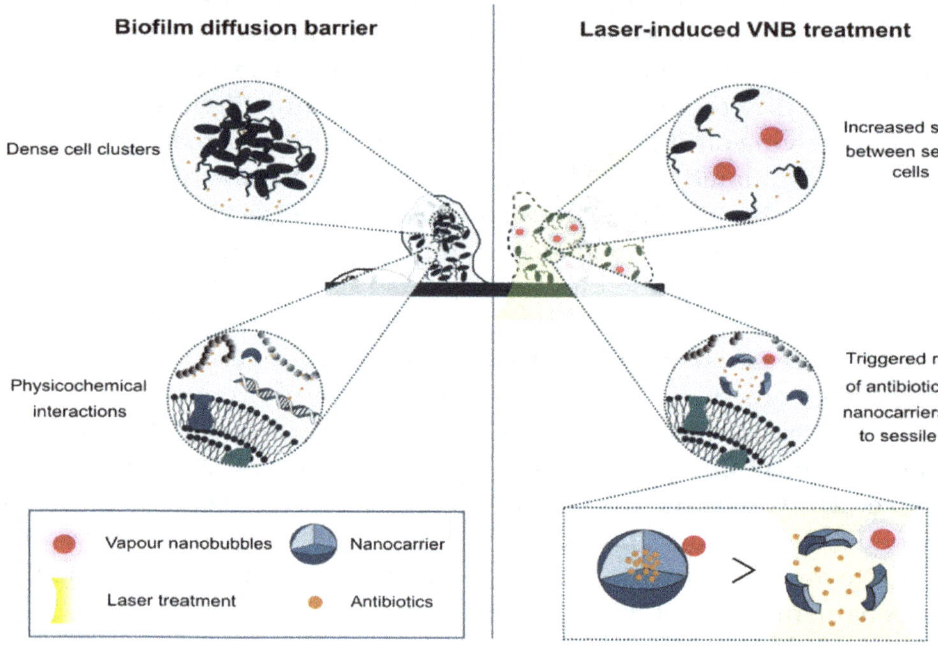

Figure 1. Biofilm diffusion barrier and the potential of laser-induced vapor nanobubbles (VNB) to improve antibiotic delivery to biofilms. Impaired biofilm diffusion is caused by the fact that sessile cells cluster together into dense aggregates of hundreds of micrometres in size and because of the multi-component nature of the biofilm matrix which can trap molecules in their passage through biofilms. The mechanical impact of laser-induced VNB can on the one hand increase the space between sessile cells leading to a better flux and effectivity of antimicrobial agents and on the other hand their mechanical force can trigger antibiotic release from nanocarriers close to sessile bacteria.

2. Materials and Methods

2.1. Materials and Strains

P. aeruginosa LESB58 (LMG 27622) was used for all experiments. Lysogeny Agar/Broth was purchased from Lab M Limited (Lancashire, UK), NaCl from Applichem (Darmstadt, Germany) and tobramycin from Tokyo Chemical Industry (Zwijndrecht, Belgium). Hydrogen peroxide (H_2O_2), fluorescamine, dimethyl sulfoxide (DMSO), chloroform, sucrose, 4-(2-hydroxyethyl)piperazine-1-ethanesulfonic acid (HEPES) and Triton X-100 were obtained from Sigma-Aldrich (St. Louis, MO, USA). The phospholipids DOPC and DPPG were purchased from Avanti® Polar Lipids (Alabaster, AL, USA).

2.2. *Synthesis of Gold Nanoparticles (AuNP) and Graphene Quantum Dots (GQD)*

Gold nanoparticles were prepared in house using the Turkevich method [18], in which gold ions were reduced by citrate. A 150 mL 0.2 mM chloroauric acid solution ($HAuCl_4$) was heated and stirred for 30 min in the presence of 0.5 mL 0.01 M citrate solution (corresponding to a 1:1 Au/citrate molar ratio). The particles were overgrown to the desired size of 70 nm by addition of Au^{3+} and ascorbate solutions in equimolar concentrations (0.005 M). A layer of poly (diallyldimethylammonium chloride) was adsorbed onto the synthesized AuNP using a solution 20 wt.% in water (final concentration of 0.06 mg mL^{-1}) of the polymer. The polymer was added for at least 2 h at room temperature to allow complete functionalization, followed by a centrifugal washing step at 5000 rcf for 5 min. Determination of the particles size, zeta potential and concentration was done by combining UV/VIS-spectroscopy (NanoDrop 2000c spectrophotometer, Thermo Scientific, Rockford, IL, USA), Transmission Electron Microscopy imaging (JEM 1400 plus transmission electron microscope, JEOL, Tokyo, Japan), Dynamic Light Scattering (DLS) and electrodynamic modelling using the Mie theory.

To prepare GQD, 100 mg reduced graphene oxide (rGO, Graphitene, UK) was dispersed in 100 mL of 30% (*w*/*v*) H_2O_2 and ultrasonicated for 30 min. The solution was kept refluxing for 12 h at 60 °C. Next, purification by filtration (Whatman® Puradisc syringe filter 0.2 µm, Sigma, Overijse, Belgium) and dialysis was done.

The size and zeta potential of GQD particles were measured in triplicate by Nanoparticle Tracking Analysis (NTA) and Dynamic Light Scattering (DLS), respectively. After diluting the particles 1:10,000 in ultrapure water, 1 mL was inserted into the NTA chamber (Nanosight LM10, Malvern, UK) and the movement of each particle was captured by the camera. Through analysis of the Brownian motion, the average particle size could be calculated. To measure the zeta potential, 1 mL of the diluted sample was transferred in a folded capillary cell and after applying an electric field trough the Zetasizer Nano-ZS (Malvern, Worcestershire, UK), the particles in the solution migrated with a certain velocity towards the counter electrode which enabled to calculate the zeta potential of those particles.

2.3. *Preparation of Tobramycin-Loaded Liposomes*

Negatively charged liposomes consisting of the neutral phospholipid 1,2-dioleoyl-*sn*-glycero-3-phosphocholine (DOPC) and the anionic phospholipid 1,2-dipalmitoyl-*sn*-glycero-3-phospho-(1′-*rac*-glycerol) (DPPG) were prepared by the Thin Film Hydration (TFH) method as described before [19]. After mixing the two lipids in a molar ratio of 8:2 and final lipid concentration of 20 mg mL^{-1}, a thin lipid film was created by rotary evaporation (Vaccubrand PC 2001, Wertheim, Germany) at 50 °C for 15 min. Next, the lipid film was hydrated with a 80 mg mL^{-1} tobramycin solution for 30 min in a warm water bath at 50 °C (IKA® HB10, Staufen, Germany). To obtain a monodisperse population, the liposomes were sonicated with a pulsed tip sonicator (Branson Digital Sonifier, Danbury, CT, USA) for 1 min at 10% amplitude. In order to prevent overheating of particles, every 10 s of sonication was followed by a 15 s pause (total sonication time = 1 min). As purification, tobramycin-loaded liposomes were subjected to 2 rounds of ultracentrifugation at 35,000 rpm for 1 h. The second class of DOPC/DPPG liposomes were prepared by the Dehydration-Rehydration Vesicles (DRV) method as described before [20,21]. After hydrating the DOPC/DPPG lipid film with a 2 mL distilled water/sucrose solution (1:1 *w*/*w* sucrose to lipid), for stabilization during freeze drying, the particles were subjected to 3 rounds of vortexing and 5 min sonication in an ultrasonic bath. Next, the particles were mixed with 1 mL of a 80 mg mL^{-1} tobramycin solution and the suspension was freeze-dried in an Amsco FINN-AQUA GT4 freeze-dryer (GEA, Köln, Germany). Therefore, the sample was transferred into 10R vials (Schott, Müllheim, Germany) and placed on a precooled shelf at 3 °C. To ensure complete solidification, the plate temperature was gradually lowered at a rate of 1 °C min^{-1} to −40 °C for 185 min. Then, the pressure was decreased to 100 µbar while the plate temperature was increased to −25 °C for 15 h as primary drying step. To get rid of residual moisture, the shelf temperature was further increased to 10 °C at a rate of 1 °C min^{-1}. At the end of the process, the chamber was aerated with nitrogen gas while the vials were closed with bromobutyl rubber stoppers

(West Pharmaceutical Co., Lionville, PA, USA). For the rehydration step, the powder was incubated with 200 μL distilled water for 30 min at 50 °C. This step was repeated twice for another 30 min at 50 °C with 200 μL and 1.6 mL HEPES-buffer (20 mM, pH 7.4), respectively. Then, 2 rounds of ultracentrifugation at 35,000 rpm for 1 h was done to separate the tobramycin-loaded liposomes from the unbound tobramycin. Size and zeta potential of the liposomes was measured by DLS in triplicate.

2.4. Quantification of Tobramycin Content by High Performance Liquid Chromatography (HPLC)–UV

The amount of encapsulated tobramycin inside liposomes was determined by LC2010-HT HPLC (Shimadzu, Tokyo, Japan) equipped with a 5 μm QS Uptishere® 300 Å, 250 × 4.6 mm silica-C4 column (Interchim, Montluçon, France) heated to 40 °C. For the mobile phase, a mixture of eluent A (trifluoroacetic acid 0.05% in water) and eluent B (trifluoroacetic acid 0.05% in acetonitrile) at a flow rate of 1 mL min^{-1} was used. First, isocratic flow (eluent A) was done for 5 min, then solution B was increased gradually from 0 to 80% during 10 min and finally 80% of eluent B was done for 5 min. Detection was performed at 215 nm. A calibration curve was generated by injecting 40 μL of a series of tobramycin solutions with known concentrations (5–200 μg mL^{-1}). The area under the curve was plotted against the tobramycin concentration and fitted using a linear curve. After rupturing the liposomes with 10% Triton X-100, 40 μL was injected into the HPLC column and the resulting tobramycin concentration was calculated by making use of the calibration curve. Tobramycin loading capacity was determined according to Equation (1):

$$\text{Tobramycin loading capacity} = \frac{c_{\text{Triton X-100}}}{c_0} \times 100\% \quad (1)$$

$c_{\text{Triton X-100}}$ = [tobramycin] after rupturing the liposomes with Triton X-100
c_0 = [tobramycin] added initially

2.5. Biofilm Formation

Twenty-four-hour-old mature biofilms were grown aerobically in 96-well SensoPlates™ (Greiner Bio-One, Monroe, NC, USA) with microscopy grade borosilicate glass bottom at 37 °C. *P. aeruginosa* cultures were grown in Lysogeny Broth at 37 °C with shaking at 250 rpm until stationary phase, after which 100 μL was added to the wells of the 96-well SensoPlate. After 4 h incubation at 37 °C, the adhered cells were washed with physiological saline (0.9% NaCl (*w*/*v*)), covered with Lysogeny Broth and incubated for another 20 h at 37 °C.

2.6. Effect of Laser-Irradiated Tobramycin Loaded Liposomes

After 24 h of growth, 100 μL supernatant was removed and biofilms were incubated with 100 μL tobramycin at 16 μg mL^{-1}, tobramycin-loaded DRV liposomes (corresponding to 16 μg mL^{-1} tobramycin) or AuNP functionalized DRV liposomes (corresponding to 16 μg mL^{-1} tobramycin) for 24 h. AuNP functionalized liposomes were made by adding positively charged AuNP in a 1:1 liposome:AuNP ratio to the negatively charged tobramycin loaded DRV liposomes via electrostatic binding. A home-made optical set-up was used to generate VNB inside the biofilms. The set-up is built around an inverted TE2000 epi-fluorescence microscope (Nikon, Nikon BeLux, Brussels, Belgium) equipped with a Plan Fluor 10 × 0.3 NA objective lens (Nikon). An Optical Parametric Oscillator laser (Opelette™ HE 355 LD, OPOTEK Inc., Faraday Ave, CA, USA) produces laser pulses of 7 ns tuned to 561 nm in order to excite the gold nanoparticles, while at the same time being compatible with optical filters in the set-up. The energy of each laser pulse is monitored with an energy meter (J-25MB-HE&LE, Energy Max-USB/RS sensors, Coherent, Santa Clara, CA, USA) synchronized with the pulsed laser. Biofilms were irradiated with laser pulses at a laser fluence of 1.69 J cm^{-2}. An automatic Prior Proscan III stage (Prior scientific Ltd., Cambridge, UK) was used to scan the sample through the 150 μm diameter laser beam (firing at 20 Hz) line by line.

After incubation for 24 h at 37 °C, the sessile cells were washed with physiologic saline and harvested by 2 rounds of 5 min vortexing (900 rpm, Titramax 1000, Heidolph Instruments, Schwabach, Germany) and 5 min sonication (Branson 3510, Branson Ultrasonics Corp., Danbury, CT, USA). Next, the number of CFU/biofilm per condition was determined by plating ($n = 3 \times 3$).

2.7. Evaluation of AuNP-Triggered Tobramycin Release from Liposomes

After functionalizing the liposomes with AuNP in 1:1 ratio at different incubation times (15–120 min), liposomes were separated from the supernatant containing the released tobramycin by Vivaspin® 500, 30,000 MWCO (Sartorius, Stonehouse, UK) centrifugation at 13.5 × 1000 rpm for 5 min. As a positive control, AuNP-functionalized liposomes were completely lysed by adding 10% Triton X-100. 40 μL filtrate was measured by HPLC analysis and the resulting tobramycin concentration was determined using the tobramycin calibration curve. Tobramycin release was calculated according to Equation (2):

$$\text{Tobramycin release } (\%) = \frac{c_{\text{supernatant}}}{c_{\text{Triton X-100}}} \times 100\% \quad (2)$$

$c_{\text{supernatant}}$ = [tobramycin] released into the supernatant
$c_{\text{Triton X-100}}$ = [tobramycin] after rupturing the liposomes with Triton X-100

2.8. GQD-Induced VNB Formation and Tobramycin Treatment in *P. aeruginosa* Biofilms

After cultivation of 24 h-old *P. aeruginosa* biofilms in 50 mm glass bottom dishes (No. 1.5 coverslip) (MatTek Corporation, Ashland, OR, USA), the supernatant was removed and biofilms were incubated with 1.87×10^{10} GQD mL^{-1} for 15 min at room temperature. Biofilms were irradiated with laser pulses at a laser fluence of 2.00 J cm^{-2}. As VNB efficiently scatter light, the generation of VNB inside biofilms could be detected by dark-field microscopy. Because of the short nature of VNB generation (lifetime < 1 μs), the camera (EMCCD camera, Cascade II: 512, Photometrics, Tucson, AZ, USA) was synchronized with the pulsed laser by an electronic pulse generator (BNC575, Berkeley Nucleonics Corporation, San Rafael, CA, USA). Dark-field pictures were taken before, during VNB formation and immediately after illumination, in order to elucidate any conformational changes in the biofilm structure. After loading the biofilms with GQD and irradiation with pulsed laser light, as described above, 100 μL supernatant was removed and 100 μL tobramycin (at 16 μg mL^{-1}) or control solution (0.9% NaCl (*w*/*v*)) was added for 24 h at 37 °C. Then, the sessile cells were washed with physiologic saline and harvested by 2 rounds of 5 min vortexing and 5 min sonication followed by plate counting ($n = 3 \times 3$).

2.9. Preparation of Tobramycin-Loaded GQD

GQD and tobramycin were mixed in a 1:2 GQD:tobramycin weight ratio and stirred in water for 1.5 h at room temperature. To separate the unbound tobramycin, the particles were washed with ultrapure water by centrifugation at 13.5 × 1000 rpm for 30 min. The loading capacity of GQD for tobramycin was calculated according to Equation (3):

$$\text{Tobramycin loading capacity} = \frac{c_0 - c_{\text{supernatant}}}{c_0} \times 100\% \quad (3)$$

c_0 = [tobramycin] added initially
$c_{\text{supernatant}}$ = [tobramycin] in the supernatant after centrifugation

Tobramycin concentration was quantified fluorometric by using the reactive compound fluorescamine. Therefore, 3 mg mL^{-1} fluorescamine (DMSO) was added to a series of tobramycin solutions with known concentrations and after reacting with the primary amines of tobramycin, a fluorescent product was formed that could be measured using the VICTOR3 1420-012 fluorescence microplate reader with 355/460 nm excitation/emission (Perkin Elmer, Boston, MA, USA). Next, the data was plotted and fitted into a quadratic curve, which could then be used to calculate the tobramycin content in the supernatant of the GQD-tobramycin constructs.

2.10. The Effect of Laser-Irradiated GQD-Tobramycin Particles in P. aeruginosa Biofilms

24 h-old *P. aeruginosa* biofilms were treated with 100 µL of 16 µg mL^{-1} tobramycin, GQD-tobramycin (corresponding to 16 µg mL^{-1} tobramycin) or control solution (0.9% NaCl (*w*/*v*)), with and without laser irradiation, as described above, to generate VNB. After 24 h incubation at 37 °C, the number of CFU/biofilm per condition was determined by plating ($n = 3 \times 3$).

2.11. Evaluation of VNB-Triggered Tobramycin Release from GQD

To evaluate VNB mediated tobramycin release, 100 µL of GQD-tobramycin particles were placed into a Grace Bio-Labs CoverWell^{TM} perfusion chamber (Sigma-Aldrich, St. Louis, MO, USA) and illuminated with pulsed laser light at a laser fluence of 2.00 J cm^{-2}. Then, the solution was centrifuged at 13.5 × 1000 rpm for 30 min so that GQD-tobramycin particles were separated from the supernatant containing the released tobramycin. Tobramycin content was measured fluorometric by using fluorescamine. Tobramycin release was quantified according to Equation (4):

$$\text{Tobramycin release } (\%) = \frac{c_{supernatant}}{c_{pellet}} \times 100\% \quad (4)$$

$c_{supernatant}$ = [tobramycin] in the supernatant after centrifugation
c_{pellet} = [tobramycin] in the pellet

Repeated VNB formation was tested by illuminating the particles with 3 laser pulses instead of 1 at 2.00 J cm^{-2}. The influence of continuous laser irradiation was investigated by irradiation with a continuous mode laser (Gbox model, Fournier Medical Solution, Bondues, France) with an output light at 980 nm at various power densities (1–4 W cm^{-2}) for 10 min. Thermal images were captured by an Infrared Camera (Thermovision A40, Goleta, CA, USA) and treated using ThermaCam Researcher Pro 2.9 software.

2.12. Statistical Analysis

SPSS Statistics 24 (SPSS, Chicago, IL, USA) was used to analyse the data. The Shapiro–Wilk test was used to test the normality of the data sets. The one-way analysis of variance test and independent samples *t*-test were used for normal distributed data. The Kruskal–Wallis test and Mann–Whitney U test were used for non-normally distributed data. Differences with a p-value < 0.05 were considered significant.

3. Results

3.1. Development of Tobramycin-Loaded Liposomes

The first set of tobramycin loaded DOPC/DPPG liposomes were prepared via the Thin Film Hydration (TFH) method and had an average size and zeta potential of 214 ± 84 nm and −41 ± 15 mV, respectively. Tobramycin loading capacity was determined after complete liposome rupture with 10%

Triton X-100 by measuring the tobramycin content with High Performance Liquid Chromatography (HPLC) with UV detection (Supplementary Figure S1). The preparation of liposomes via the TFH method resulted in rather low encapsulation efficiencies for tobramycin (0.33%), as reported by other groups as well [22]. The Dehydration Rehydration Vesicles (DRV) method has been shown to enhance liposomal entrapment [20,23]. Indeed, when liposomes were prepared via the DRV method, tobramycin loading capacity increased to 13%. The size and zeta potential of these liposomes were 99 ± 60 nm and −40 ± 12 mV before freeze drying and increased to 182 ± 102 nm and −9.97 ± 0.72 mV after freeze drying. Due to the higher loading efficiency, further experiments were performed with the DRV liposomal formulation.

3.2. *The Effect of Tobramycin-Loaded Liposomes and Laser-Generated VNB in P. aeruginosa Biofilms*

First, the efficacy of the DRV liposomal tobramycin formulation was evaluated in *P. aeruginosa* biofilms. Twenty four hours treatment with tobramycin in DOPC/DPPG liposomes already had a greater effect on cell viability as compared to the same concentration of free tobramycin (Figure 2a) ($p = 0.041$). It shows that these liposomes can prevent to a certain extent the inactivation of tobramycin by physicochemical interactions with the biofilm matrix and release at least a part of the encapsulated tobramycin close to the sessile cells. The next step was to further functionalize the liposomal formulation with AuNP and evaluate if the formation of VNB can further enhance this release. Cationic AuNP (70 nm, + 55 mV) were electrostatically coupled to tobramycin-loaded liposomes in a 1:1 ratio (zeta potential increased from −9.97 ± 0.72 mV to +20.93 ± 0.69 mV). When added to the *P. aeruginosa* biofilms, biofilm survival was decreased further compared to liposomes alone, indicating that the presence of AuNP already had an additional effect, possibly due to these positively charged nanocarriers interacting more strongly with the negative cell surface of *P. aeruginosa* pathogens and enhancing the level of local release. Upon laser irradiation to form VNB, however, no further biofilm eradication was achieved. This observation was rather surprising, indicating that something did not work as hypothesized. We considered the following possibilities: (1) the laser light may (partly) inactivate tobramycin, (2) VNB are not (as efficiently) formed when AuNP are attached to liposomes, (3) AuNP functionalization of tobramycin loaded liposomes destabilizes the liposomes and prematurely releases tobramycin. We consequently tested each of these hypotheses via the following experiments. First, we checked if tobramycin is damaged upon laser irradiation and VNB formation by simultaneously incubating biofilms with AuNP and tobramycin and irradiating with pulsed laser light to form VNB (Supplementary Figure S2a). A similar enhanced anti-biofilm effect was observed as previously reported when biofilms were first treated separately with VNB before adding tobramycin [10]. This confirms that laser irradiation and VNB formation in the presence of tobramycin does not alter its antibacterial efficacy. The second hypothesis was that VNB formation could be possibly not as effective when created around AuNP attached to liposomes compared to free AuNP. To this end, we added empty AuNP functionalized liposomes to the biofilms and applied laser irradiation together with co-administered tobramycin. Again an enhanced effect of tobramycin was found similar to what was previously found with AuNP alone, thus confirming successful VNB formation and ruling out this hypothesis as well (Supplementary Figure S2b). Thirdly, we tested if tobramycin was prematurely released from the liposomes upon functionalization with AuNP. This turned out to be the case, with already ~ 50% tobramycin released after 2 h in buffer solution (Figure 2b). We conclude that very likely most of the tobramycin had already leaked out of the liposomes upon addition to the biofilms, explaining why no additional effect of VNB mediated release could be obtained.

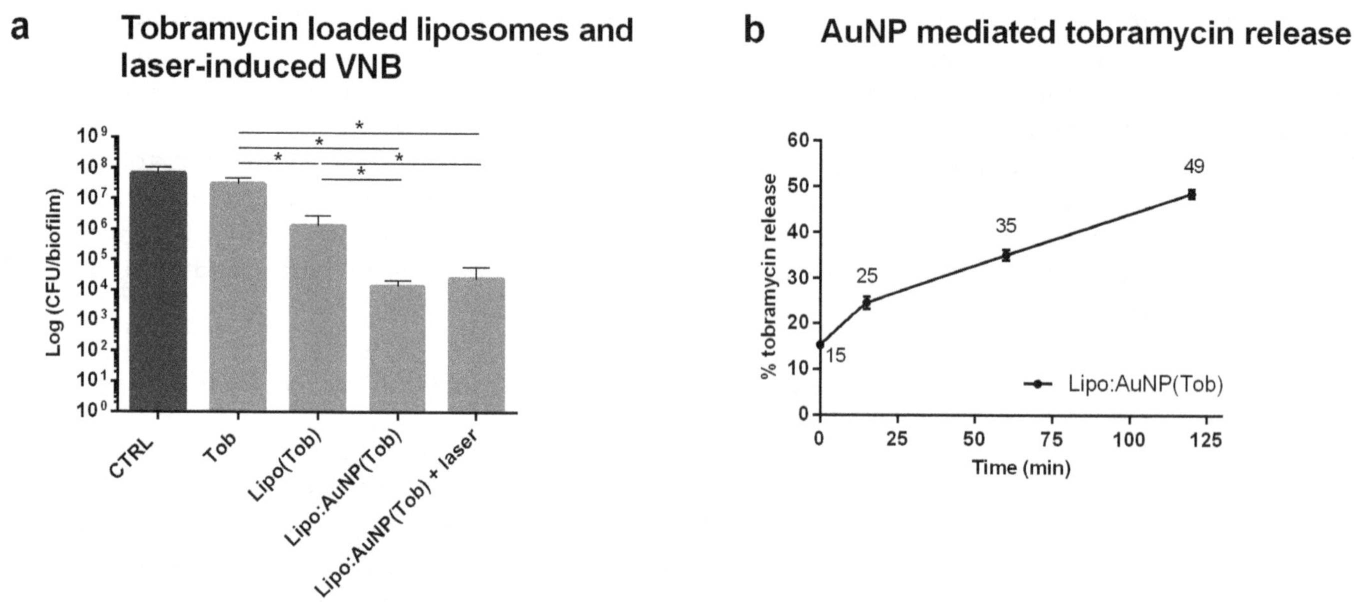

Figure 2. Evaluation of combining tobramycin loaded liposomes with laser-induced VNB for *P. aeruginosa* biofilm treatment. (**a**) Anti-biofilm effect of tobramycin loaded liposomes and laser-induced VNB in *P. aeruginosa* biofilms (average ± SD). CTRL: 0.9% NaCl (*w*/*v*), Tob: tobramycin at 16 μg mL^{-1}, Lipo(Tob): DOPC/DPPG liposomes containing tobramycin at 16 μg mL^{-1}, Lipo:AuNP(Tob): AuNP functionalized tobramycin loaded DOPC/DPPG liposomes at 16 μg mL^{-1}, laser: pulsed laser irradiation at 1.69 J cm^{-2} ($n = 3 \times 3$) (p-values < 0.05 were considered significant). (**b**) Tobramycin release from AuNP functionalized liposomes as a function of increasing liposome:AuNP incubation time (min) normalized to maximal release after Triton X-100 treatment (average ± SD).

3.3. VNB Formation from Graphene Quantum Dots for Biofilm Disruption

Due to the stability issues encountered with AuNP functionalized liposomes, we switched to graphene quantum dots (GQD) as alternative nanocarriers of which we have recently demonstrated that they can generate VNB upon pulsed laser irradiation as well [24]. Their large surface area and various functional groups enable outstanding potential as a drug delivery vehicle making it ideally suited for direct drug loading [15,17]. Moreover, it has been documented that photothermal heating of these particles with a 980 nm continuous laser can successfully trigger the release of adsorbed molecules upon laser irradiation [16,25]. First, we evaluated whether VNB originating from GQD can increase the space between sessile *P. aeruginosa* cells and enhance tobramycin diffusion, similar to what we demonstrated before with AuNP [10]. *P. aeruginosa* biofilms were incubated with GQD for 15 min (39 ± 14 nm, −30 ± 1.7 mV) and the effect on sessile clusters was visualized by dark field microscopy before, during and immediately after irradiation with a single laser pulse (7 ns, 561 nm). Clear biofilm deformation was observed, confirming successful VNB formation from GQD in biofilms (Figure 3a). As shown in Figure 3b, treatment with GQD alone or GQD-induced VNB did not alter *P. aeruginosa* viability. Incubating the biofilms with GQD followed by the addition of tobramycin (without laser irradiation) lead to a potentiating effect of ~ 20 times on the activity of tobramycin. However, when tobramycin was added to the biofilms after first forming laser-induced VNB, its effect was enhanced further to ~ 90 times as compared to tobramycin alone ($p = 0.006$). It shows that VNB generated from GQD can enhance tobramycin diffusion and efficacy, similar to AuNP.

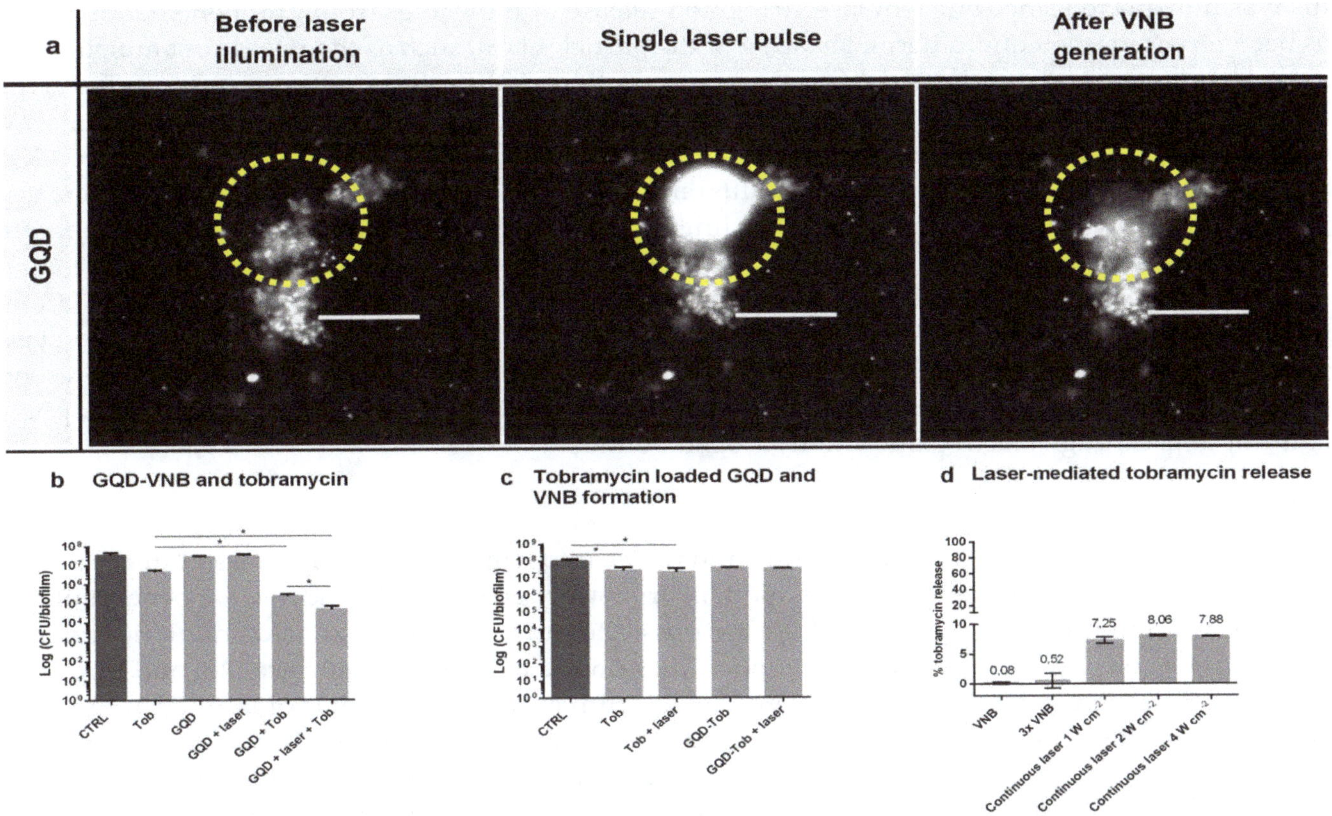

Figure 3. Evaluation of combining tobramycin loaded GQD with laser-induced VNB for *P. aeruginosa* biofilm treatment. (**a**) VNB formation around GQD in *P. aeruginosa* biofilms. Dark field pictures were taken before, during and immediately after a single nanosecond laser pulse (561 nm, 7 ns). The yellow circle indicates the laser beam area. Scale bar = 100 μm. (**b**) The effect of GQD-induced VNB on tobramycin in the treatment of *P. aeruginosa* biofilms (average ± SD). CTRL: 0.9% NaCl (*w*/*v*), Tob: tobramycin at 16 μg mL^{-1}, GQD: only addition of GQD, laser: pulsed laser treatment. ($n = 3 \times 3$) (*p*-values < 0.05 were considered significant). (**c**) Anti-biofilm effect of laser-irradiated GQD loaded with tobramycin in *P. aeruginosa* biofilms (average ± SD). CTRL: 0.9% NaCl (*w*/*v*), Tob: tobramycin 16 μg mL^{-1}, laser: pulsed laser treatment, GQD-Tob: GQD containing tobramycin at 16 μg mL^{-1} ($n = 3 \times 3$) (*p*-values < 0.05 were considered significant). (**d**) Tobramycin release from GQD-tobramycin nanoparticles was quantified for different laser settings: single and repeated (3) VNB formation at a laser fluence of 2.00 J cm^{-2}, and continuous laser illumination at 980 nm for 10 min at 1, 2 and 4 W cm^{-2} (mean ± SD).

3.4. Development of Tobramycin-Loaded GQD

Having confirmed that GQD are suitable for VNB treatment of biofilms, the next step was to adsorb tobramycin onto GQD, which was done by mixing of the 2 compounds for 1.5 h at room temperature. A decrease of negative charge of the particles from −30 ± 1.7 mV for GQD to −8.4 ± 0.50 mV indicated that tobramycin was successfully loaded onto GQD. The tobramycin loading capacity was found to be 73 ± 0.84%, as evaluated by determining the concentration of unreacted tobramycin in the supernatant by fluorescamine fluorimetry after removing GQD-tobramycin nanoparticles by centrifugation (Supplementary Figure S3a).

Treatment of *P. aeruginosa* biofilms with tobramycin-loaded GQD for 24 h did not have a significant effect on biofilm viability, indicating that tobramycin was not spontaneously released (Figure 3c). Unfortunately, however, after laser irradiation and VNB formation no reduction in cell viability was obtained either. Therefore, we checked if pulsed laser irradiation was indeed able to release tobramycin from GQD in suspension, which turned out not to be the case (Figure 3d). Even when the laser irradiation procedure was repeated three times, no significant amount of tobramycin was released.

This was unexpected since efficient laser-triggered release of molecules from graphene nanoparticles has been reported upon photothermal heating of the particles [16], such as the release of ampicillin and cefepime from reduced graphene oxide nanoconstructs [25]. A difference with previous reports is that we used pulsed laser irradiation (561 nm laser) instead of the more traditionally used continuous wave laser irradiation (980 nm laser). Therefore, in a final attempt we irradiated tobramycin loaded GQD with continuous wave laser irradiation at different intensities (1, 2 and 4 W cm^{-2}) which increased the temperature of the GQD dispersion according to expectations (Supplementary Figure S3b). After 10 min of irradiation, a slightly higher amount of tobramycin was indeed found in the supernatant but still > 90% was not released. Together it shows that, while GQD are suitable for VNB mediated biofilm disruption, tobramycin is too strongly associated so that it is not efficiently released upon laser irradiation. The numerous positively charged amine groups on tobramycin together with the presence of hydroxyl groups could account for the high binding affinity between tobramycin and graphene quantum dots through electrostatic and hydrogen bounds.

4. Discussion

In recent years, interest in encapsulating antibiotics into nanocarriers has increased tremendously as they hold the potential to enhance antibiotic delivery towards bacteria [7]. Indeed, nanoencapsulation can reduce systemic degradation [13], offers the possibility to guide encapsulated antibiotics towards specific target cells by including targeting modalities on the nanoparticle surface [26] and can shield antibiotics from detrimental interactions with the biofilm matrix [7]. The use of laser light to trigger release of molecules from nanocarriers has attracted increasing attention [27]. Zhao et al., for instance, documented successful eradication of *P. aeruginosa* biofilms by making use of continuous wave near infrared laser light which triggered tobramycin release from photo responsive liposomes close to the sessile cells [28]. Another example is that by Meeker et al. who showed that continuous wave near infrared laser light was able to activate and release daptomycin from gold nanocages thereby efficiently killing *S. aureus* biofilms [29]. While in those cases continuous wave laser irradiation was clearly effective in releasing the encapsulated drugs from the nanocarriers, substantial heat generation can be damaging to healthy tissue while it does not interfere with the biofilm structure itself. Therefore, in this study, we explored the use of pulsed laser light with photoresponsive nanocarriers that can form VNB, a phenomenon of which we have recently shown that it can interfere with the biofilm structure and improve drug diffusion without heating up the environment [10]. We started to evaluate this concept with AuNP functionalized liposomes since AuNP are very well suited to form VNB, while liposomes have demonstrated advantages as antibiotic drug carriers, such as good biocompatibility and ability to penetrate biofilms [13,14]. Unfortunately, laser irradiation of tobramycin loaded AuNP-liposomes did not result in an increased anti-biofilm efficacy as compared to the effect of tobramycin loaded liposomes alone. We found that this was due to rapid leakage of tobramycin from the liposomes upon addition of AuNP so that disruption of liposomes by laser-induced VNB did not produce a significant additional effect. AuNP-mediated leakage of cargo was also reported by Wang et al. who found that adsorption of AuNP to DOPC liposomes resulted in release of the encapsulated compounds [30]. Yet, stable integration of AuNP onto liposomes without cargo leakage has already been successfully accomplished by others [27]. Lajunen et al. for example successfully loaded hydrophilic gold nanorods (width 25 nm, length 60 nm) and gold nanostars (50–60 nm in diameter) into the liposomal lumen and documented efficient triggered release of encapsulated calcein upon visible and near infrared light irradiation [31]. In future research it will be of interest to re-evaluate the concept put forward in our current study on such types of liposomal formulations.

Due to the stability issues with AuNP functionalized liposomes, we changed to GQD which can be used as carriers for tobramycin due to their large surface area and various functional groups [15]. In addition, we have recently shown that VNB can be formed from GQD with pulsed laser irradiation of sufficient intensity [24]. The GQD by themselves did not alter the viability of *P. aeruginosa* biofilms, which is in line with a previous study where it was found that GQD prepared from graphene oxide—as in our case—lacked antibacterial activity [32]. Upon irradiation with pulsed laser light we could confirm by dark field microscopy that the structure of cell clusters is altered, without affecting the biofilm's viability. Next we tested the combination with tobramycin, finding that GQD had a synergistic effect on the efficiency of tobramycin. This is similar to what has been reported by Fan et al. who also found a synergistic effect of polyethyleneimine-graphene oxide on daptomycin in the treatment of *Staphylococcus aureus* [33]. When we combined VNB pre-treatment of *P. aeruginosa* biofilms with subsequent addition of tobramycin, a significant effect on biofilm viability was found, confirming that VNB from GQD can enhance the diffusion of tobramycin and enhance its effectivity, similar to what we have shown before with AuNP [10]. Next, we tested tobramycin loading on GQD for light triggered release. Similarly as reported in literature [34], we noticed the superior capability of GQD to load molecular agents, as a 73% tobramycin encapsulation efficiency was obtained. Tobramycin loaded GQD by themselves did not have any anti-biofilm effect, likely since tobramycin is not spontaneously released. Unfortunately, also after pulsed laser irradiation and VNB formation, no decrease in biofilm viability was found. Further investigations showed that tobramycin could not be released by pulsed laser irradiation. This was rather surprising as previous studies did report laser-assisted release of molecules from graphene upon photothermal heating with continuous wave laser irradiation [16,25]. A possible explanation is that the very short rise in temperature upon pulsed laser irradiation was not sufficient to interfere with the interactions between GQD and tobramycin. Indeed, as reported by Teodorescu et al., generating sufficient heat by long-term continuous wave laser irradiation has been found to be a critical step for triggered release of molecules, as shown for the release of ondansetron (anti-nausea drug) from reduced graphene oxide sheets [35]. Therefore, as a final test we tested irradiation with continuous laser light for 10 min as well. Although we found that GQD-tobramycin particles exhibited good photothermal heating, with suspension temperatures increasing by ~30 °C after 10 min, also in that case less than 10% tobramycin was released into the supernatant, far below the expectations according to literature [16]. In summary, most of tobramycin remained bound on GQD, even after pulsed or continuous laser irradiation, which explains its lack of anti-biofilm effect in *P. aeruginosa* biofilms. A possible explanation for the strong interaction between tobramycin and GQD is the high positive charge of tobramycin at physiologic pH due to its protonated amine groups (pKa ranging from 7.52 to 9.66) and the numerous hydroxyl groups present on its surface. These functional groups enable strong binding with graphene through electrostatic interactions and hydrogen bonds. In future studies it would be of interest to investigate whether VNB are able to release antibiotics which are less strongly bound to graphene such as ampicillin and cefepime [25]. For these kind of molecules, less electrostatic and hydrophobic bonds are formed with graphene (being zwitterionic) while pi-pi stacking becomes an important interaction due to their aromatic ring. It has been shown that irradiation with light can successfully interfere with these kind of interactions thereby triggering antibiotic release from graphene carriers.

5. Conclusions

In conclusion, while we showed that the anti-biofilm efficacy of tobramycin could be improved by liposomal encapsulation, functionalization with AuNP resulted in premature leakage of tobramycin. Consequently, laser-irradiation and VNB-formation did not further improve *P. aeruginosa* biofilm eradication. Attaching tobramycin onto GQD on the other hand did result in stable formulations with high encapsulation efficiency. However, even though laser-induced VNB around GQD resulted in biofilm disruption, enhanced anti-biofilm effect could not be accomplished as tobramycin was not released from GQD upon laser irradiation. Altogether, our work shows that there is a delicate balance between stability and ability to release encapsulated antibiotics from light-responsive nanocarriers upon VNB formation and future research should re-evaluate the concept in more suitable nanocarriers.

Supplementary Materials:
Figure S1. Tobramycin calibration curve by measuring the tobramycin content by HPLC-UV. (a) A series of tobramycin solutions ranging from 5–200 μg mL^{-1} was analyzed by HPLC-UV. (b) The standard curve was

generated by plotting the Area Under Curve to the corresponding tobramycin concentration and fitting to a linear curve (average ± SD). Figure S2. (a) Investigating the effect of generating VNB in the presence of tobramycin (average ± SD). Tobramycin was added simultaneously with AuNP and laser treatment was performed so that VNB were created in close proximity of tobramycin. After 24 h incubation at 37 °C, cell survival was quantified by plate counting. AuNP + Tob: simultaneous addition of a 50 μL double concentrated gold nanoparticle solution and 50 μL double concentrated tobramycin, AuNP + Tob + laser: subsequent laser irradiation generated VNB in the presence of tobramycin. (b) Formation of VNB around AuNP that were attached to empty DOPC/DPPG liposomes (loaded with HEPES-buffer) instead of using free AuNP and its effect on additional tobramycin treatment (average ± SD). HEPES-loaded liposomes were prepared similarly as stated above, except using HEPES-buffer instead of tobramycin. Lipo:AuNP(HEPES): AuNP functionalized DOPC/DPPG liposomes containing HEPES-buffer, Lipo:AuNP(HEPES) + laser (+ Tob): laser irradiation resulted in generation of VNB around AuNP attached to DOPC/DPPG liposomes (+ tobramycin treatment) ($n = 3 \times 3$) (p-values < 0.05 were considered significant). Figure S3. (a) Tobramycin calibration curve by measuring the fluorescamine fluorescence of a series of tobramycin concentrations (1–100 μg mL^{-1}) by a fluorescence plate reader (355/460 nm) and fitting into a quadratic curve (mean ± SD) (b) Photothermal heating curve of GQD-tobramycin particles using a 980 nm continuous wave laser at 1, 2 and 4 W cm^{-2} (mean ± SD).

Author Contributions: K.B. and T.C. developed the conceptual ideas, directed the project and worked on the manuscript. S.C.D.S., R.B. and S.S. aided in interpreting the results and helped in writing the manuscript. E.T. carried out the experiments, analyzed the data, and wrote the manuscript with input from all authors. A.B., J.L., J.C.F., T.L., R.X., K.F., C.L. and A.U. were involved in the experimental design, analysis, and writing of the manuscript.

Acknowledgments: We would like to acknowledge the laboratory of Pharmaceutical Technology, University Ghent for performing the freeze-drying experiments

References

1. Van Acker, H.; Van Dijck, P.; Coenye, T. Molecular mechanisms of antimicrobial tolerance and resistance in bacterial and fungal biofilms. *Trends Microbiol.* **2014**, *22*, 326–333. [CrossRef]
2. Flemming, H.-C.; Wingender, J.; Szewzyk, U.; Steinberg, P.; Rice, S.A.; Kjelleberg, S. Biofilms: An emergent form of bacterial life. *Nat. Rev. Microbiol.* **2016**, *14*, 563–575. [CrossRef] [PubMed]
3. Flemming, H.-C.; Wingender, J. The biofilm matrix. *Nat. Rev. Microbiol.* **2010**, *8*, 623. [CrossRef]
4. Bjarnsholt, T.; Alhede, M.; Eickhardt-Sørensen, S.; Moser, C.; Kühl, M.; Jensen, P.; Høiby, N. The in vivo biofilm. *Trends Microbiol.* **2013**, *21*, 466–474. [CrossRef]
5. Allison, D.G.; Gilbert, P.; Lappin-Scott, H.M.; Wilson, M. *Community Structure and Co-Operation in Biofilms*; Cambridge University Press: Cambridge, UK, 2000.
6. Stoodley, P.; Wilson, S.; Hall-Stoodley, L.; Boyle, J.D.; Lappin-Scott, H.M.; Costerton, J.W. Growth and detachment of cell clusters from mature mixed-species biofilms. *Appl. Environ. Microbiol.* **2001**, *67*, 5608–5613. [CrossRef]
7. Forier, K.; Raemdonck, K.; De Smedt, S.C.; Demeester, J.; Coenye, T.; Braeckmans, K. Lipid and polymer nanoparticles for drug delivery to bacterial biofilms. *J. Control. Release* **2014**, *190*, 607–623. [CrossRef] [PubMed]
8. Meers, P.; Neville, M.; Malinin, V.; Scotto, A.W.; Sardaryan, G.; Kurumunda, R.; Mackinson, C.; James, G.; Fisher, S.; Perkins, W.R. Biofilm penetration, triggered release and in vivo activity of inhaled liposomal amikacin in chronic Pseudomonas aeruginosa lung infections. *J. Antimicrob. Chemother.* **2008**, *61*, 859–868. [CrossRef]
9. Horev, B.; Klein, M.I.; Hwang, G.; Li, Y.; Kim, D.; Koo, H.; Benoit, D.S.W. pH-Activated Nanoparticles for Controlled Topical Delivery of Farnesol To Disrupt Oral Biofilm Virulence. *ACS Nano* **2015**, *9*, 2390–2404. [CrossRef] [PubMed]

10. Teirlinck, E.; Xiong, R.; Brans, T.; Forier, K.; Fraire, J.; Van Acker, H.; Matthijs, N.; De Rycke, R.; De Smedt, S.C.; Coenye, T.; et al. Laser-induced vapour nanobubbles improve drug diffusion and efficiency in bacterial biofilms. *Nat. Commun.* **2018**, *9*, 4518. [CrossRef]
11. Lapotko, D. Plasmonic nanoparticle-generated photothermal bubbles and their biomedical applications. *Nanomedicine* **2009**, *4*, 813–845. [CrossRef]
12. Xiong, R.; Joris, F.; Liang, S.; De Rycke, R.; Lippens, S.; Demeester, J.; Skirtach, A.; Raemdonck, K.; Himmelreich, U.; De Smedt, S.C.; et al. Cytosolic Delivery of Nanolabels Prevents Their Asymmetric Inheritance and Enables Extended Quantitative in Vivo Cell Imaging. *Nano Lett.* **2016**, *16*, 5975–5986. [CrossRef] [PubMed]
13. Rukavina, Z.; Vanić, Ž. Current Trends in Development of Liposomes for Targeting Bacterial Biofilms. *Pharmaceutics* **2016**, *8*, 18. [CrossRef] [PubMed]
14. Forier, K.; Messiaen, A.-S.; Raemdonck, K.; Nelis, H.; De Smedt, S.; Demeester, J.; Coenye, T.; Braeckmans, K. Probing the size limit for nanomedicine penetration into Burkholderia multivorans and Pseudomonas aeruginosa biofilms. *J. Control. Release* **2014**, *195*, 21–28. [CrossRef] [PubMed]
15. Liu, J.; Cui, L.; Losic, D. Graphene and graphene oxide as new nanocarriers for drug delivery applications. *Acta Biomater.* **2013**, *9*, 9243–9257. [CrossRef] [PubMed]
16. Teodorescu, F.; Oz, Y.; Quéniat, G.; Abderrahmani, A.; Foulon, C.; Lecoeur, M.; Sanyal, R.; Sanyal, A.; Boukherroub, R.; Szunerits, S. Photothermally triggered on-demand insulin release from reduced graphene oxide modified hydrogels. *J. Control. Release* **2017**, *246*, 164–173. [CrossRef] [PubMed]
17. Yang, C.; Chan, K.K.; Xu, G.; Yin, M.; Lin, G.; Wang, X.; Lin, W.-J.; Birowosuto, M.D.; Zeng, S.; Ogi, T.; et al. Biodegradable Polymer-Coated Multifunctional Graphene Quantum Dots for Light-Triggered Synergetic Therapy of Pancreatic Cancer. *ACS Appl. Mater. Interfaces* **2019**, *11*, 2768–2781. [CrossRef] [PubMed]
18. Turkevich, J.; Stevenson, P.C.; Hillier, J. A study of the nucleation and growth processes in the synthesis of colloidal gold. *Discuss. Faraday Soc.* **1951**, *11*, 55. [CrossRef]
19. Forier, K. *Overcoming Biological Barriers to Nanomedicines for the Treatment of Pulmonary Biofilm Infections in Cystic Fibrosis*; Ghent University: Ghent, Belgium, 2014.
20. Mugabe, C.; Azghani, A.O.; Omri, A. Preparation and characterization of dehydration–rehydration vesicles loaded with aminoglycoside and macrolide antibiotics. *Int. J. Pharm.* **2006**, *307*, 244–250. [CrossRef]
21. Messiaen, A.-S.; Forier, K.; Nelis, H.; Braeckmans, K.; Coenye, T. Transport of Nanoparticles and Tobramycin-loaded Liposomes in Burkholderia cepacia Complex Biofilms. *PLoS ONE* **2013**, *8*, e79220. [CrossRef] [PubMed]
22. Lagacé, J.; Dubreuil, M.; Montplaisir, S. Liposome-encapsulated antibiotics: Preparation, drug release and antimicrobial activity against Pseudomonas aeruginosa. *J. Microencapsul.* **1991**, *8*, 53–61. [CrossRef]
23. Kirby, C.; Gregoriadis, G. Dehydration-Rehydration Vesicles: A Simple Method for High Yield Drug Entrapment in Liposomes. *Nat. Biotechnol.* **1984**, *2*, 979–984. [CrossRef]
24. Liu, J.; Xiong, R.; Brans, T.; Lippens, S.; Parthoens, E.; Zanacchi, F.C.; Magrassi, R.; Singh, S.K.; Kurungot, S.; Szunerits, S.; et al. Repeated photoporation with graphene quantum dots enables homogeneous labeling of live cells with extrinsic markers for fluorescence microscopy. *Light Sci. Appl.* **2018**, *7*, 47. [CrossRef]
25. Altinbasak, I.; Jijie, R.; Barras, A.; Golba, B.; Sanyal, R.; Bouckaert, J.; Drider, D.; Bilyy, R.; Dumych, T.; Paryzhak, S.; et al. Reduced Graphene-Oxide-Embedded Polymeric Nanofiber Mats: An "On-Demand" Photothermally Triggered Antibiotic Release Platform. *ACS Appl. Mater. Interfaces* **2018**, *10*, 41098–41106. [CrossRef]
26. Koo, H.; Allan, R.N.; Howlin, R.P.; Stoodley, P.; Hall-Stoodley, L. Targeting microbial biofilms: Current and prospective therapeutic strategies. *Nat. Rev. Microbiol.* **2017**, *15*, 740–755. [CrossRef]
27. Mathiyazhakan, M.; Wiraja, C.; Xu, C. A Concise Review of Gold Nanoparticles-Based Photo-Responsive Liposomes for Controlled Drug Delivery. *Nano-Micro Lett.* **2018**, *10*, 10. [CrossRef]
28. Zhao, Y.; Dai, X.; Wei, X.; Yu, Y.; Chen, X.; Zhang, X.; Li, C. Near-Infrared Light-Activated Thermosensitive Liposomes as Efficient Agents for Photothermal and Antibiotic Synergistic Therapy of Bacterial Biofilm. *ACS Appl. Mater. Interfaces* **2018**, *10*, 14426–14437. [CrossRef] [PubMed]
29. Meeker, D.G.; Jenkins, S.V.; Miller, E.K.; Beenken, K.E.; Loughran, A.J.; Powless, A.; Muldoon, T.J.; Galanzha, E.I.; Zharov, V.P.; Smeltzer, M.S.; et al. Synergistic Photothermal and Antibiotic Killing of Biofilm-Associated Staphylococcus aureus Using Targeted Antibiotic-Loaded Gold Nanoconstructs. *ACS Infect. Dis.* **2016**, *2*, 241–250. [CrossRef] [PubMed]

30. Wang, F.; Liu, J. Self-healable and reversible liposome leakage by citrate-capped gold nanoparticles: Probing the initial adsorption/desorption induced lipid phase transition. *Nanoscale* **2015**, *7*, 15599–15604. [CrossRef]
31. Lajunen, T.; Viitala, L.; Kontturi, L.-S.; Laaksonen, T.; Liang, H.; Vuorimaa-Laukkanen, E.; Viitala, T.; Le Guével, X.; Yliperttula, M.; Murtomäki, L.; et al. Light induced cytosolic drug delivery from liposomes with gold nanoparticles. *J. Control. Release* **2015**, *203*, 85–98. [CrossRef]
32. Hui, L.; Huang, J.; Chen, G.; Zhu, Y.; Yang, L. Antibacterial Property of Graphene Quantum Dots (Both Source Material and Bacterial Shape Matter). *ACS Appl. Mater. Interfaces* **2016**, *8*, 20–25. [CrossRef]
33. Fan, Z.; Po, K.H.L.; Wong, K.K.; Chen, S.; Lau, S.P. Polyethylenimine-Modified Graphene Oxide as a Novel Antibacterial Agent and Its Synergistic Effect with Daptomycin for Methicillin-Resistant Staphylococcus aureus. *ACS Appl. Nano Mater.* **2018**, *1*, 1811–1818. [CrossRef]
34. Turcheniuk, K.; Khanal, M.; Motorina, A.; Subramanian, P.; Barras, A.; Zaitsev, V.; Kuncser, V.; Leca, A.; Martoriati, A.; Cailliau, K.; et al. Insulin loaded iron magnetic nanoparticle-graphene oxide composites: Synthesis, characterization and application for in vivo delivery of insulin. *RSC Adv.* **2014**, *4*, 865–875. [CrossRef]
35. Teodorescu, F.; Quéniat, G.; Foulon, C.; Lecoeur, M.; Barras, A.; Boulahneche, S.; Medjram, M.S.; Hubert, T.; Abderrahmani, A.; Boukherroub, R.; et al. Transdermal skin patch based on reduced graphene oxide: A new approach for photothermal triggered permeation of ondansetron across porcine skin. *J. Control. Release* **2017**, *245*, 137–146. [CrossRef] [PubMed]

4

High Ultraviolet Absorption in Colloidal Gallium Nanoparticles Prepared from Thermal Evaporation

Flavio Nucciarelli [1,2,*], Iria Bravo [3,4], Sergio Catalan-Gomez [2], Luis Vázquez [5], Encarnación Lorenzo [3,4,6] and Jose Luis Pau [2]

1 Physics Department, Lancaster University, Lancaster LA1 4YB, UK
2 Grupo de Electrónica y Semiconductores, Departamento de Física Aplicada, Universida Autónoma de Madrid, 28049 Madrid, Spain; sergio.catalan@uam.es (S.C.-G.); joseluis.pau@uam.es (J.L.P.)
3 Departamento de Química Analítica y Análisis Instrumental, Universidad Autónoma de Madrid, Cantoblanco, 28049 Madrid, Spain; iria.bravo@uam.es (I.B.); encarnacion.lorenzo@uam.es (E.L.)
4 Instituto Madrileño de Estudios Avanzados en Nanociencia (IMDEA-Nanociencia), Faraday, 9, Campus UAM, Cantoblanco, 28049 Madrid, Spain
5 Materials Science Factory, Instituto de Ciencia de Materiales de Madrid, CSIC, 28049 Madrid, Spain; lvb@icmm.csic.es
6 Institute for Advanced Research in Chemical Sciences (IAdChem), Universidad Autónoma de Madrid, 28049 Madrid, Spain
* Correspondence: nccflv@gmail.com;

Abstract: New methods for the production of colloidal Ga nanoparticles (GaNPs) are introduced based on the evaporation of gallium on expendable aluminum zinc oxide (AZO) layer. The nanoparticles can be prepared in aqueous or organic solvents such as tetrahydrofuran in order to be used in different sensing applications. The particles had a quasi mono-modal distribution with diameters ranging from 10 nm to 80 nm, and their aggregation status depended on the solvent nature. Compared to common chemical synthesis, our method assures higher yield with the possibility of tailoring particles size by adjusting the deposition time. The GaNPs have been studied by spectrophotometry to obtain the absorption spectra. The colloidal solutions exhibit strong plasmonic absorption in the ultra violet (UV) region around 280 nm, whose width and intensity mainly depend on the nanoparticles dimensions and their aggregation state. With regard to the colloidal GaNPs flocculate behavior, the water solvent case has been investigated for different pH values, showing UV-visible absorption because of the formation of NPs clusters. Using discrete dipole approximation (DDA) method simulations, a close connection between the UV absorption and NPs with a diameter smaller than ~40 nm was observed.

Keywords: gallium; nanoparticle; colloid; AZO; tetrahydrofuran; thermal evaporation; DDA simulation

1. Introduction

Insulating, metal and semiconducting nanoparticles (NPs) have played a crucial role in the development of nanotechnology during the last two decades. The driving force in the field comes from the large surface-to-volume ratio and the manifestation of quantum effects that make the physical and chemical properties of these particles different from those found in bulk materials. Due to their applicability in different areas such as drug delivery [1], disinfection [2], photovoltaics [3], (bio)sensing [4,5], and catalysis [6,7], many studies have addressed the need for reproducible and reliable methods for the preparation of NPs. One of the main goals has been the production of colloidal suspensions in a liquid medium to ease the manipulation, storage, chemical modification and administration of the NPs in many practical cases.

Metal nanoparticles can be prepared as colloidal suspensions following bottom-up or top-down approaches. After Turkevich's work in the early fifties on the synthesis of gold NPs in aqueous solution at boiling temperature, one of the most popular bottom-up methods for producing metal NPs became the reduction of metal salts solved in a liquid phase [8,9]. Other liquid-phase methods commonly used for the fabrication of metal NPs have been magnetic-microwave heating [10], template synthesis [11] and electrodeposition [12]. They typically require the use of toxic reagents, which remain adsorbed on the surface after the NP synthesis and have potential adverse effects on human health [13]. On the other hand, gas phase methods are based on the nucleation and condensation of the gas molecules after supersaturation [14]. Examples of these methods are laser ablation, spray pyrolysis and furnace evaporation. Generally, size-selective precipitation is needed in liquid and gas phase methods to produce narrow size distributions [15].

Metal NPs are highly soluble in nonpolar organic solvents where, due to the low dielectric constant of the medium, the solvent molecules are not able to screen the surface charges around the particle, keeping a repulsive force between the NPs [16]. However, in polar solvents, the electrostatic surface interactions between the particles tend to produce their condensation and precipitation, giving rise to disordered aggregates that are not easily resoluble [17]. Those interactions are dominated by Van der Waals forces that increase inversely with the sixth power of distance between them [18]. The light-cluster interaction will depend on the number of agglomerated NPs, their special arrangement and the surface-environment interplay [19]. For that reason, the aqueous colloids must be stabilized to reduce surface interactions between NPs through the formation of self-assembled monolayers, polymeric coating or the use of ionic liquids [20,21]. The stabilization of the NPs is therefore considered a key task in the preparation of NPs, and the steps followed to achieve this are intimately involved in the fabrication process.

Gallium (Ga) is a low melting point metal whose interesting properties have attracted much attention in recent years. Colloidal NPs of this material with sizes lower than 50 nm have been characterized, exhibiting strong plasmonic absorption bands in the ultraviolet region [22,23], which makes them very attractive for surface-enhanced Raman scattering and fluorescence spectroscopy under UV excitation. They are in liquid state at room temperature surrounded by a thin gallium oxide layer that keeps them stable for months at ambient conditions [23]. The NPs have also shown a large charge storage capacity, fostering their investigation as one of the components in lithium ion batteries. Thanks to their fast reaction in the acidic environment found around tumors, they have also performed optimally for drug delivery purposes in cancer treatment [24]. Indeed, in vivo experiments in mice have demonstrated the reduction of tumors through the release of doxorubicin in the affected area without clear signs of toxicity. For this application, the size of the NPs must be very specific to allow surpassing of the cell barrier and delivery of the drug inside the cell to provoke the apoptosis of the tumoral cells.

Monodisperse colloidal Ga NPs have been synthesized using Ga alkylamides precursors in liquid-phase chemistry [23]. Another method based on the co-deposition of Ga atoms and solvent molecules at 77 K has been reported, yielding colloidal NPs in different organic solvents like tetrahydrofuran (THF), 2-propanol and acetone [22]. Furthermore, taking advantage of the liquid state of the Ga-In eutectic alloy, ultrasound sonication of bulk pieces has also enabled the production of large concentrations of NPs in a controlled manner [24]. In this work, we propose a bottom-up method for the production of GaNP colloids from the physical vapor deposition (PVD) of Ga under vacuum conditions on a solid substrate that contains a metal oxide expendable layer. The method provides a coating layer of self-assembled NPs without photolithographic steps.

The fabrication process enables the synthesis of colloids with a quite uniform NP size in polar protic and aprotic solvents after etching the oxide layer in an acidic solution. The aggregation of the NPs in THF and aqueous solutions is investigated through ultraviolet/visible spectrophotometry. The Ga NPs absorbance spectrum is usually found in the UV range [2] and it has its origin in the high plasmon frequency of the material. When a photon with the resonance energy impinges on the particle, a localized surface wave is built and the resultant energy can be absorbed or reemitted as scattered light. Additionally, the wave gives rise to a near-field enhancement around the structure. The nanoparticle size distribution can be tuned by changing the evaporation time of the gallium target. Furthermore, the use of physical vapor deposition methodologies reduces the cost, improves the reproducibility of the NP preparation, and enables pre-functionalization and size tuning separately from the selected solvent. The method can be easily scaled to large coverage areas to increase the fabrication yield. Moreover, in comparison to other methods, it produces a minimum amount of contaminant wastes.

2. Results and Discussion

2.1. Colloidal Synthesis Optimization

A colloidal solution of gallium nanoparticles was prepared following the procedure as shown in Figure 1. The step-by-step process will be analyzed in the methods and materials section, while the technological problems and the colloid opto-chemical features are presented here.

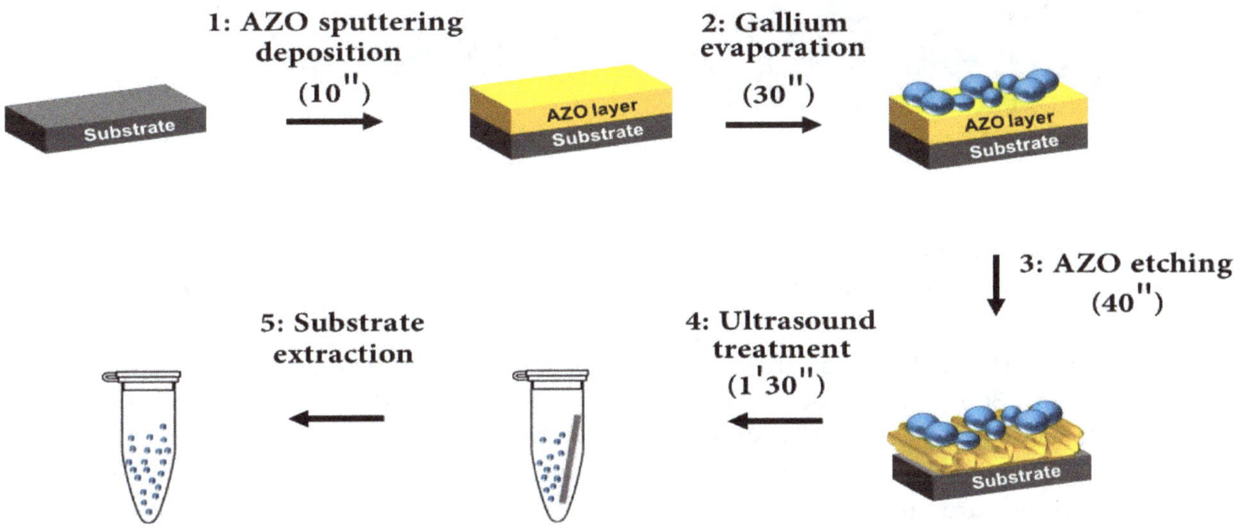

Figure 1. Colloidal Ga NPs synthesis. Step 1: about 300 nm of AZO expendable layer deposition on silicon substrate; Step 2: Ga NPs evaporation on the AZO layer; Step 3: the expendable layer is etched until NPs almost detached from the surface; Step 4: by means of ultrasound treatment, the NPs are transfer into the solution; Step 5: extraction of the substrate from the as-synthetized colloidal solution.

The endurance of the Ga nanoparticles in acidic environments was studied after their evaporation on a bare glass substrate. The substrates were immersed in a phosphoric acid/acetic acid/deionized water (1:1:75) bath for various times, ranging from 1 min to 8 h. The NP size distribution of each SEM image was determined and compared, in order to study the etching rate of the NPs. After a 1 min etch (Figure 2b) the NPs size did not change significantly, revealing a similar distribution as the un-etched sample (Figure 2a). This is a remarkable result, considering that the AZO layer has a total etching time of less than 1 min. Clearly, after 2 h (Figure 2c) small NPs started to disappear, as the biggest ones reduced their dimension, showing an increase of the number of NPs with an average size of 90 nm. After 8 h (not shown), all the NPs dissolved completely, leaving no residual of Ga on the glass surface.

In acidic medium, the NPs' oxide shell did not endure more than a few minutes [25,26], provoking the exposure of the gallium to the chemical solution. As time passed, the metal kept oxidizing slowly, and the new oxide layers were quickly dissolved until all the inner metal gallium disappeared. The comparison between histograms of 1 min and 2 h etched samples (Figure 2d) shows a decrease in the smaller NP population. For this reason, the etching process in our synthesis has been kept under 1 min, to avoid changes in the NPs' morphology.

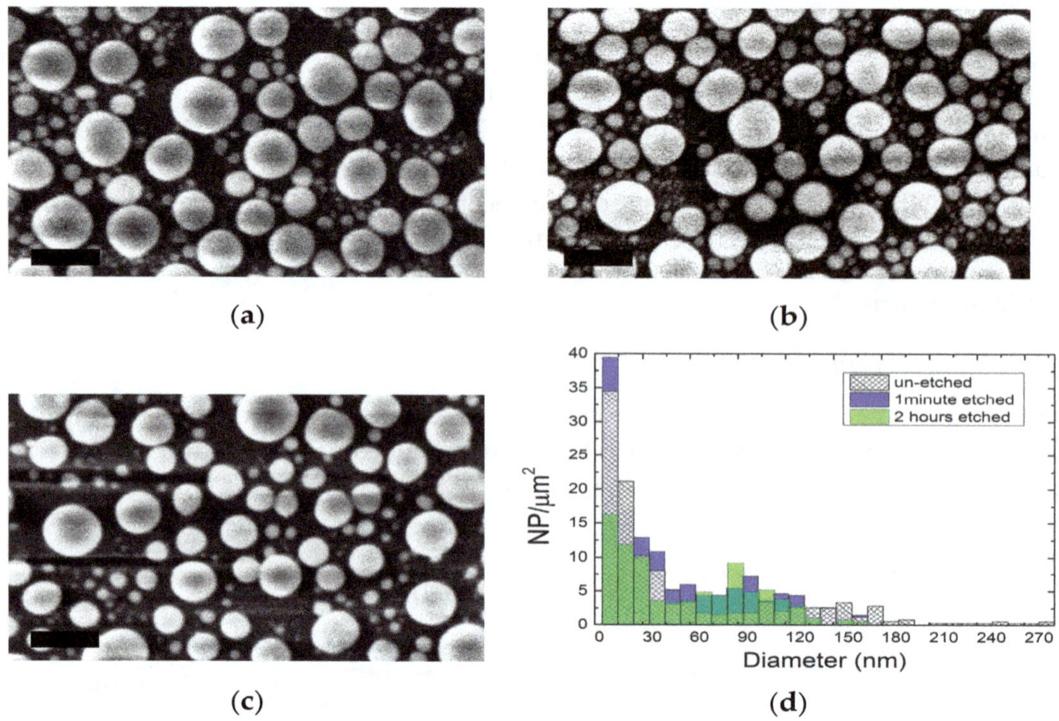

Figure 2. (**a**) Ga NPs evaporated on a glass substrate and immersed in an acidic bath for (**b**) 1 min; (**c**) 2 h. After 2 h, many of the smallest NPs have disappeared and the biggest ones have reduced their dimensions. (**d**) Histograms obtained from the SEM images. Scale bars are all 200 nm in length.

The AZO expendable layer in the preparation scheme (Figure 1) was deposited at room temperature (RT) and 300 °C in order to compare possible structural differences of the two surfaces and find the best conditions for the Ga NP deposition. As atomic force microscopy (AFM) analysis shows (Figure 3), the room temperature (RT) sample exhibited a mean surface roughness of 6 nm, while, for high-temperature growth, this value doubled to 13.6 nm. The images clearly show a smaller grain size for the RT layer, compared to the 300 °C sample.

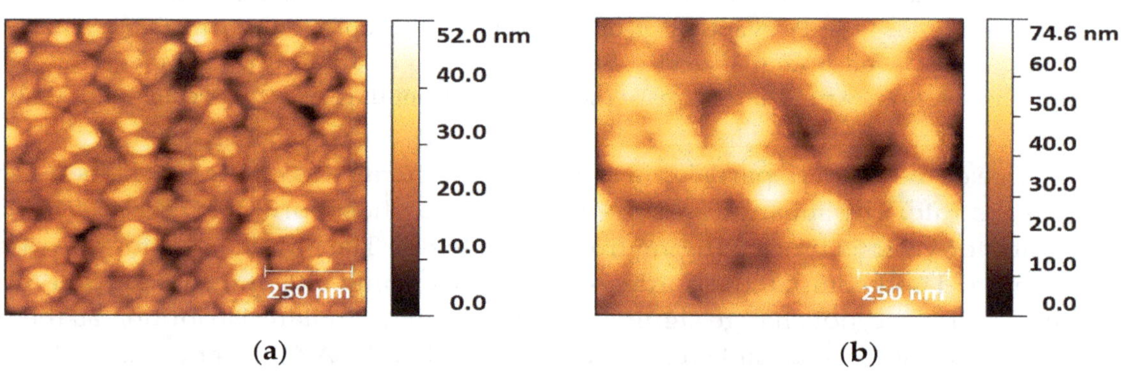

Figure 3. AFM images of the surface of AZO layer deposited at (**a**) RT and (**b**) 300 °C.

In order to identify the most suitable candidate for our process, Ga was evaporated on both AZO surfaces. Figure 4a,b show the as-evaporated distributions, where the first column is centered at a diameter of 12 nm with a width of ±6 nm, and includes the largest number of NPs in both cases. Comparing the RT and 300 °C histograms, the NPs' dimensions are not affected by the deposition temperature of the AZO, but their concentration is. In particular, the higher the AZO grown temperature, the higher the number of particles obtained per square micron. This increase in the number of particles might be related to the faceting of the AZO surface upon growth at higher temperature, and the larger surface to volume ratio in those samples.

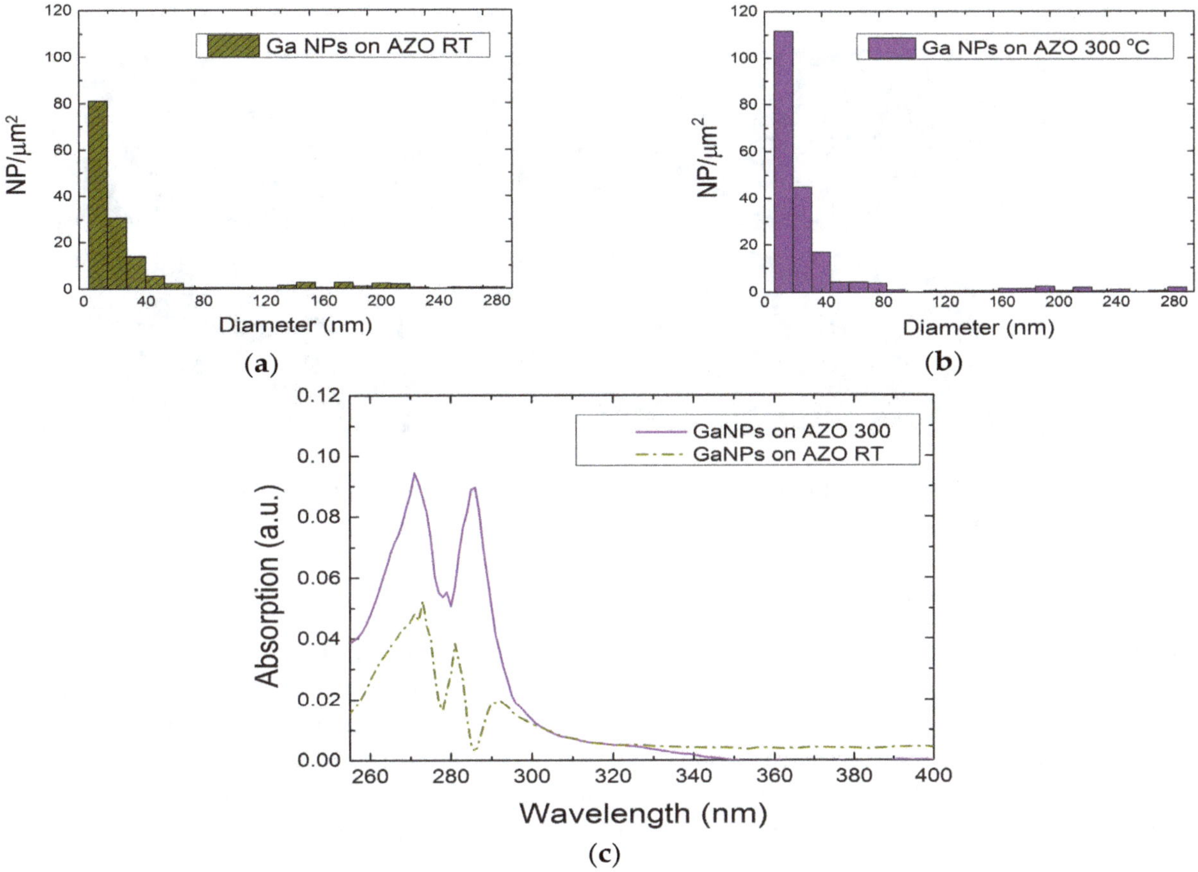

Figure 4. As-evaporated distributions of Ga NPs on (**a**) an AZO layer deposited at RT and (**b**) AZO layer deposited at 300 °C. (**c**) Absorption spectra in THF solvent.

In addition, the entire colloidal synthesis for both types of expendable layers was performed in order to study possible changes in the optical characteristics. For that aim, the absorption spectroscopy analysis between 200 nm and 1000 nm was carried out in THF solvent. A larger absorption in the UV spectra was observed for both samples (Figure 4c) and similar experiments have been conducted in sets of different AZO thickness. As expected, higher reproducibility and larger absorption was obtained in the solution prepared from the layers grown at 300 °C.

The expendable layer etching rate was also determined for AZO layers deposited at 300 °C. Layers of 300 nm were grown on silicon for that purpose. By measuring the etching depth as a function of time, the etching rate was found to be 18 nm/s. Similar samples with evaporated Ga NPs were also investigated, and the etching rate in this case was estimated to be 6 nm/s, three times slower than the uncovered case.

Further investigations of the evaporated Ga NPs on AZO layers grown at RT and 300 °C were carried out. The samples were etched in a phosphoric acid/acetic acid/deionized water (1:1:75) solution for 5 s, 15 s and 20 s (Figure 5). Scanning electron microscopy was performed to study the etching evolution of the expendable layer in order to obtain information on the minimum time to assure the NPs detachment from the hard support. As the AZO layer gradually disappears (dark zone indicated by arrows) the particles have higher probability to be dispersed in the solution by means of ultrasound treatment. After 5 s etching (Figure 5a,d), the layer was not dissolved and no significant changes were produced. Between 15 and 20 s, the NPs were less bonded to the expendable layer, and significant void areas are found between the largest NPs. Thus, the etching time for colloidal synthesis was chosen to be 40 s, in order to assure the highest NP detachment rate while preserving the NP size obtained after the evaporation.

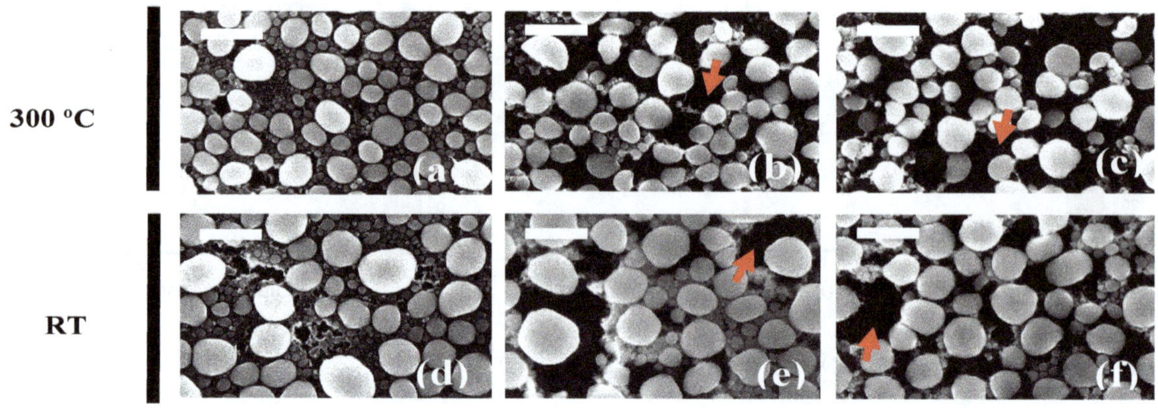

Figure 5. Ga NP/AZO/Si sample immersed in water/phosphoric acid/acetic acid bath for (**a**,**d**) 5 s (**b**,**e**) 15 s and (**c**,**f**) 20 s. Scale bar is 500 nm in length in all the pictures.

2.2. Optical Characteristics of Ga NPs

In order to study the interactions between the nanoparticles and the surrounding environment, two different solvents were used to prepare the Ga NPs colloids: deionized water (DIW) and tetrahydrofuran (THF). By means of aqueous solution, we studied how colloidal Ga NPs behave at different pH levels, while tetrahydrofuran was used to test the sample in a polar aprotic environment. Table 1 shows their chemical and optical features, which have also been used to study and simulate the developed samples. The protic and aprotic nature of the solvents influences the Ga NPs agglomeration status, as will be discussed later. The refractive index values were used to simulate the stand-alone and cluster nanoparticle status in both solvents with the use of the discrete dipole approximation (DDA) method. Finally, considering that both solvents heavily absorb light in the UV range, only the data obtained above their cut-off wavelength were analyzed.

Table 1. Solvent properties. Optical characteristics were extracted from [27].

Solvent	Class	Refractive Index @ 270 nm	Solvent λ Cut-Off (nm)
Water	Polar protic	1.33	190
THF	Polar aprotic	1.40	212

The stability of NPs in a solution depends on the interface between the surrounding media and the nanoparticle. In the case of colloids, the force balance between close particles may be expressed in consideration of different contributions such as gravitational, inertial, electrical and chemical reactivity [28]. Since the first two may be neglected for nanoparticles smaller than 0.5 μm [28,29], according to the Derjaguin, Landau, Vervey, and Overbeek (DLVO) theory [30,31] the electrostatic (repulsive) and Van der Waals (attractive) forces have a primary role in the inter-particle interaction. Recently, an extended DLVO theory (XDLVO) [32] demonstrated that the colloid's stability also takes into account other parameters, such as the ion concentration in the solution and the NP's hydrophobicity, which are relevant to our case of study.

2.2.1. Ga NPs in THF Solvent

The Ga NPs colloids in THF solution were prepared and optically characterized in the UV/visible range. Different NPs' size distributions were found using 30 s, 45 s and 60 s evaporation time. Figure 6 shows the related histograms of the three samples obtained from scanning electron microscopy (SEM) images. In the case of 30 s evaporation, a quasi-unimodal distribution was obtained, where the density of NPs with diameters lower than 40 nm density was higher than in the other two samples. Furthermore, SEM investigation of the tilt drop-cast sample shows that our colloidal Ga NPs have a hemispherical structure similar to that obtained by other authors [33,34]. During the Ga thermal evaporation, the NP's shape strongly depends of the nucleation process, which is related to the surface wettability of the substrate material. When the NPs' outer surface meets oxygen, an oxide shell covers the metal core and preserves the obtained geometry. The NPs also keep this geometry after being transferred to the solvent.

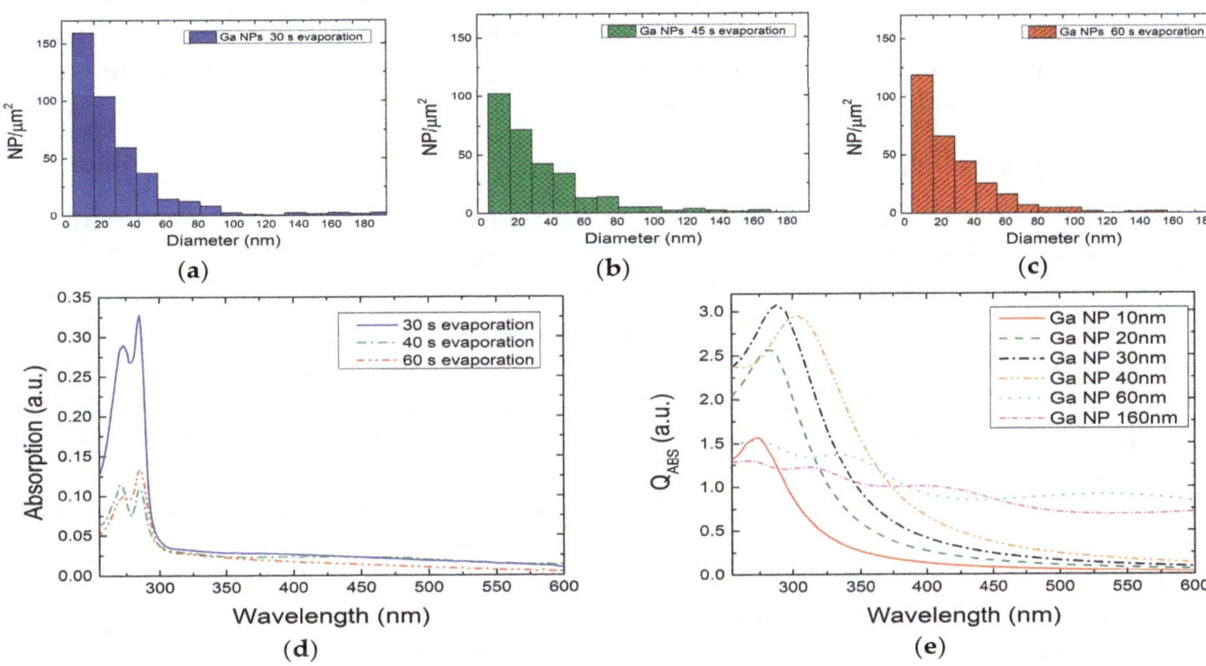

Figure 6. Ga NP distributions for (**a**) 30 s; (**b**) 45 s and (**c**) 60 s evaporation time; (**d**) The optical absorption was measured after colloidal preparation in THF; (**e**) Numerical simulation of the absorption efficiency (QABS) in structures with different diameters was carried out in order to find a relationship between the measured spectra and the NPs distributions.

The experimental absorption spectra of the three samples are shown in Figure 6d. As already discussed, THF has a cut-off absorbance wavelength of 212 nm, and the measurements were considered reliable only for data above that value. The curves have a similar shape, and exhibit a main absorption band between 260–300 nm with peaks centered at 273 nm and 285 nm. According to the Beer-Lambert's law, the measured optical signal is strictly related with the concentration of the smallest Ga NPs in the solution, which scales well for the exhibited distributions. Bigger NPs may contribute to the broad band between 300–600 nm.

In order to further understand the relationship between the experimental absorption and the Ga NP distribution, the light-matter interaction was theoretically studied through discrete-dipole approximation implemented by DDSCAT software (Department of Astrophysical Sciences, Princeton University, U.S.) [35]. The simulations consisted of hemispherical NPs of liquid gallium, with a 2 nm native oxide shell in THF solvent. The liquid gallium and gallium oxide permittivities were extracted from Knight et al. [34] and Rebiena et al. [36], respectively, whereas solvent refractive index refers to the value in Table 1. In order to reproduce the experimental conditions, the diameter of the NPs varies between 10 and 160 nm. Their optical behavior was studied for wavelengths ranging from 255 to 800 nm. In addition, a circular polarized light beam was set to emulate the un-polarized beam from the spectrophotometer source. Interaction cut-off and error tolerance parameters were set as high as possible, with values of 3×10^3 and 10^{-4}, respectively. The simulation results were expressed in terms of absorption efficiency (Q_{ABS}) and scattering efficiency (Q_{SCAT}), both of which depend on the target cross-sectional area. Note that the absorption coefficient is directly proportional to the particle diameter, while the scattering is proportional to the fourth power of it. Figure 6e shows Q_{ABS} for different NP diameters, where 30 nm has the highest value in the UV region. Thus, the experimental absorption band is likely related to absorption NPs of smaller diameters (10–40 nm). The biggest NPs contribute less to the absorption at low wavelengths, but they can be responsible for the absorption at higher wavelengths, according to the simulations.

It is believed that the stability of the Ga NPs is high, and does not show agglomeration effects. The outer gallium oxide shell may confer hydrophobic behavior, preventing agglomerative clustering. Similar results have been found by Vasiliev [37] during the investigation of polymer-coated Ag nanoparticles, where different agglomeration statuses for Ag—functionalized and unfunctionalized colloidal—were verified both in water and THF.

2.2.2. Ga NPs in Aqueous Solution

The behavior of the Ga NP colloids was also studied in the case of aqueous solution under different pH conditions. The acid/base level of the sample was achieved by adding NaOH 10^{-1} M and HCl 10^{-1} M solutions to reach the target acidity. Generally, the NPs' flocculation behavior is related to their surface charge, estimated from the zeta potential (ζ) measurement. The latter calculates the electrokinetic potential of the colloid and the further the value is from zero, the less the NPs aggregate. In the case of Ga oxide NPs, the zeta potential zero value—the so-called point of zero charge (PZC)—is set between pH 7.5–8.5 [38], and because of the Ga NPs oxide shell, it was assumed that our colloidal nanoparticles would have the same PZC value.

Figure 7a shows the comparison of colloidal absorption spectra for different pHs. The experiment was carried out on 3 mL of colloidal solution ranging in pH from 2.8 to 8.5, as described in the methods section. As the pH shifts from acidic to basic, the absorption decreases when the pH approaches 7.5 (near the PZC of the Ga oxide particle), and it starts rising again at a value of 8.5. The signal tends to decrease, getting close to the PZC pH value because of cluster formation, which reduces the colloidal absorption in the observed range. All the curves show a characteristic absorption band between 250 nm and 300 nm, which is related to the colloidal Ga NP size distribution as in the THF case.

Further simulation on NP agglomeration and comparison between the aqueous and the THF case absorption peak were investigated. To evaluate the Ga NPs cluster absorption trend in aqueous solution, different structures made from 8 to 64 sphere nanoparticles were simulated by the DDA method (Figure 7b,c) [39]. Usually, the light interaction with an NP cluster generates a higher scattering contribution than absorption according to the Mie theory and both contributions are red-shifted compared to the single particle characteristic. When more than 16 nanoparticles of 20 nm diameter agglomerate, the absorption decreases drastically, as shown in Figure 7b. A similar result was found for the 30 nm nanoparticle cluster, where the maximum agglomeration level before the absorption falls was 16 NPs, as well. For this reason, the decreasing trend of the absorption for the pH change may be explained by the agglomeration theory. The closer the pH is to the PZC, the higher the agglomeration occurring between NPs, which leads to a lower absorption signal. In addition, the NP plasmon resonance condition for the aqueous and THF solutions was compared. As expected, the nanoparticle absorption peak shifts in value depending on the medium permittivity (Figure 7d). The comparison of 30 nm Ga hemisphere with 2 nm oxide shell in THF (n = 1.4) and aqueous solution (n = 1.33) shows a red-shifted curve in the case of the higher refractive index solution, with absorption peaks displayed at 285 nm and 273 nm, respectively. Later, these results were compared with the measured absorption band and good agreement was observed.

In conclusion, the Ga NPs' oxide shell likely acts as a hydrophilic material in water, provoking the agglomeration phenomenon. Also, by means of different pH, the ion concentration around the colloidal NPs can be varied and the cluster formation may change because of it.

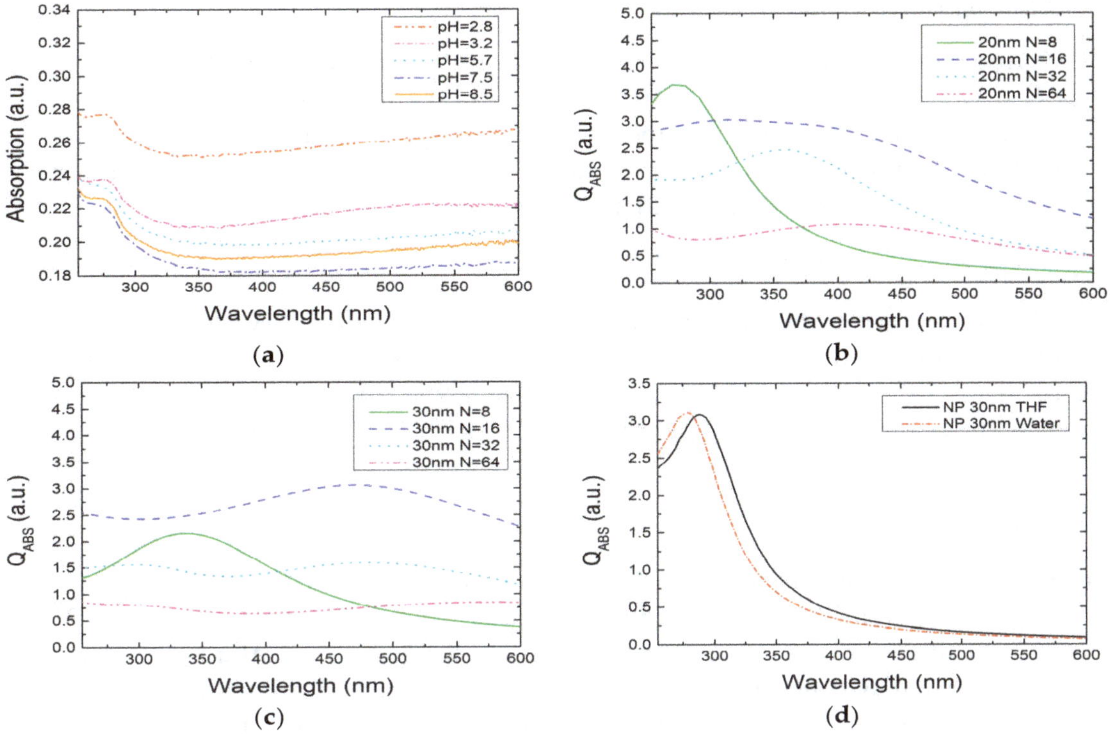

Figure 7. (**a**) Absorption measurements of aqueous colloidal solutions for different pH levels ranging from 2.8 to 8.5. Results of the simulations for NP clusters made of N number of agglomerated spheres with (**b**) 20 nm and (**c**) 30 nm diameter. (**d**) Calculated QABS of NPs in THF and aqueous solution.

3. Materials and Methods

3.1. Ga NPs Synthesis

A colloidal solution of gallium nanoparticles was prepared following the procedure as shown in Figure 1. First, a substrate of silicon with an area of 0.5 cm × 2 cm was cleaved and cleaned using an aqueous solution of 40% hydrofluoric acid in order to remove the native oxide. The AZO [40] expendable layer was deposited using an Alcatel A450 radio frequencies (RF) sputtering system. For the sake of comparison, the layers were prepared depositing at room temperature and 300 °C. The system comprises an RF source set at 150 W and a 50 sccm Ar flow to generate the plasma that sputters the AZO target (Kurt J. Lesker ZnO/Al_2O_3, 2% Standard Doping). Prior to deposition, the target was sputtered for 1 min to remove impurities. The deposition time for the AZO layer was 10 min under a pressure of 10^{-2} mbar to obtain a 300 nm thick layer. The AZO was chosen taking into account its fast etching in moderately acidic solutions.

Gallium was evaporated [41] on the expendable layer using a Joule-effect Edwards E306 evaporation system (Moorfield, Knutsford, UK). For our process, 0.28 g of solid Ga (99.9999%) was heated for 30 s with a 50 W power under 10^{-6} Torr pressure. The distance from the material heater to the sample was set at 20 cm. An ice cooling system was employed to keep the substrate temperature as low as possible, in order to limit the metal surface mobility during the nucleation process. During the growth, the lower the substrate temperature the less NPs coarsening occurs.

To prepare the colloidal solutions, several vials of 3 mL volume were filled with the following solvents: DIW and THF. After Ga deposition and extraction from the thermal evaporation system, the sample was immersed in a phosphoric acid/acetic acid/deionized water (1:1:75) bath for 40 s to partially etch the AZO layer and weaken the structural support of the NPs. Later, it was rinsed in water and promptly inserted into the selected solvent. To allow the NPs transfer from the sample to the solution, an ultrasound treatment of 1′30″ was used.

3.2. Scanning Electron Microscopy (SEM)

The SEM investigation was carried out using a Philips XL30 S-FEG microscope (Philips, Amsterdam, The Netherlands) under a 10^{-3} bar pressure at room temperature. The colloidal solution was drop cast on a clean silicon substrate, and promptly analyzed in order to avoid possible contamination effects. After the investigation, images were post-processed by Gwyddion open-source software to estimate nanoparticle size and distribution [42].

3.3. Atomic Force Microscopy (AFM)

In order to characterize the sputtered AZO layer surface, an Agilent PicoPlus 5500 AFM (Agilent Technologies Inc., Santa Clara, CA, USA) was used operating in dynamic mode. The analyzed samples comprised a 300 nm thick AZO layer grown on a silicon substrate at room temperature and 300 °C. Images were analyzed and post-processed by Gwyddion open source software to investigate the surface morphology of both samples.

3.4. pH Measurement

Colloidal sample pH was varied by adding NaOH 10^{-1} M and HCl 10^{-1} M solutions to achieve the target acidity. The total added liquid did not exceed 0.1% of the original volume (3 mL), in order to avoid changes of the colloid concentration and, therefore, the optical absorption signal. For all solutions, the pH was measured before and after the spectrophotometry analysis to rule out pH changes during measurement due to rearrangement of ions in the solution.

3.5. UV-Visible Spectrophotometry

UV-visible spectra of the different colloidal samples were acquired using a Thermo Scientific GO spectrophotometer. For the analysis, differential optical absorption was measured on the colloidal solution poured in a 1.0 cm quartz cuvette using the same colloidal solvent as reference. By means of the equipment, temperature was fixed at 25 °C and exposed to a light ranging from 200 nm to 1000 nm in wavelength, with a system resolution of 1 nm.

4. Conclusions

We investigated the properties of the colloidal Ga NPs in THF and aqueous solvents with the use of SEM, AFM and UV spectrophotometer. The colloidal solutions were prepared from the evaporation of nanoparticles on an expandable layer, which gave plenty of possible solutions (such as ion implantation or thermal annealing) for the modification of physico-chemical properties. The AZO expandable layer growth was optimized in order to achieve the highest yield and reproducibility of the synthesis. The NPs' endurance during the etch step of the process was also proved. The colloidal Ga NPs were surrounded by GaOx, and had different agglomeration status depending on the solvent. In the aqueous solution case, the oxide shell had a hydrophilic behavior and NPs tended to agglomerate promptly, depending on the pH. A broad absorption along the UV-visible spectrum due to cluster formation was observed. In the THF solvent, the gallium oxide shell instead acted as a hydrophobic interface, and colloidal flocculation was mostly prevented. In that case, a strong and quite narrow UV absorption band was measured. Later, colloidal absorption bands were explained by DDA numerical simulations. Jointly with the use of the centrifugation process, it will be possible to select different absorption bands, depending on the evaporated nanoparticles' dimensions. Future works may use these results to investigate and develop new medical and innovative applications based on Ga NPs.

Acknowledgments: The authors would to thank Eduardo Ruiz Martin for helping with the clean room processes and for fruitful discussions. We are also grateful to the international PROMIS project, framed in the Horizon 2020 research and innovation program under the Marie Sklodowska-Curie grant agreement No. 641899. This research is supported by the MINECO (CTQ2014-53334-C2-2-R, MAT2014-54231-C4-1-P and MAT2016-80394-R) and Comunidad de Madrid (NANOAVANSES ref. S2013/MIT-3029) project. I.B. gratefully acknowledges the FPI-2012 Grant from Spanish Ministerio de Economía y Competitividad.

Author Contributions: F.N. and J.L.P. conceived and designed the experiments; F.N. performed the experiments; F.N. and J.L.P. analyzed the data; S.C.-G., I.B., L.V., and E.L. contributed reagents/materials/analysis tools; F.N. wrote the paper.

References

1. Dreaden, E.C.; Austin, L.A.; Mackey, M.A.; El-Sayed, M.A. Size matters: Gold NPs in targeted cancer drug delivery. *Ther. Deliv.* **2012**, *3*, 457–478. [CrossRef] [PubMed]
2. Yuan, Z.; Chen, Y.; Li, T.; Yu, C.-P. Reaction of silver NPs in the disinfection process. *Chemosphere* **2013**, *93*, 619–625. [CrossRef] [PubMed]
3. Wang, P.H.; Millard, M.; Brolo, A.G. Optimizing Plasmonic Silicon Photovoltaics with Ag and Au Nanoparticle Mixtures. *J. Phys. Chem.* **2014**, *118*, 5889–5895. [CrossRef]
4. Doria, G.; Conde, J.; Veigas, B.; Giestas, L.; Almeida, M.; Assunção, M.; Rosa, J.; Baptista, P.V. Noble Metal NPs for Biosensing Applications. *Sensors* **2012**, *12*, 1657–1687. [CrossRef] [PubMed]
5. Tiwari, P.M.; Vig, K.; Dennis, V.A.; Singh, S.R. Functionalized Gold Nanoparticles and Their Biomedical Applications. *Nanomaterials* **2011**, *1*, 31–63. [CrossRef] [PubMed]
6. Corti, C.W.; Holliday, R.J.; Thompson, D.T. Progress towards the commercial application of gold catalysts. *Top. Catal.* **2007**, *44*, 331–343. [CrossRef]
7. Hudson, R.; Hamasaka, G.; Osako, T.; Yamada, Y.M.A.; Li, C.-J.; Uozumi, Y.; Moores, A. Highly efficient iron(0) nanoparticle-catalyzed hydrogenation in water in flow. *Green Chem.* **2013**, *15*, 2141–2148. [CrossRef]
8. Kimling, J.; Maier, M.; Okenve, B.; Kotaidis, V.; Ballot, H.; Plech, A. Turkevich Method for Gold Nanoparticle Synthesis Revisited. *J. Phys. Chem.* **2006**, *110*, 15700–15707. [CrossRef] [PubMed]
9. Turkevich, J.; Stevenson, P.C.; Hillier, J. A study of the nucleation and growth processes in the synthesis of colloidal gold. *Discuss. Faraday Soc.* **1951**, *11*, 55–75. [CrossRef]
10. Chikan, V.; McLaurin, E.J. Rapid Nanoparticle Synthesis by Magnetic and Microwave Heating. *Nanomaterials* **2016**, *6*, 85. [CrossRef] [PubMed]
11. McCaffrey, R.; Long, H.; Jin, Y.; Sanders, A.; Park, W.; Zhang, W. Template Synthesis of Gold NPs with an Organic Molecular Cage. *J. Am. Chem. Soc.* **2014**, *136*, 1782–1785. [CrossRef] [PubMed]
12. Hezard, T.; Fajerwerg, K.; Evrard, D.; Collière, V.; Behra, P.; Gros, P. Gold NPs electrodeposited on glassy carbon using cyclic voltammetry: Application to Hg(II) trace analysis. *J. Electroanal. Chem.* **2012**, *664*, 46–52. [CrossRef]
13. Bhau, B.S.; Ghosh, S.; Puri, S.; Borah, B.; Sarmah, D.K.; Khan, R. Green synthesis of gold NPs from the leaf extract of Nepenthes khasiana and antimicrobial assay. *Adv. Mater. Lett.* **2015**, *6*, 55–58. [CrossRef]
14. Kruis, F.E.; Fissan, H.; Peled, A. Synthesis of NPs in the gas phase for electronic, optical and magnetic applications—A review. *J. Aerosol Sci.* **1998**, *29*, 511–535. [CrossRef]
15. Kowalczyk, B.; Lagzi, I.; Grzybowski, B.A. Nanoseparations: Strategies for size and/or shape-selective purification of NPs. *Curr. Opin. Colloid Interface Sci.* **2011**, *16*, 135–148. [CrossRef]
16. Markovich, G.; Collier, C.P.; Henrichs, S.E.; Remacle, F.; Levine, R.D.; Heath, J.R. Architectonic Quantum Dot Solids. *Acc. Chem. Res.* **1999**, *32*, 415–423. [CrossRef]
17. Collier, C.P.; Vossmeyer, T.; Heath, J.R. Nanocrystal superlattices. *Annu. Rev. Phys. Chem.* **1998**, *49*, 371–404. [CrossRef] [PubMed]
18. Fendler, J.H. Colloid Chemical Approach to Nanotechnology. *Korean J. Chem. Eng.* **2001**, *18*, 1–13. [CrossRef]
19. Tomalia, D.A.; Khanna, S.N. A Systematic Framework and Nanoperiodic Concept for Unifying Nanoscience: Hard/Soft Nanoelements, Superatoms, Meta-Atoms, New Emerging Properties, Periodic Property Patterns, and Predictive Mendeleev-like Nanoperiodic Tables. *Chem. Rev.* **2016**, *116*, 2705–2774. [CrossRef] [PubMed]
20. Ulman, A. Formation and structure of self-assembled monolayers. *Chem. Rev.* **1996**, *96*, 1533–1554. [CrossRef] [PubMed]
21. Sakai, T.; Alexandridis, P. Single-Step Synthesis and Stabilization of Metal NPs in Aqueous Pluronic Block Copolymer Solutions at Ambient Temperature. *Langmuir* **2004**, *20*, 8426–8430. [CrossRef] [PubMed]
22. Meléndrez, M.F.; Cárdenas, G.; Arbiol, J. Synthesis and characterization of gallium colloidal NPs. *J. Colloid Interface Sci.* **2010**, *346*, 279–287. [CrossRef] [PubMed]

23. Yarema, M.; Wörle, M.; Rossell, M.D.; Erni, R.; Caputo, R.; Protesescu, L.; Kravchyk, K.V.; Dirin, D.N.; Lienau, K.; von Rohr, F.; et al. Monodisperse Colloidal Gallium NPs: Synthesis, Low Temperature Crystallization, Surface Plasmon Resonance and Li-Ion Storage. *J. Am. Chem. Soc.* **2014**, *136*, 12422–12430. [CrossRef] [PubMed]
24. Lu, Y.; Hu, Q.; Lin, Y.; Pacardo, D.B.; Wang, C.; Sun, W.; Ligler, F.S.; Dickey, M.D.; Gu, Z. Transformable liquid-metal nanomedicine. *Nat. Commun.* **2014**, *136*, 12422–12430. [CrossRef] [PubMed]
25. Ohira, S.; Arai, N. Wet chemical etching behavior of β-Ga_2O_3 single crystal. *Phys. Status Solidi C* **2008**, *5*, 3116–3118. [CrossRef]
26. Junga, Y.; Ahna, J.; Baikb, K.H.; Kimc, D.; Peartond, S.J.; Rene, F.; Kima, J. Chemical Etch Characteristics of N-Face and Ga-Face GaN by Phosphoric Acid and Potassium Hydroxide Solutions. *J. Electrochem. Soc.* **2012**, *159*, H117–H120. [CrossRef]
27. Snyder, L.R.; Kirkland, J.J.; Glajch, J.L. *Practical HPLC Method Development*, 2nd ed.; John Wiley & Sons: Hoboken, NJ, USA, 1997.
28. Ring, T.A. *Fundamentals of Ceramic Powder Processing and Synthesis*; Academic Press Inc.: New York, NY, USA, 1996.
29. Tsuda, A.; Henry, F.S.; Butler, J.P. Particle transport and deposition: Basic physics of particle kinetics. *Compr. Physiol.* **2013**, *3*, 1437–1471. [PubMed]
30. Verwey, E.J.; Overbeek, J.T.G. *Theory of the Stability of Lyophobic Colloids*; Elsevier: Amsterdam, The Netherlands, 1948.
31. Derjaguin, B.V.; Lanadau, L. Theory of the stability of strongly charged lyophobic sols and of the adhesion of strongly charged particles in solution of electrolytes. *Acta Physicochim. USSR* **1941**, *14*, 633–662. [CrossRef]
32. Hotze, E.M.; Phenrat, T.; Lowry, G.V. Nanoparticle Aggregation: Challenges to Understanding Transport and Reactivity in the Environment. *J. Environ. Qual.* **2010**, *39*, 1909–1924. [CrossRef] [PubMed]
33. Losurdo, M.; Suvorova, A.; Rubanov, S.; Hingerl, K.; Brown, A.S. Thermally stable coexistence of liquid and solid phases in gallium nanoparticles. *Nat. Mater.* **2016**, *15*, 995–1002. [CrossRef] [PubMed]
34. Knight, M.W.; Coenen, T.; Yang, Y.; Brenny, B.J.M.; Losurdo, M.; Brown, A.S.; Everitt, H.O.; Polman, A. Gallium Plasmonics: Deep Subwavelength Spectroscopic Imaging of Single and Interacting Gallium Nanoparticles. *ACS Nano* **2015**, *9*, 2049–2060. [CrossRef] [PubMed]
35. Draine, B.T.; Flatau, P.J. Discrete dipole approximation for scattering calculations. *J. Opt. Soc. Am. A* **1994**, *11*, 1491–1499. [CrossRef]
36. Rebiena, M.; Henrion, W.; Hong, M.; Mannaerts, J.P.; Fleischer, M. Optical properties of gallium oxide thin films. *Appl. Phys. Lett.* **2002**, *81*, 250. [CrossRef]
37. Vasiliev, A.N.; Gulliver, E.A.; Khinast, J.G.; Riman, R.E. Highly dispersible polymer-coated silver Nanoparticle. *Surf. Coat. Technol.* **2009**, *203*, 2841–2844. [CrossRef]
38. Kosmulski, M. Pristine Points of Zero Charge of Gallium and Indium Oxides. *J. Colloid Interface Sci.* **2001**, *238*, 225–227. [CrossRef] [PubMed]
39. Shen, Y.; Draine, B.T.; Johnson, E.T. Modeling Porous Dust Grains with Ballistic Aggregates. I. Geometry and Optical Properties. *Astrophys. J.* **2008**, *689*, 260–275. [CrossRef]
40. Minami, T.; Nanot, H.; Takata, S. Highly Conductive and Transparent Aluminum Doped Zinc Oxide Thin Films Prepared by RF Magnetron Sputtering. *Jpn. J. Appl. Phys.* **1984**, *23*, 776–779. [CrossRef]
41. Marín, A.G.; Hernández, M.J.; Ruiz, E.; Abad, J.M.; Lorenzo, E.; Piqueras, J.; Pau, J.L. Immunosensing platform based on gallium nanoparticle arrays on silicon substrates. *Biosens. Bioelectron.* **2015**, *74*, 1069–1075. [CrossRef] [PubMed]
42. Nečas, D.; Klapetek, P. Gwyddion: An open-source software for SPM data analysis. *Cent. Eur. J. Phys.* **2012**, *10*, 181–188. [CrossRef]

5

Stealth and Cationic Nanoliposomes as Drug Delivery Systems to Increase Andrographolide BBB Permeability

Vieri Piazzini [1], Elisa Landucci [2], Giulia Graverini [1], Domenico E. Pellegrini-Giampietro [2], Anna Rita Bilia [1] and Maria Camilla Bergonzi [1,*]

1 Department of Chemistry, University of Florence, Via Ugo Schiff 6, Sesto Fiorentino, 50019 Florence, Italy; vieri.piazzini@unifi.it (V.P.); giulia.graverini@stud.unifi.it (G.G.); ar.bilia@unifi.it (A.R.B.)
2 Department of Health Sciences, Section of Clinical Pharmacology and Oncology, University of Florence, Viale Pieraccini 6, 50139 Florence, Italy; elisa.landucci@unifi.it (E.L.); domenico.pellegrini@unifi.it (D.E.P.-G.)
* Correspondence: mc.bergonzi@unifi.it;

Abstract: (1) Background: Andrographolide (AG) is a natural compound effective for the treatment of inflammation-mediated neurodegenerative disorders. The aim of this investigation was the preparation of liposomes to enhance the penetration into the brain of AG, by modifying the surface of the liposomes by adding Tween 80 (LPs-AG) alone or in combination with Didecyldimethylammonium bromide (DDAB) (CLPs-AG). (2) Methods: LPs-AG and CLPs-AG were physically and chemically characterized. The ability of liposomes to increase the permeability of AG was evaluated by artificial membranes (PAMPA) and hCMEC/D3 cells. (3) Results: Based on obtained results in terms of size, homogeneity, ζ-potential and EE%. both liposomes are suitable for parenteral administration. The systems showed excellent stability during a month of storage as suspensions or freeze-dried products. Glucose resulted the best cryoprotectant agent. PAMPA and hCMEC/D3 transport studies revealed that LPs-AG and CLPs-AG increased the permeability of AG, about an order of magnitude, compared to free AG without alterations in cell viability. The caveolae-mediated endocytosis resulted the main mechanism of up-take for both formulations. The presence of positive charge increased the cellular internalization of nanoparticles. (4) Conclusions: This study shows that developed liposomes might be ideal candidates for brain delivery of AG.

Keywords: liposomes; brain delivery; surfactant; cationic liposomes; andrographolide; PAMPA; hCMEC/D3 cells

---

1. Introduction

The major hindrance in the treatment of brain disorders is the blood–brain barrier (BBB), which prevents the transfer of most drugs, peptides and large molecules across the endothelial cell lining to protect the brain from undesirable side effects. To overcome such problems various approaches are used.

The liposomes offer a promising tool to resolve the low permeability and high selectivity of the BBB.

Liposomes are non-toxic, biocompatible and biodegradable drug carrier systems. Their structure which is composed of phospholipids with an aqueous reservoir allows the encapsulation of a wide variety of hydrophilic and hydrophobic agents [1–4]. Their phospholipid bilayer structure, similar to physiological membranes, makes them more compatible with the lipoid layer of BBB and increase the permeability of the drug.

Liposomes allow relatively higher intracellular uptake than other particulate systems, due to their sub-cellular size. They are highly studied for the treatment of central nervous system's pathologies such as infections, cerebral ischemia, brain tumors and neurodegenerative diseases, for instance Parkinson's and Alzheimer's [5,6]. Several studies have reported an increased transport across the BBB of encapsulated drugs both through intracerebral and intravenous administration [7].

The surface can be modified with functional ligands to enhance the brain targeting. The functionalized nanoparticles with structures able to interact with targets on the surface of the BBB represents a tool of enormous potentiality to ameliorate the bioavailability and to reduce side effects. Several studies on animal models of Alzheimer's disease demonstrated the efficacy of functionalized liposomes to cross BBB and ameliorate impaired cognitions [8–10].

In a previous research studies, the authors developed solid lipid nanoparticles [11] and polymeric nanoparticles [12] to deliver the andrographolide (AG), a natural compound, through the central nervous system and ameliorate its biopharmaceutical characteristics.

AG is one of the characteristic diterpenoids from *Andrographis paniculata* with a wide spectrum of biological activities, being anti-inflammatory, anticancer, hepatoprotective and antihyperlipidemic. AG is involved in oxidative stress-related pathways implicated in stroke pathogenesis and it protects against ischemic stroke [13]. Furthermore, it has shown protection against damage induced by amyloid-β oligomers in vitro, it reduces amyloid-β levels and tau phosphorylation in mice, it modulates the formation of amyloid plaques and it retrieves spatial memory functions in Alzheimer's disease transgenic mouse model [14]. The high lipid solubility of AG would permit its penetration of the BBB but its poor water solubility and stability reduces its bioavailability: indeed, these factors are the greatest drawbacks for clinical application [15,16].

In recent years, surfactants such as Tween 80 have been studied for the application in liposomal formulations. The sterically stabilized liposomes exhibited a superior entrapment stability compared with surfactant-free liposomes [17]. The surfactant during preparation of liposomes helps in efficient emulsification resulting in decreasing the size of vesicles and promotes the flexibility of the vesicle to penetrate the biological cell membranes. Tween 80 was also able to enhance liposomes half-life [18] and, in addition, has interesting properties including the formation of a superficial coating on liposomes that can produce "stealth" nanocarriers. Tween 80 can adsorb ApoE, which subsequently binds to its specific LDL receptor by increasing carrier endocytosis at the level of cerebral endothelial cells [4,19–22]. Finally, this surfactant is also an inhibitor of the P-gp effluent pump [23].

Another approach is the use of the cationic liposomes, able to cross the BBB via absorption-mediated transcytosis [24]. Several studies have shown that these cationic nanocarriers are more efficient vehicles for drug delivery to the brain than conventional, neutral, or anionic liposomes, possibly due to the electrostatic interactions between the cationic liposomes and the negatively charged cell membranes, enhancing nanoparticle uptake. In particular, this kind of liposome interacts with the endothelial cells of microvessels rich in lecithin, which binds positively charged material and induces its cell internalization process through endocytosis [6,24]. Furthermore, the cationic liposomes very easily fuse with cells.

The aim of the present study was the formulation of nano-sized liposomes of AG for brain targeting. Tween 80 alone or in combination with Didecyldimethylammonium bromide (DDAB) were considered to investigate the effects, on chemical and physical aspects, stability, release characteristics, in vitro uptake and permeability of the AG liposomes and to ameliorate the loading and the solubility of AG.

Liposomes were evaluated for various formulation parameters (size, polydispersity, ζ-potential, morphology, chemical and physical stability, in vitro release) and the optimized formulations were studied and characterized with in vitro tests. The ability of liposomes to increase the permeability of AG was evaluated by a Parallel Artificial Membrane Permeability Assay (PAMPA) [25]. Furthermore, the uptake of liposomes as well as their permeability across hCMEC/D3 monolayer cells, as an in vitro BBB model [11,26,27], were considered. Cell viability and cytotoxicity studies were also conducted.

2. Materials and Methods

2.1. Materials

Egg phosphatidylcholine (Phospholipon 90G) was purchased from Lipoid AG, Cologne, Germany with the support of its Italian agent AVG srl, Milan, Italy. Andrographolide, Cholesterol $\geq$95%, Didecyldimethylammonium bromide (DDAB, 98%), Coumarin-6 (6C), Fluorescein sodium salt (NaF), Human Serum Albumin (HSA), Phosphate Buffered Saline (PBS 0.01 M) powder (29 mM NaCl, 2.5 mM KCl, 7.4 mM $Na_2HPO_4{\cdot}7H_2O$, 1.3 mM KH_2PO_4) pH 7.4 and Tween 80 were from Sigma Aldrich, Milan, Italy. Glucose anhydrous and sucrose came from Merck, Darmstadt, Germany. 96-well Multi-Screen PAMPA filter plate (pore size 0.45 μm) were purchased from Millipore Corporation, Tullagreen, Carrigtwohill, County Cork, Ireland. Porcine polar brain lipid was obtained from Avanti Polar Lipids, Inc., Alabaster, AL, USA. All the solvents used (acetonitrile, dichloromethane, dodecane, ethanol, formic acid, methanol) were HPLC grade from Sigma Aldrich, Milan, Italy. Water was purified by Millipore, Milford, MA, USA, Milli-Qplus system. Phosphotungstic acid (PTA) was from Electron Microscopy Sciences, Hatfield, PA, USA.

2.2. Preparation of Liposomal Carriers

Stealth liposomes containing Tween 80 (LPs) and cationic liposomes (CLPs) with Tween 80 and DDAB were prepared according to the thin layer evaporation method [28]. For LPs, 160 mg of egg phosphatidylcholine (P90G) and 10 mg of cholesterol (CHOL) were dissolved in dichloromethane. The organic solvent was vacuum evaporated, and the dry lipid film was hydrated by adding 10 mL PBS containing Tween 80 at a concentration of 3% w/v. The aqueous dispersion was shaken with a mechanical stirrer for 30 min in a water bath at the constant temperature of 37 °C. In order to obtain small unilamellar vesicles from multilamellar vesicles, an ultrasonication probe was used for 10 min (with pulsed duty cycles of $\frac{1}{2}$ s on and $\frac{1}{2}$ s off, amplitude 50%) with the sample in an ice bath to prevent lipid degradation [29]. Finally, a gentle centrifugation of 1 min at 1205× g was performed to remove possible metallic particles released by the ultrasonic probe inside the liposomal dispersion [30].

In addition, for CLPs, 10 mg of DDAB were weighted together with P90G and CHOL and then vesicles were prepared by hydrating the dry lipid film with 10 mL PBS containing 3% of Tween 80 [31].

AG-loaded LPs (LPs-AG) and AG-loaded CLPs (CLPs-AG) were prepared with the same method described above, adding 8.5 mg of AG (0.85 mg/mL, corresponding to 5% of the weight of the lipid component) together with P90G, CHOL, DDAB in the case of CLPs-AG and 1–2 mL of methanol with dichloromethane to completely dissolve AG.

Coumarin-6-loaded liposomes (LPs-6C and CLPs-6C) were prepared using the same method, adding 5 mg of the probe (λ_{max} = 444, λ_{ex} = 420 nm, λ_{em} = 505 nm, green), corresponding to 3% of the weight of the lipid component, to the organic phase.

2.3. Physical and Morphological Characterization

Liposomes' hydrodynamic diameter, size distribution and ζ-potential were measured by Light Scattering (LS), using a Zsizer Nano series ZS90 (Malvern Instruments, Malvern, UK) outfitted with a JDS Uniphase 22 mW He-Ne laser operating at 632.8 nm, an optical fiber-based detector, a digital LV/LSE-5003 correlator and a temperature controller (Julabo water-bath) set at 25 °C. Time correlation functions were analyzed by the Cumulant method, to obtain the hydrodynamic diameter of the vesicles ($Z_{average}$) and the particle size distribution (polydispersity index, PdI) using the ALV-60 × 0 software V.3.X provided by Malvern. ζ-potential, instead, was calculated from the electrophoretic mobility, using the Henry correction to Smoluchowski's equation. The samples were diluted 100-fold in distilled water and an average of three measurements at stationary level was taken. A Haake temperature controller kept the temperature constant at 25 °C.

Liposomes were also analyzed in terms of morphology, shape, and dimensions by the transmission electron microscopy (TEM). The aqueous dispersion was diluted 10-fold in PBS and 5 μL were applied to a carbon film-covered copper grid. Most of the sample was blotted from the grid with filter paper to form a thin film. After the adhesion of liposomes, 5 μL of phosphotungstic acid solution (1% *w/v* in sterile water) were dropped onto the grid as a staining medium and the excess solution was removed with filter paper. Samples were dried for 3 min, after which they were examined with a JEOL 1010 electron microscope and then photographed at an accelerating voltage of 64 kV.

2.4. Chemical Characterization of Formulations

The percentage of the AG or 6C entrapped into liposomes in respect to the amount of substances initially used in the liposomal preparation was expressed as encapsulation efficiency (EE%) and calculated using the direct method. Free AG or 6C was removed by means of dialysis. 2 mL of liposomal suspensions were transferred in a dialysis bag (cut-off 3500–5000 Dalton), which was stirred in 1 L of water at room temperature for 1 h [29]. The content of AG or 6C entrapped within liposomes was quantified by HPLC-DAD analysis, respectively after disruption with methanol of purified liposomes (placed in the ultrasonic bath for 30 min) and ultracentrifugation for 10 min at 11,330× *g*.

LC% for liposomal formulations was calculated using the following Equation (1):

$$LC\% = \frac{\text{Total amount of determined drug}}{\text{Weight of liposomes}} \times 100 \quad (1)$$

The Recovery% was carried out with the same procedure but without initial dialysis and was calculated using the following Formula (2):

$$\text{Recovery}\% = \frac{\text{Total amount of determined drug}}{\text{Initial amount of drug loading}} \times 100 \quad (2)$$

2.5. HPLC-DAD and HPLC-FLD Methods

An HP 1100 liquid chromatograph equipped with a DAD detector was used to carry out the quali-quantitative determinations of AG. A 150 mm × 4.6 mm i.d., 5 μm Zorbax Eclipse XDB, RP18 column (Agilent Technologies, Santa Clara, CA, USA) was employed. The mobile phases were (A) CH_3CN and (B) formic acid/water pH 3.2. Flow rate was 0.8 mL/min and temperature were set to 27 °C. The following gradient profile was utilized: 0–2 min, 5–15% A, 95–85% B; 2–5 min, 15% A, 85% B; 5–7 min 15–50% A, 85–50% B; 7–12 min, 50% A, 50% B; 12–15 min, 50–30% A, 50–70% B; 15–20 min, 30% A, 70% B; 20–25 min, 30–5% A, 70–95% B with equilibration time of 5 min. Injection volume was 10 μL. The UV/vis spectra were recorded in the range 200–800 nm and the chromatograms were acquired at 223 nm.

6C characterization was performed using an HP 1200 liquid chromatograph with Luna RP18 column (4.6 mm × 250 mm i.d., 5 μm) maintained at 25 °C. The mobile phase was composed of (A) CH_3CN and (B) formic acid/water pH 3.2 with a flow rate of 1 mL/min. The gradient profile was: 0–2 min, 30% A, 70% B; 2–26 min 30–100% A, 70–0% B; 26–29 min 100% A, 0% B; 29–35 min 100–30% A, 0–70% B with post-time of 5 min. Chromatograms were acquired at 444 nm.

An HP 1200 liquid chromatograph equipped with a FLD detector was used for the quantification of NaF probe (λ_{ex} = 460 nm, λ_{em} = 515 nm, green). The column was a Kinetex C18 (4.6 mm × 150 mm i.d., 5 μm) maintained at 27 °C. The mobile phases were (A) CH_3CN and (B) formic acid/water pH 3.2. Flow rate was 0.8 mL/min and the injection volume was 10 μL. The following gradient profile was utilized: 0–3 min, 20% A, 80% B; 3–23 min, 20–80% A, 80–20% B; 23–25 min 80–100% A, 20–0% B; 25–27 min, 100–20% A, 0–80% B with equilibration time of 5 min.

Diluting stock solutions in CH_3OH (0.5 mg/mL for AG and 0.1 mg/mL for 6C) and in H_2O (0.1 mg/mL for NaF), standard solutions were freshly prepared. To quantify each compound, an external standard method was applied using a regression curve and analyses were performed in triplicate. Results were expressed as the mean ± SD of the 3 experiments.

All the compounds showed a linear response: AG from 0.05 to 25 μg/mL, NaF from 0.05 to 46 μg/mL and 6C from 0.515 to 51.5 μg/mL. All the curves had coefficients of linear correlation $R^2 \geq 0.999$.

Progressive dilutions of standard solutions were used to calculate the limit of detection LOD (S/N $\geq$ 3) and the limit of quantification LOQ (S/N $\geq$ 10). LOD and LOQ for AG were 2.6 ng and 5.3 ng, respectively.

2.6. Stability Studies

The stability of empty and AG-loaded liposomes was studied for one month. Aqueous dispersions were kept at 4 °C and, at fixed time intervals, their physical and chemical stabilities were assayed: physical stability was checked by monitoring sizes, polydispersity index and ζ-potential, while chemical stability was determined by quantification of encapsulated drug by HPLC-DAD analysis.

The freeze-drying process in the absence of cryoprotectant and in the presence of 1% *w/v* of glucose or sucrose was also considered. Afterwards, lyophilization physical stability was checked for one month at 25 °C.

200 μL of LPs and CLPs dispersions were incubated at body temperature with a solution of human serum albumin (HSA, 40 mg/mL in PBS) for two hours under magnetic stirring to mimic in vivo conditions [32,33]. Physical stability of the formulations was evaluated using Dynamic Light Scattering, by controlling liposomes sizes at regular intervals.

The yield of the preparation of freeze-dried LPs-AG and CLPs-AG was calculated as the weight of the product obtained after the freeze-drying, compared to the weight of the components used in the reaction (3):

$$\text{Yield\%} = \frac{\text{real weight (mg)}}{\text{teoric weight (mg)}} \times 100 \tag{3}$$

2.7. In Vitro Release

AG in vitro release from liposomes was performed using a dialysis membrane (cut-off 3000–5000 Dalton) in PBS at 37 °C. Two mL of AG solution (0.85 mg/mL in methanol), LPs and CLPs suspensions were filled in pre-soaked dialysis tubes and placed in 200 mL of release medium using a magnetic stirrer. An aliquot of 1 mL of release medium was removed at pre-determined time intervals and replaced with 1 mL of fresh PBS maintained at 37 °C [34]. AG concentration at different times was calculated using HPLC analyses: the mean of triplicate drug release and standard deviation (mean $\pm$ SD, $n = 3$) was used to draw the drug release profiles.

The following Formula (4) was applied to calculate the percentage of AG released in the medium at pH 7.4 at each time interval (0, 30, 60, 120, 240, 360 and 1440 min):

$$\%\ \text{drug released} = \frac{\text{drug(t) (mg)}}{\text{total drug (mg)}} \times 100 \tag{4}$$

To evaluate the kinetics and mechanism of drug release from the liposomes, the Korsmeyer–Peppas model, Hixson Crowell model, Higuchi model, first order and zero order mathematical models were used and the best fitted model was selected based on high regression coefficient (R^2) value for the release data.

2.8. PAMPA Studies

PAMPA studies for LPs-AG and CLPs-AG were carried out using the method previously published [11]. A solution (2% *w/v*) of Porcine Polar Brain Lipid (PBL) in n-dodecane was prepped and the mixture was sonicated. PBL solution (5 μL) was added to each donor plate well [16]. Right after the application of the artificial membrane, 250 μL of formulation were added to each donor compartment, whilst the acceptor compartment was filled with PBS/Ethanol solution. Then the drug-filled donor compartment was installed into the acceptor plate. After incubation for 18 h, the donor and acceptor plate samples were withdrawn and analyzed by HPLC-DAD analyses for quantification of AG concentration: 150 μL were taken from both compartments, later diluted with methanol, placed in the ultrasonic bath for 30 min and finally ultra-centrifuged for 10 min at 11,330× *g* (4 °C). The permeability of AG was calculated using the following Formula (5) [35]:

$$P_e = -\ln\left[1 - C_A(t)/C_{equilibrium}\right]/A \times (1/V_D + 1/V_A) \times t \quad (5)$$

where P_e is permeability in the unit of cm/s, effective filter area (A) = f × 0.3 cm^2, where f = apparent porosity of the filter, $C_A(t)$ = compound concentration in receptor well at time t, V_D = donor well volume (mL), V_A = receptor well volume (mL), t = incubation time (s), $C_D(t)$ = compound concentration in donor well at time t, and (6)

$$C_{equilibrium} = [C_D(t) \times V_D + C_A(t) \times V_A]/(V_D + V_A) \quad (6)$$

The experiments were performed in triplicate.

2.9. hCMEC/D3 Cell Culture

This cell line (Millipore Cat. # SCC066) derives from human temporal lobe micro-vessels isolated from tissue excised during surgery for epilepsy control. Cells were seeded in a concentration of 2.5 × 10^4 cells/cm^2 and grown at 37 °C in an atmosphere of 5% CO_2 in 25 cm^2 rat tail collagen type I coated culture flasks. EndoGRO^{TM}-MV Complete Media Kit (Cat. # SCME004) supplemented with 1 ng/mL FGF-2 (Cat. #GF003) was changed every three days and cells were grown until they were 90% confluent. Cells were passaged at least twice before use. Confluent hCMEC/D3 cells were split by Accumax^{TM} Cell Counting Solution in DPBS.

2.10. 3-(4,5-Dimethylthiazol-2-yl)-2,5-diphenyltetrazolium Bromide (MTT) Assay

To assess cell viability after AG and LPs-AG and CLPs-AG exposure, an MTT assay was performed [36,37]. Cells were seeded in a 24-well plate (6 × 10^4 cells/cm^2) pre-coated with Collagen Type I, Rat Tail (Cat. #08–115) and grown at 37 °C in an atmosphere of 5% CO_2 in EndoGRO^{TM} Basal Medium (EBM-2). When the cells were approximately 70–80% confluent they were incubated with different concentrations of AG (10 and 100 μM), LPs-AG (0.085 and 0.0085 mg/mL) and CLPs-AG (0.085 and 0.0085 mg/mL), obtained by dilution (1:10 and 1:100) of the formulation in EBM-2 for 2, 4 and 24 h. The liposome formulations were previously filtered through 0.4 μm sterile filter units. The medium of each well was separated from the cells and stored for lactate dehydrogenase (LDH) assay, and cells were treated with 1 mg/mL of MTT for 1 h at 37 °C and 5% CO_2. Finally, DMSO was added to dissolve MTT formation and absorbance was measured at 550 and 690 nm. Cell viability was expressed as a percentage compared to the cells incubated only with EBM-2 (positive control). Triton X-100 was used in the MTT assay as the negative control since its detergent action disrupts the cells.

2.11. LDH Assay

Cytotoxicity after AG and liposomes exposure was verified with LDH assay. The medium resulting from incubation of AG and liposomes with cells was centrifuged (250× *g*, 10 min at RT) and the supernatant separated from the deposited cells in each well. This centrifugation process allowed us to remove any waste and cellular debris as well as AG and liposomes. The release of LDH into culture supernatants was detected by adding catalyst and dye solutions of a Cytotoxicity Detection Kit (LDH) (Roche Diagnostics, Indianapolis, IN, USA). The absorbance values were recorded at 490 nm and 690 nm. Cytotoxicity was expressed as a percentage compared to the maximum LDH release in the presence of triton X-100 (positive control). EBM-2 was used as negative control since no cytotoxicity was detected in such conditions.

2.12. hCMEC/D3 Cell Culture for Transwell Permeability Studies

High density pore (2×10^6 pores/cm^2) transparent PET membrane filter inserts (0.4 µm, 23.1 mm diameter, Falcon, Corning BV, Amsterdam, Netherlands) were used in 6-well cell culture plates (Falcon, Corning, Amsterdam, Netherlands) for all transcytosis assays. The transparent PET membrane filter inserts were coated with rat tail collagen type I at a concentration of 0.1 mg/mL and incubated at 37 °C for 1 h prior to cell barrier coating. Inserts were subsequently washed with PBS and incubated for 1 h, after which PBS was removed and replaced with the assay medium. The inserts were calibrated for at least 1 h with assay medium at 37 °C. Optimum media volumes were calculated to be 1 mL and 1.2 mL respectively for apical and basolateral chambers. The transwell inserts were calibrated with assay medium for 1 h, then the medium was removed and hCMEC/D3 cells were seeded onto the apical side of the inserts at a density of 6×10^4 cells/cm^2 in 1 mL assay media. 1.2 mL of fresh medium was added to the basolateral chamber. The assay medium was changed every 3 days following transwell apical insert seeding with hCMEC/D3. For seven days, cells were grown to confluence. hCMEC/D3 monolayers were used as a permeability assay for AG and AG-loaded liposomes. Fluorescein sodium salt (NaF) was considered at a concentration of 10 µg/mL as an integrity control marker with a known permeability coefficient (P_{app}) for this cell line [19]. The integrity of monolayer cells was confirmed also by observation of cultures under phase-contrast microscopy or under bright-field optics using of transparent membranes. The image was observed using an inverted microscope (Olympus IX-50; Solent Scientific, Segensworth, Fareham, UK) with a low-power objective (20X). The images were digitized using a video image obtained with a CCD camera (Diagnostic Instruments Inc., Sterling Heights, MI, USA) controlled by software (InCyt Im1TM; Intracellular Imaging Inc., Cincinnati, OH, USA).

For permeability studies, AG (10, and 100 µM), LPs-AG and CLPs-AG (0.085 mg/mL, corresponding to AG 240 µM) obtained by dilution 1:10 of the formulation in EBM-2 were tested and incubated for 1, 2, 3 and 4 h in the apical donor compartment. At the end of the incubation, the amount of NaF and AG were quantified both in apical and basolateral compartments by HPLC-FLD or HPLC-DAD method. In the case of the formulation, EBM-2 was diluted with methanol and placed in the ultrasonic bath for 30 min and then ultra-centrifuged for 1 h at 11,330× *g* (4 °C). The apparent permeability coefficients (P_{app}) of free AG and AG encapsulated in LPS and CLPs were calculated according to the Equation (7):

$$P_{app}\ (\text{cm/s}) = V_D/(A \cdot M_D) \times (\Delta M_R/\Delta t) \quad (7)$$

where: V_D = apical (donor) volume (cm^3), M_D = apical (donor) amount (mol), $\Delta M_R/\Delta t$ = change in amount (mol) of compound in receiver compartment over time.

The recovery for AG and NaF was calculated according to the Equation (8) [19]:

$$\text{Recovery}\ (\%) = C_{Df} \cdot V_D + C_{Rf} \cdot V_R/(C_{D0} \cdot V_D) \times 100 \quad (8)$$

where C_{Df} and C_{Rf} are the final compound concentrations in the donor and receiver compartments, C_{D0} is the initial concentration in the donor compartment and V_D and V_R are the volumes in the donor and receiver compartments, respectively. All experiments were performed at least in triplicate.

2.13. Cellular Uptake of LPs-6C and CLPs-6C

For the evaluation of the intracellular content of 6-Coumarin, hCMEC/D3 cells (1×10^4) were exposed for 2 h to the LPs-6C and CLPs-6C loaded with 0.5 mg/mL of 6C and diluted 1:100 into EBM-2, and to a saturated solution of fluorescent probe. To elucidate the endocytic uptake mechanisms, these experiments were carried out in presence/absence of endocytic inhibitors. Control cells were exposed to liposomal formulations without any agent pre-treatment and their uptake was assumed to be 100%. A second group of cells was pre-treated with 15 μM chlorpromazine for 30 min followed by incubation with liposomes. A third group of cells was pre-treated with 25 μM of indomethacin for 30 min; and, finally, a fourth group of cells was maintained at 4 °C during the LPs-6C and CLPs-6C exposure to observe the effect of low temperature, a general metabolic inhibitor.

At the end of the treatments, the amount of 6C was quantified on cellular lysate by HPLC. For control cells and cells maintained at 4 °C during exposure, a morphological evaluation of cellular uptake was also performed: hCMEC/D3 cells were cultured on histological slides, treated as described above, fixed in 4% formaldehyde in 0.1 mol/L phosphate buffer, pH 7.4, for 10 min then stained with Fluoro scheld with DAPI (Sigma, Milan, Italy) to display the nucleus and observed by fluorescence microscopy (Labophot-2 Nikon, Tokyo, Japan). Ten photomicrographs were randomly taken for each sample.

Cellular uptake was investigated by confocal microscopy Nikon Eclipse Ti using liposomes labeled with 6C, with S Fluor 20x, NA = 0.75 high pressure Hg vapor lamp (Intensilight, Nikon, Tokyo, Japan).

Filter set: excitation 365 nm emission 400 nm hi-pass DAPI, excitation 485 nm emission 524 nm 6Co and CCD camera: Coolsnap HQ^2, Princeton instruments, Trenton, NJ, USA, 1392 × 1040, 6.45 um square pixels.

2.14. *Statistical Analysis*

The experiments were repeated three times and results expressed as a mean ± standard deviation. Statistical significance of hCMEC/D cell viability and cellular uptake was analyzed using one-way ANOVA followed by the post hoc Tukey's w-test for multiple comparisons. All statistical calculations were performed using GRAPH-PAD PRISM v. 5 for Windows (GraphPad Software, San Diego, CA, USA). A probability value (p) of <0.05 was considered significant.

3. Results and Discussion

3.1. *Preparation and Characterization of Liposomes*

LPs were prepared by using P90G, CHOL and Tween 80. This compound was selected as a coating agent to increase the stability of the formulation, to produce "stealth" nanovesicles and to promote endocytosis of the carrier at the level of cerebral endothelial cells [23]. Various ratios of the two lipid constituents were tested to obtain small sizes, good polydispersity and favorable ζ-potential. In particular, the ratios P90G:CHOL 18:1, 16:1, 14:1, 12:1, and 10:1 were considered. The best ratio resulted to be 16:1, corresponding to 160 mg of P90G and 10 mg of CHOL. Then, 3% *w/v* of Tween 80 was added (LPs). Furthermore, different sonication times were tested to optimize LPs physical characteristics. The selected conditions consisted in two cycles of 5 min of sonication, each including 0.5 s of sonication alternating with 0.5 s of pause, as reported in the materials and methods section. LPs were nanosized unilamellar vesicles, with a PdI less than 0.25 and a ζ-potential, around −20 mV (Table 1), confirming a homogeneous and stable dispersion. LC% was 2.28% ± 0.22. The mean vesicle sizes and the width of the particle distribution are important parameters as they govern physical stability and permeation through BBB [38]. Moreover, the vesicles sizes highly affected the interaction of the liposomes with the hCMEC/D3 cellular model [39,40].

AG does not influence the stability of the formulation (Table 1); when LPs were loaded with AG, LPs-AG showed the same physical parameters as LPs. The electron microscope analysis confirmed the liposomal structure; the results evidenced the presence of spherical vesicles, with a defined phospholipid bilayer, well separated, due to the presence of the surfactant that prevents agglomeration, and with dimensions around 100 nm, confirming the DLS results (Figure 1a).

Next, LPs were functionalized with positive surface charges by using DDAB (cationic liposomes, CLPs) in the same amount of CHOL (10 mg in the total formulation). In this case, ζ-potential resulted positive, indicating the presence of positive charges on the surface of the carrier.

Then, CLPs loaded with 8.5 mg of AG (corresponding to 5% of the weight of the lipid component) were prepared (CLPs-AG); the presence of DDAB and AG did not modify the physical characteristics of the formulation (Table 1). LC% was 3.08% ± 0.21. TEM analysis showed well separated spherical shape vesicles, with a distinct phospholipid bilayer (Figure 1b).

The compound 6-Coumarin (6C), a lipophilic fluorescent dye, was incorporated into liposomes to investigate the ability of nanoparticles to penetrate into hCMEC/D3 cells, as BBB-model, and to elucidate trans-endothelial transport in vitro. The preparation of fluorescent liposomes was performed as reported for LPs and CLPs, by adding 6C (0.5 mg/mL) to the organic phase. Their physical and chemical parameters are shown in Table 1. The same dimensions of the two types of liposomes, was very important to interact with the HCMEC/D3 equally [39]. LPs-6C and CLPs-6C resulted larger but useful for a parenteral administration. AG and 6C are lipophilic compounds and there are inserted in the bilayer, but the effect on the sizes of nanoparticles is different due to their unlike chemical structure. The high ζ-potential of all formulations is indicative of their stability, as also supported by stability studies.

Table 1. Physical characterization of empty, andrographolide (AG) and coumarin-6 (6C) loaded liposomes.

Sample	Size (nm)	PdI	ζ-Potential	EE%	Recovery%
LPs	80.2 ± 3.6	0.22 ± 0.03	−20.4 ± 4.1	-	-
CLPs	84.6 ± 8.1	0.23 ± 0.02	20.7 ± 4.7	-	-
LPs-AG	96.4 ± 9.5	0.23 ± 0.03	−22.8 ± 1.2	44.7 ± 3.2	91.1 ± 5.3
CLPs-AG	82.1 ± 9.3	0.25 ± 0.01	20.3 ± 3.7	47.5 ± 3.3	94.9 ± 4.7
LPs-6C	193.1 ± 3.0	0.21 ± 0.02	−27.4 ± 0.4	46.0 ± 1.4	71.2 ± 4.2
CLPs-6C	197.1 ± 1.4	0.27 ± 0.03	31.1 ± 0.6	63.1 ± 0.1	80.6 ± 5.0

LPs: liposomes with Tween 80, CLPs: liposomes with Tween 80 and DDAB. Data displayed as mean ± SD; n = 3.

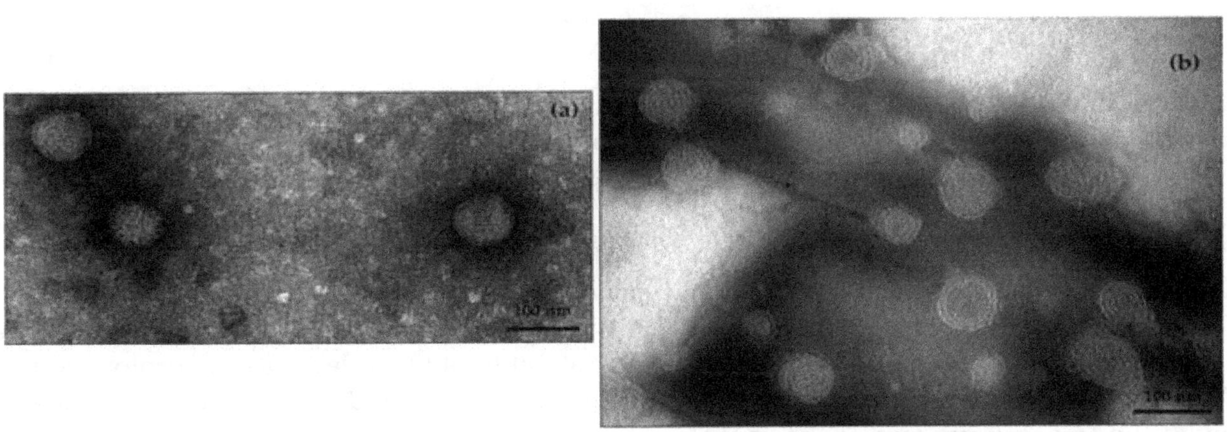

Figure 1. TEM images of LPs-AG (**a**) and CLPs-AG (**b**) (scale 100 nm).

3.2. Stability Studies

Liposomes stability was evaluated both as a colloidal dispersion and in the freeze-dried form. The ability of the aqueous dispersions to maintain their physicochemical properties in terms of particle size, PdI, surface charge and drug entrapment was assessed after 1-month storage at 4 °C and the Light Scattering analyses were performed to control the stability over time. No significant changes were observed in physical parameters of empty or LPs-AG and CLPs-AG dispersions (Figure 2). The presence of non-ionic surfactant is expected to reduce the agglomeration between liposomes via steric repulsion. Also, the presence of DDAB on the surface of liposomes prevented the aggregation and the precipitation of the vesicles and increased the systems stability. In addition, the entrapment efficiency remained constant, around 45%.

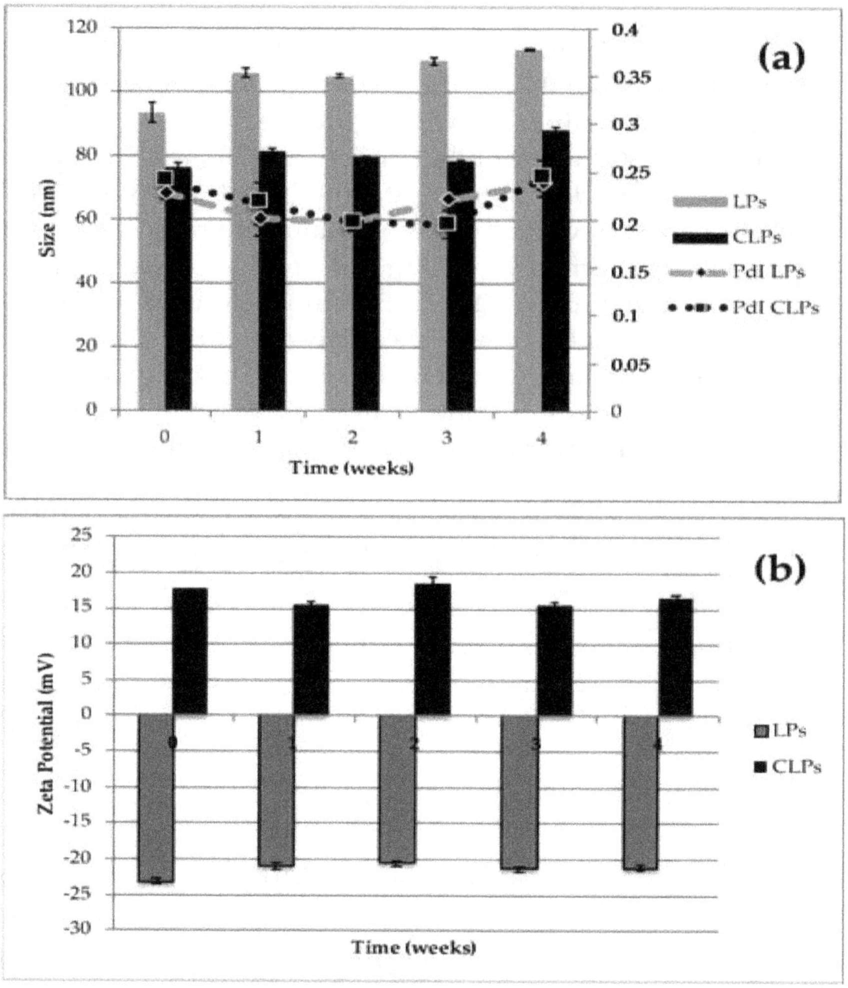

Figure 2. Particle size, polydispersity index (PdI) (**a**) and zeta-potential (**b**) of LPs-AG and CLPs-AG as dispersion after one-month storage at 4 °C. (Data displayed as mean ± SD; $n = 3$).

The major limitation to liposomes use is due to their physical and chemical instability, when the aqueous suspension is stored for an extended period. The poor stability in an aqueous medium forms a real obstacle against the clinical application of nanoparticles.

To improve the physical and chemical stability, water needs to be removed. Freeze-drying is a good technique to enhance the chemical and physical stability of formulations over prolonged periods.

The stability of LPs-AG and CLPs-AG with time was evaluated also in the freeze-dried form. However, the freezing process of the sample might cause problems of possible structural and/or functional damages of the system, and/or subsequent difficulties in sample re-solubilization, due to particle aggregation phenomena. The addition of cryoprotectants improves the quality of the dehydrated product, decreases particle aggregation phenomena and allows to obtain an easier re-dispersion of the freeze-dried product.

Therefore, to estimate the effect of the presence and type of cryoprotectant, empty, LPs-AG and CLPs-AG formulations were freeze-dried with and without sucrose or glucose (1% *w*/*v*). After the lyophilization process, all formulations were dispersed in PBS and analyzed by DLS and ELS (Table 2). As shown in Table 2, the drying process produced an increase in terms of size and PdI, respect to the values reported before the freeze-drying process (Table 1). However, all liposomes maintained characteristics suitable for parenteral administration. The best freeze-drying process was obtained in the presence of glucose both for LPs-AG and CLPs-AG. The EE% remained almost constant around 43%. The yield % of the preparation process was also calculated, in this case without addition of the cryoprotectant, and resulted 69.5% ± 0.1 for LPs and 71.2% ± 0.1 for CLPs (mean ± SD; $n = 3$). After a month of storage at 25 °C the freeze-dried product retained the starting characteristics.

Table 2. Physical parameters of andrographolide loaded liposomes, after the freeze-drying process with and without cryoprotectant, 1% w/v of sucrose or glucose.

LPs-AG	No Cryoprotector	Glucose	Sucrose
Size (nm)	148.8 ± 1.4	135.0 ± 0.9	147.5 ± 1.2
PdI	0.32 ± 0.03	0.25 ± 0.02	0.35 ± 0.01
ζ (mV)	−21.3 ± 0.9	−19.4 ± 1.1	−18.5 ± 1.0
CLPs-AG			
Size (nm)	144.6 ± 2.2	131.3 ± 5.1	149.3 ± 1.2
PdI	0.38 ± 0.02	0.28 ± 0.01	0.29 ± 0.01
ζ (mV)	+28.6 ± 0.9	+27.0 ± 0.8	+26.5 ± 0.9

LPs-AG: liposomes with Tween 80 loaded with AG, CLPs-AG: liposomes with Tween 80 and DDAB loaded with AG. Data displayed as mean ± SD; $n = 3$.

A drawback to the use of nanocarriers, in particular cationic nanocarriers, for brain delivery is their binding to serum proteins that attenuates their surface charge. Therefore, the stability of LPs-AG and CLPs-AG in presence of human serum albumin (HSA) at physiological concentration was also tested. After 2 h of incubation, DLS analyses confirmed that sizes were not affected by the presence of HSA and therefore revealed coexistence of free serum proteins and optimized nanocarrier without any protein corona effect (Table 3).

Table 3. Physical stability of LPs-AG and CLPs-AG in presence of human serum albumin.

	LPs-AG		CLPs-AG	
Time	**Size (nm)**	**Pd**	**Size (nm)**	**Pd**
0	94.8 ± 2.4	0.23 ± 0.02	76.4 ± 1.2	0.24 ± 0.01
30′	103.8 ± 2.0	0.39 ± 0.01	82.9 ± 0.5	0.41 ± 0.02
1 h	97.2 ± 3.2	0.39 ± 0.02	83.5 ± 4.8	0.40 ± 0.01
2 h	99.1 ± 5.1	0.39 ± 0.01	81.9 ± 3.4	0.43 ± 0.02

LPs-AG: liposomes with Tween 80 loaded with AG, CLPs-AG: liposomes with Tween 80 and DDAB loaded with AG. Data displayed as mean ± SD; $n = 3$.

3.3. *In Vitro Release*

AG in vitro release at 37 °C from LPs-AG and CLPs-AG was evaluated for 24 h by using a dialysis bag and PBS as receptor medium to mimic sink conditions. The release profiles of AG from AG solution, LPs-AG and CLPs-AG were reported in Figure 3. The result indicated that the release of AG from methanol solution through the dialysis membrane was much faster, with a fast release during the first 2 h and approximately 100% of the drug released within 6 h. In contrast, the immediate release of the drug (burst effect) does not occur in the case of LPs-AG and CLPs-AG. The percentages of AG released from LPs and CLPs were gradual: only 56.8% and 69.7% of drug was released within 6 h, respectively. The percentages rose to 83.5% and 77.4%, after 24 h, respectively. The almost linear and gradual trend of the release indicated that the liposomal systems can release AG for prolonged periods and in greater quantities compared to the saturated aqueous solution, were the solubility of AG resulted very low (0.05 mg/mL). Optimized liposomal formulations are able to solubilize 0.85 mg/mL of drug.

Different theoretical models were considered to examine the nature of release. The drug release mechanism was defined by fitting AG release data with various kinetics models. By comparing the regression coefficient values, the Higuchi model (R^2 = 0.8366 and 0.9264, respectively, Table 4) resulted as the best to describe the kinetics of these two types of liposomes. Thus, the liposomal membrane disruption controlled the release mechanism [41].

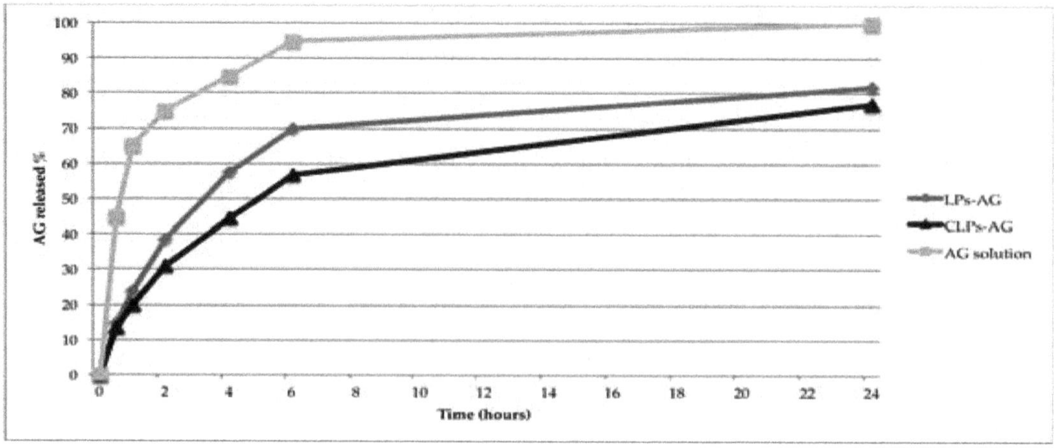

Figure 3. In vitro release profiles of LPs-AG and CLPs-AG in PBS. (each data point represents the average of three samples).

Table 4. Regression coefficient (R^2) obtained in different kinetics models for AG release from LPs-AG and CLPs-AG.

Release Kinetics	LPs-AG	CLPs-AG
Zero order	0.5722	0.7079
First order	0.7685	0.8816
Korsmeyer-Peppas	0.4552	0.4980
Hixson	0.7033	0.8292
Higuchi	0.8366	0.9264

LPs-AG: liposomes with Tween 80 loaded with AG, CLPs-AG: liposomes with Tween 80 and DDAB loaded with AG.

Due to the very low solubility of AG in water and the related problems of bioavailability, both the liposomal formulations allow the administration of a high amount of solubilized molecule according to the requirements for parenteral preparations.

3.4. PAMPA Study

Parallel Artificial Membrane Permeability Assay (PAMPA) was performed to estimate passive transcellular permeability. It is a non-cell-based permeability model because it lacks transporter- and pore-mediated permeability, but is considered robust, reproducible and it results in a helpful complement to the cellular permeability model for its speed, low cost and versatility, and readily provides information about passive transport permeability.

AG is a molecule with low BBB permeability (effective permeability, P_e value of $0.49 \pm 0.16 \times 10^{-6}$ cm/s [11] and therefore liposomal formulation could represent a useful tool to improve its permeation. P_e of AG-loaded liposomes resulted as increased, in particular $3.94 \pm 0.60 \times 10^{-6}$ cm/s for LPs-AG and $3.87 \pm 0.36 \times 10^{-6}$ cm/s for CLPs-AG. These values confirmed that LPs-AG and CLPs-AG increased the permeability of the drug, of about an order of magnitude, compared to the aqueous solution.

Though this test does not discriminate the different behavior of the two systems because the artificial membrane fails to mimic all properties of a cell, a mechanism of permeation through the artificial membrane was hypothesized. An interaction between the phospholipid bilayer, which is a flexible system, with the lipid that covers the artificial membrane, similar to one of mechanisms of liposome-cell interaction.

3.5. MTT and LDH Assays

MTT and LDH assays were performed in the hCMEC/D3 cell line to evaluate the effect of AG and LPs-AG and CLPs-AG in cell viability and cytotoxicity, and permeability studies were also conducted in transwell devices using the same cell line. The in vitro cytotoxicity of the developed LPs-AG and CLPs-AG and AG was assessed by cell viability determination and membrane integrity evaluation using the hCMEC/D3 cell line in MTT and LDH assays, respectively (Figure 4). When cells were exposed to different concentrations of AG (10 and 100 μM) and LPs-AG and CLPs-AG (0.0085 and 0.085 mg/mL) for 2 (Figure 4a) and 4 h (Figure 4b), no significant changes were observed in MTT metabolization, except for LPs-AG and CLPs-AG (0.085 mg/mL) or LDH release when compared to cells exposed to the EBM-2 medium alone, indicating that AG and LPs-AG and CLPs-AG affected neither the metabolic activity of the cells nor the membrane integrity at these time points. On the other hand, when the cells were incubated for 24 h with AG at a dose of 100 μM, LPs-AG (0.085 mg/mL) and CLPs-AG (0.0085 and 0.085 mg/mL) we observed a significant reduction of cell viability and an increase in cytotoxicity compared to the control (Figure 4c).

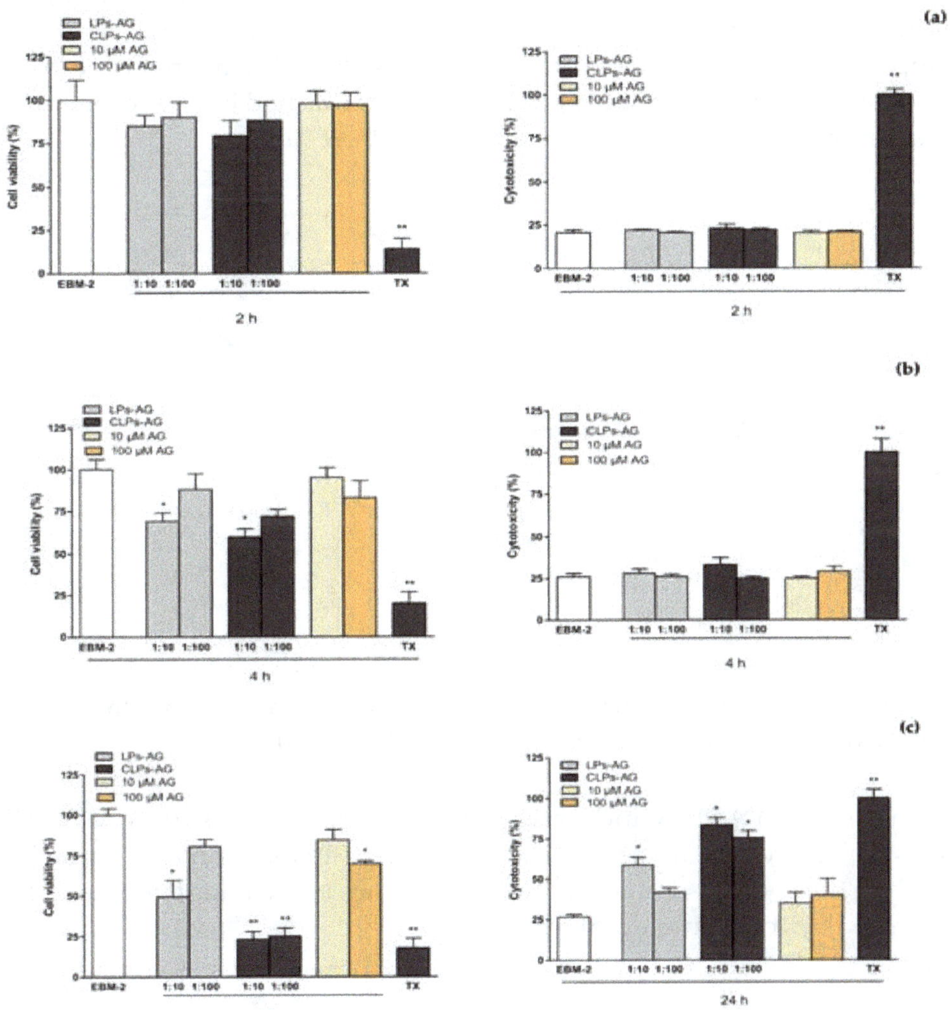

Figure 4. hCMEC/D3 cell viability evaluated by MTT assay (left panel) and cytotoxicity by LDH assay (right panel) when exposed for 2 h (**a**), 4 h (**b**) and 24 h (**c**) to AG (10 and 100 μM) or LPs-AG and CLPs-AG (0.0085 and 0.085 mg/mL). Data is expressed as percentage of control (EBM-2 medium) and Triton-X (TTX) which represent, respectively, the maximum cell viability and cell cytotoxicity. Values represent the mean ± SEM of at least three experiments performed in triplicate. * $p < 0.05$ and ** $p < 0.01$ vs. EBM-2 alone.

3.6. BBB Permeability Studies

hCMEC/D3 brain microvascular endothelial cell line is a model of human BBB utilized to study the drug transport mechanisms [18,42]. The cells retain the expression of most transporters and receptors expressed in vivo in the human BBB. hCMEC/D3 apparent permeability coefficient (P_{app}) correlates well with in vivo permeability data, and therefore permeability studies were performed to predict the permeability of free AG and LPs-AG and CLPs-AG across the BBB. NaF was used as the negative control and its P_{app} was determined during all transport experiments to monitor the integrity of the cell layer. This aspect was also been checked by phase-contrast microscopy [11].

P_{app} of NaF was $8.27 \pm 1.81 \times 10^{-6}$ cm/s, in agreement with the literature values [11,12,19]. This value remained constant during the permeability assay, and demonstrates the confluence of the monolayer and assesses the tight junction integrity. P_{app} of LPs-AG and CLPs-AG were only slightly higher than the P_{app} values of the free AG for the first 3 h. However, at 4 h, the P_{app} value for both LPs-AG and CLPs-AG was significantly higher (about double) than that of the free AG (P_{app} of AG: $8.67 \pm 0.95 \times 10^{-6}$ cm/s; P_{app} LPs-AG: $16.8 \pm 1.70 \times 10^{-6}$ cm/s; P_{app} CLPs-AG: $17.2 \pm 1.43 \times 10^{-6}$ cm/s). The amount of AG that permeated when loaded into liposomes increased about 200 times in respect to the free molecule, as confirmed by the increase of the P_{app} values during the time reported in Figure 5. AG transport across the cell was in a time-dependent manner. The obtained P_{app} data are useful for in vitro prediction, as confirmed by the recovery value, which was above 80% in all experiments. The data agrees with PAMPA results.

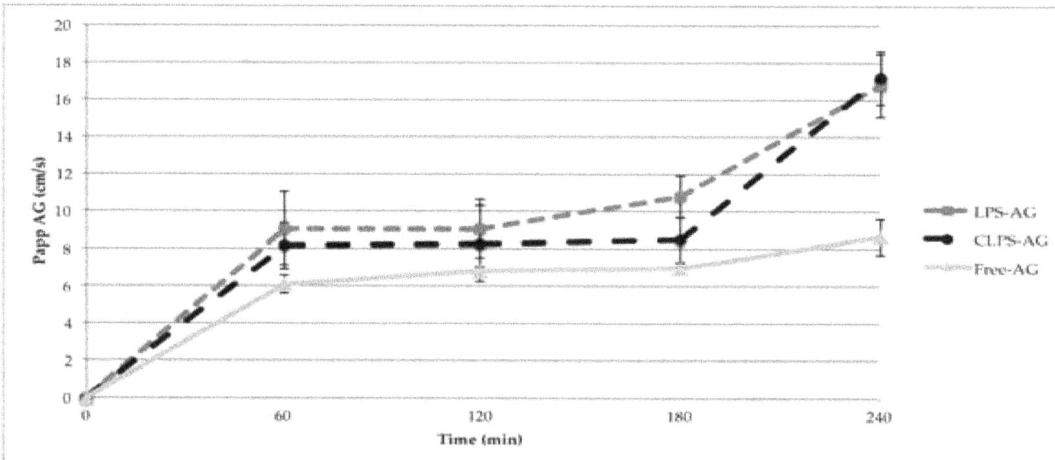

Figure 5. The apparent permeable coefficient of different liposomal formulations for different treatment time in the in vitro BBB model. (Data represent means ± S.D, $n = 3$).

A combination assay of PAMPA and unidirectional (apical to basal) hCMEC/D3 permeability model can synergistically provide invaluable permeability/absorption assessment of AG. The P_{app} values are greater than those of P_e, due to the presence of an active endocytic mechanism in addition to a passive one, as seen by following uptake studies.

3.7. Liposome Uptake by hCMEC/D3 Cells

Figure 6 shows the fluorescence images of hCMEC/D3 cells treated with LPs-6C and CLPs-6C after 2 h of incubation. The images revealed that the probe was internalized and LPs-6C and CLPs-6C were punctually concentrated in intracellular vesicles (endosomes or lysosomes) which can be related to their endocytic mechanism of uptake [42]. Besides their cytoplasmic location, green fluorescence indicates that nanoparticles were also transported to the perinuclear area. This is an important finding for pharmaceutical drug delivery research, since the nucleus is the target site for several drugs [43].

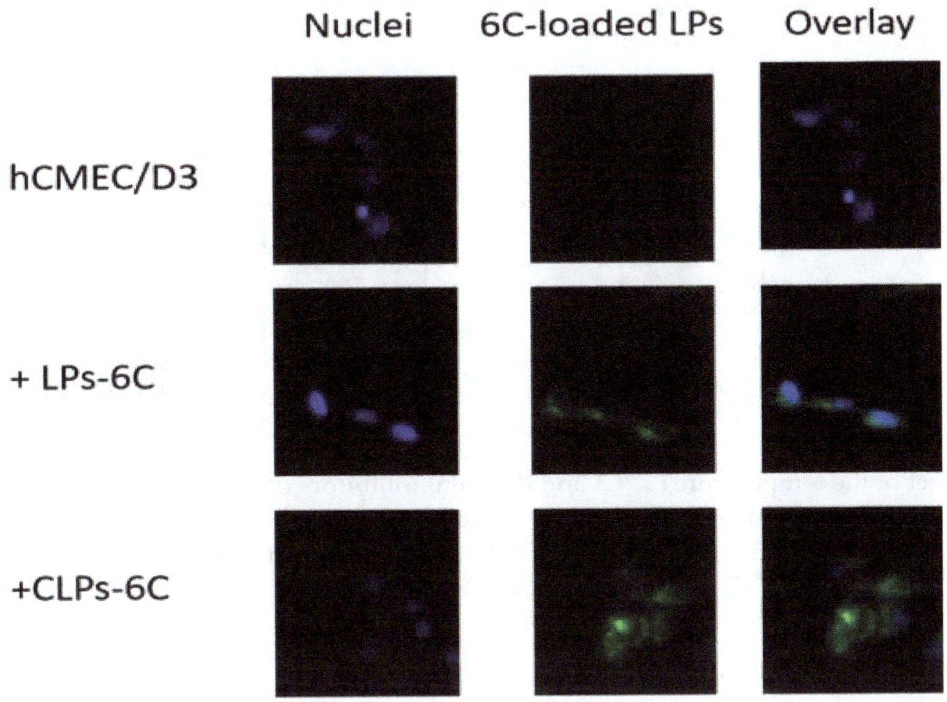

Figure 6. Cellular uptake of LPs-6C and CLPs-6C by hCMEC/D3 cells after 2 h incubation at 37 °C. Images of nuclei stained with DAPI (blue), 6-Coumarin (green) and their overlay. Scale bar: 20 μm.

Concerning the uptake of liposomes by hCMEC/D3 cells, it was different for both liposomes LPs-6C and CLPs-6C: 6.4% and 14.0%, respectively. The result proves that the internalization ability of liposomes increases in the presence of positive charge on the bilayer that improves the binding affinity between carrier and cellular membrane [31].

Furthermore, a group of cells was maintained at 4 °C in the presence of LPs-6C and CLPs-6C, to observe the effect of low temperature, a general metabolic inhibitor. The fluorescence of cells incubated with 6C loaded liposomes in the absence of any inhibitor was considered as 100%, while the fluorescence after incubation in the presence of inhibitors was expressed as a relative percentage compared to the cells without inhibitor. As shown in Figure 7, a significant reduction (about 80%) in hCMEC/D3 cell uptake efficiency was observed at 4 °C for all two formulations as compared with that at physiological temperature, suggesting that their uptake relied on an energy-dependent pathway and it was mediated by endocytosis [44].

To elucidate the endocytic uptake mechanisms, the experiments were also carried out in the presence of endocytic inhibitors, such as chlorpromazine, a clathrin blocker, and indomethacin, a caveolin-dependent endocytosis inhibitor.

Liposomes could be internalized into cells by different mechanisms, according to the type of cell, composition, surface charge, and size of the liposome [45–47]. In our study, the cellular association of the liposomes was significantly influenced by indomethacin, with a reduction in cellular association of about 44% and 63% for LPs-6C and CLPs-6C, respectively (Figure 7). Caveolae-mediated endocytosis is involved in the uptake of liposomes. However, it did not completely inhibit active uptake of the nanoparticles when compared with the results at 4 °C, confirming that cellular uptake of liposomes involved more that on an energy-dependent pathway. In fact, as evidenced in the Figure 7, an uptake reduction of 15% for LPs-6C and 20% for CLPs-6C was observed in the presence of chlorpromazine, even if less pronounced than with indomethacin. This indicates that clathrin-mediated endocytosis is also a mechanism involved in the uptake.

Therefore, the preferential mechanism of the liposomes uptake by hCMEC/D3 cells was found to be caveolae-mediated endocytosis, with a greater effect of inhibitors in the case of CLPs-6C.

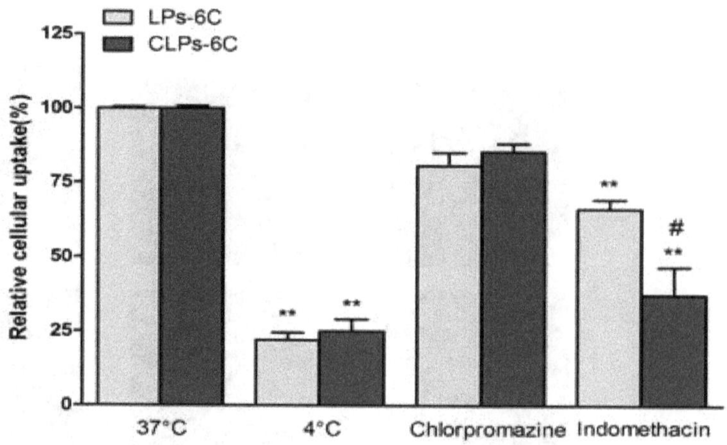

Figure 7. Effect of the temperature (4 °C) and different inhibitors on hCMEC/D3 cell internalization pathways of LPs-6C and CLPs-6C after 2 h incubation at 37 °C. (Data represent the mean ± standard deviation ($n = 3$). Bars represent the mean ± SD of at least 6 experiments ** $p < 0.01$ vs. corresponding liposome at 37 °C; # $p < 0.05$ CLPs-6C vs. LPs-6C. (ANOVA + Tukey's test).

4. Conclusions

Based on the obtained results in terms of size, homogeneity, ζ-potential and EE%, both optimized liposomal formulations of AG are suitable for parenteral administration. The systems showed excellent chemical and physical stability during a month of storage as suspensions or freeze-dried products. The optimized liposomes enhanced solubility and cellular permeability of AG, as demonstrated by in vitro tests with PAMPA and hCMEC/D3 cells. Both carriers increase the permeation of AG into the cell without alterations in cell viability and monolayer integrity. The presence of positive charge elevated the cellular internalization of liposomes. Uptake experiments suggest an energy-dependent pathway as a possible transport mechanism across the hCMEC/D3 monolayer, with caveolae-mediated endocytosis, in particular, being the main mechanism.

Author Contributions: V.P., E.L. and M.C.B. conceived and designed the experiments; V.P., E.L. and G.G. performed the experiments; V.P., E.L., G.G. and M.C.B. analyzed the data; M.C.B., E.L. and V.P. wrote the paper; M.C.B., A.R.B. and D.E.P.-G. provided materials and equipment for the experiments; A.R.B. and D.E.P.-G. reviewed and revised the paper.

Acknowledgments: Maria Cristina Salvatici, Electron Microscopy Centre "Laura Bonzi" (Ce.M.E.), ICCOM, CNR, Sesto Fiorentino, Florence, Italy and Alessio Gnerucci Department of Experimental and Clinical Biomedical Sciences, University of Florence, Florence, Italy.

References

1. Saenz del Burgo, L.; Hernández, R.M.; Orive, G.; Pedraz, J.L. Nanotherapeutic approaches for brain cancer management. *Nanomed. NBM* **2014**, *10*, e905–e919. [CrossRef] [PubMed]
2. Pattni, B.S.; Chupin, V.V.; Torchilin, V.P. New developments in liposomal drug delivery. *Chem. Rev.* **2015**, *115*, 10938–10966. [CrossRef] [PubMed]
3. Bilia, A.R.; Bergonzi, M.C.; Guccione, C.; Manconi, M.; Fadda, A.M.; Sinico, C. Vesicles and micelles: Two versatile vectors for the delivery of natural products. *J. Drug Deliv. Sc. Technol.* **2016**, *32*, 241–255. [CrossRef]
4. Grossi, C.; Guccione, C.; Isacchi, B.; Bergonzi, M.C.; Luccarini, I.; Casamenti, F.; Bilia, A.R. Development of blood–brain barrier permeable nanoparticles as potential carriers for salvianolic acid B to CNS. *Planta Med.* **2017**, *83*, 382–391. [CrossRef] [PubMed]

5. Conti, E.; Gregori, M.; Radice, I.; Da Re, F.; Grana, D.; Re, F.; Salvati, E.; Masserini, M.; Ferrarese, C.; Zola, C.P.; et al. Multifunctional liposomes interact with Abeta in human biological fluids: Therapeutic implications for Alzheimer's disease. *Neurochem. Int.* **2017**, *108*, 60–65. [CrossRef] [PubMed]
6. Agrawal, M.; Tripathi, A.D.K.; Saraf, S.; Saraf, S.; Antimisiaris, S.G.; Mourtas, S.; Margareta, H.-U.; Alexander, A. Recent advancements in liposomes targeting strategies to cross blood-brain barrier (BBB) for the treatment of Alzheimer's disease. *J. Control. Release* **2017**, *260*, 61–77. [CrossRef] [PubMed]
7. Garcia-Garcia, E.; Andrieux, K.; Gil, S.; Couvreur, P. Colloidal carriers and blood–brain barrier (BBB) translocation: A way to deliver drugs to the brain? *Int. J. Pharm.* **2005**, *298*, 274–292. [CrossRef] [PubMed]
8. Balducci, C.; Mancini, S.; Minniti, S.; La Vitola, P.; Zotti, M.; Sancini, G.; Mauri, M.; Cagnotto, A. Multifunctional liposomes reduce brain β-amyloid burden and ameliorate memory impairment in Alzheimer's disease mouse models. *J. Neurosci.* **2014**, *34*, 14022–14031. [CrossRef] [PubMed]
9. Ordóñez-Gutiérrez, L.; Re, F.; Bereczki, E.; Ioja, E.; Gregori, M.; Andersen, A.J.; Antón, M.; Moghimi, S.M.; Pei, J.J.; Masserini, M.; et al. Repeated intraperitoneal injections of liposomes containing phosphatidic acid and cardiolipin reduce amyloid-β levels in APP/PS1 transgenic mice. *Nanomedicine* **2015**, *11*, 421–430. [CrossRef] [PubMed]
10. Mancini, S.; Minniti, S.; Gregori, M.; Sancini, G.; Cagnotto, A.; Couraud, P.O.; Ordóñez-Gutiérrez, L.; Wandosell, F.; Salmona, M.; Re, F. The hunt for brain Aβ oligomers by peripherally circulating multi-functional nanoparticles: Potential therapeutic approach for Alzheimer disease. *Nanomedicine* **2016**, *12*, 43–52. [CrossRef] [PubMed]
11. Graverini, G.; Piazzini, V.; Landucci, E.; Casamenti, F.; Pantano, D.; Pellegrini-Giampietro, D.; Bilia, A.R.; Bergonzi, M.C. Solid lipid nanoparticles for delivery of andrographolide across the blood-brain barrier: In vitro and in vivo evaluation. *Colloid. Surf. B Biointerfaces* **2018**, *161*, 302–313. [CrossRef] [PubMed]
12. Guccione, C.; Oufir, M.; Piazzini, V.; Eigenmann, D.E.; Jähne, E.A.; Zabela, V.; Faleschini, M.T.; Bergonzi, M.C.; Smiesko, M.; Hamburger, M.; et al. Andrographolide-loaded nanoparticles for brain delivery: Formulation, characterisation and in vitro permeability using hCMEC/D3 cell line. *Eur. J. Pharm. Biopharm.* **2017**, *119*, 253–263. [CrossRef] [PubMed]
13. Yen, T.L.; Chen, R.J.; Jayakumar, T.; Lu, W.J.; Hsieh, C.Y.; Hsu, M.J.; Yang, C.H.; Chang, C.C.; Lin, Y.K.; Lin, K.H. Andrographolide stimulates p38 mitogen-activated protein kinase-nuclear factor erythroid-2-related factor2-heme oxygenase 1 signaling in primary cerebral endothelial cells for definite protection against ischemic stroke in rats. *Transl. Res.* **2016**, *170*, 57–72. [CrossRef] [PubMed]
14. Serrano, F.G.; Tapia-Rojas, C.; Carvajal, F.J.; Hancke, J.; Cerpa, W.; Inestrosa, N.C. Andrographolide reduces cognitive impairment in young and mature AβPPswe/PS-1 mice. *Mol. Neurodegener.* **2014**, *9*, 61. [CrossRef] [PubMed]
15. Yu, B.T.; Zhang, Z.R.; Liu, W.S.; Yang, P.W.; Wang, P. Study on stability in vitro of andrographolide. *Chin. Tradit. Pat. Med.* **2002**, *24*, 33133.
16. Wang, M.; Ren, X.L.; Gao, X.M.; Vincieri, F.F.; Bilia, A.R. Stability of active ingredients of traditional Chinese medicine (TCM). *Nat. Prod. Commun.* **2009**, *4*, 1761–1776.
17. Crosasso, P.; Ceruti, M.; Brusa, P.; Arpicco, S.; Dosio, F.; Cattel, L. Preparation characterization and properties of sterically stabilized paclitaxel-containing liposome. *J. Control. Release* **2000**, *63*, 19–30. [CrossRef]
18. Bucke, W.E.; Leitzke, S.; Diederichs, J.E.; Muller, RH. Surface-modified amikacin-liposomes: Organ distribution and interaction with plasma proteins. *J. Drug Target.* **1998**, *5*, 99–108. [CrossRef] [PubMed]
19. Gulyaev, A.E.; Gelperina, S.E.; Skidan, I.N.; Antropov, A.S.; Kivman, G.Y.; Kreuter, J. Significant transport of doxorubicin into the brain with polysorbate 80-coated nanoparticles. *Pharm. Res.* **1999**, *16*, 1564–1569. [CrossRef] [PubMed]
20. Kreuter, J.; Shamenkov, D.; Petrov, V.; Ramge, P.; Cychutek, K.; Koch-Brandt, C.; Alyautdin, R. Apolipoprotein-mediated transport of nanoparticle-bound drugs across the blood-brain barrier. *J. Drug Target.* **2002**, *10*, 317–325. [CrossRef] [PubMed]
21. Wohlfart, S.; Gelperina, S.; Kreuter, J. Transport of drugs across the blood–brain barrier by nanoparticles. *J. Control. Release* **2012**, *161*, 264–273. [CrossRef] [PubMed]
22. Kreuter, J. Mechanism of polymeric nanoparticle-based drug transport across the blood-brain barrier (BBB). *J. Microencapsul.* **2013**, *30*, 49–54. [CrossRef] [PubMed]

23. Gastaldi, L.; Battaglia, L.; Peira, E.; Chirio, D.; Muntoni, E.; Solazzi, I.; Gallarate, M.; Dosio, F. Solid lipid nanoparticles as vehicles of drugs to the brain: Current state of the art. *Eur. J. Pharm. Biopharm.* **2014**, *87*, 433–444. [CrossRef] [PubMed]
24. Wong, H.L.; Wu, X.Y.; Bendayan, R. Nanotechnological advances for the delivery of CNS therapeutics. *Adv. Drug Deliv. Rev.* **2012**, *64*, 686–700. [CrossRef] [PubMed]
25. Di, L.; Kerns, E.H.; Fan, K.; McConnell, O.J.; Carter, G.T. High throughput artificial membrane permeability assay for blood–brain barrier. *Eur. J. Med. Chem.* **2003**, *38*, 223–232. [CrossRef]
26. Weksler, B.; Romero, I.A.; Couraud, P.O. The hCMEC/D3 cell line as a model of the human blood brain barrier. *Fluids Barriers CNS* **2013**, *10*, 16. [CrossRef] [PubMed]
27. Eigenmann, D.E.; Xue, G.; Kim, K.S.; Moses, A.V.; Hamburger, M.; Oufir, M. Comparative study of four immortalized human brain capillary endothelial cell lines, hCMEC/D3, hBMEC, TY10, and BB19, and optimization of culture conditions, for an in vitro blood–brain barrier model for drug permeability studies. *Fluids Barriers CNS* **2013**, *10*, 33. [CrossRef] [PubMed]
28. Bangham, A.D.; Hill, M.W.; Miller, N.G.A. Preparation and use of liposomes as models of biological membranes. In *Methods in Membrane Biology*; Springer: Boston, MA, USA, 1974; pp. 61–68. [CrossRef]
29. Righeschi, C.; Coronnello, M.; Mastrantoni, A.; Isacchi, B.; Bergonzi, M.C.; Mini, E.; Bilia, A.R. Strategy to provide a useful solution to effective delivery of dihydroartemisinin: Development, characterization and in vitro studies of liposomal formulations. *Colloids Surf. B Biointerfaces* **2014**, *116*, 121–127. [CrossRef] [PubMed]
30. Dua, J.S.; Rana, A.C.; Bhandari, A.K. Liposome: Methods of preparation and applications. *Int. J. Pharm. Stud. Res.* **2012**, *3*, 14–20.
31. Saengkrit, N.; Saesoo, S.; Srinuanchai, W.; Phunpee, S.; Ruktanonchai, U.R. Influence of curcumin-loaded cationic liposome on anticancer activity for cervical cancer therapy. *Colloids Surf. B Biointerfaces* **2014**, *114*, 349–356. [CrossRef] [PubMed]
32. Gualbert, J.; Shahgaldian, P.; Coleman, A.W. Interactions of amphiphilic calix [4] arene-based solid lipid nanoparticles with bovine serum albumin. *Int. J. Pharm.* **2003**, *257*, 69–73. [CrossRef]
33. Koziara, J.M.; Lockman, P.R.; Allen, D.D.; Mumper, R.J. Paclitaxel nanoparticles for the potential treatment of brain tumors. *J. Control. Release* **2004**, *99*, 259–269. [CrossRef] [PubMed]
34. Righeschi, C.; Bergonzi, M.C.; Isacchi, B.; Bazzicalupi, C.; Gratteri, P.; Bilia, A.R. Enhanced curcumin permeability by SLN formulation: The PAMPA approach. *LWT-Food Sci. Technol.* **2016**, *66*, 475–483. [CrossRef]
35. Wohnsland, F.; Faller, B. High-throughput permeability pH profile and high-throughput alkane/water log P with artificial membranes. *J. Med. Chem.* **2001**, *44*, 923–930. [CrossRef] [PubMed]
36. Conti, P.; Pinto, A.; Tamborini, L.; Madsen, U.; Nielsen, B.; Bräuner-Osborne, H.; Hansen, K.B.; Landucci, E.; Pellegrini-Giampietro, D.E.; De Sarro, G.; et al. Novel 3-carboxy-and 3-phosphonopyrazoline amino acids as potent and selective NMDA receptor antagonists: Design, synthesis, and pharmacological characterization. *ChemMedChem* **2010**, *5*, 1465–1475. [CrossRef] [PubMed]
37. Landucci, E.; Lattanzi, R.; Gerace, E.; Scartabelli, T.; Balboni, G.; Negri, L.; Pellegrini-Giampietro, D.E. Prokineticins are neuroprotective in models of cerebral ischemia and ischemic tolerance in vitro. *Neuropharmacology* **2016**, *108*, 39–48. [CrossRef] [PubMed]
38. Chavan, S.S.; Ingle, S.G.; Vavia, P.R. Preparation and characterization of solid lipid nanoparticle-based nasal spray of budesonide. *Drug Deliv. Transl. Res.* **2013**, *3*, 402–408. [CrossRef] [PubMed]
39. Papadia, K.; Markoutsa, E.; Antimisiaris, S.G. How do the physicochemical properties of nanoliposomes affect their interactions with the hCMEC/D3 cellular model of the BBB? *Int. J. Pharm.* **2016**, *509*, 431–438. [CrossRef] [PubMed]
40. Markoutsa, E.; Pampalakis, G.; Niarakis, A.; Romero, I.A.; Weksler, B.; Couraud, P.-O.; Antimisiaris, S.G. Uptake and permeability studies of BBB-targeting immunoliposomes using the hCMEC/D3 cell line. *Eur. J. Pharm. Biopharm.* **2011**, *77*, 265–274. [CrossRef] [PubMed]
41. Mohan, A.; Narayanan, S.; Balasubramanian, G.; Sethuraman, S.; Krishnan, U.M. Dual drug loaded nanoliposomal chemotherapy: A promising strategy for treatment of head and neck squamous cell carcinoma. *Eur. J. Pharm. Biopharm.* **2016**, *99*, 73–83. [CrossRef] [PubMed]
42. Benfer, M.; Kissel, T. Cellular uptake mechanism and knockdown activity of siRNA-loaded biodegradable DEAPA-PVAg-PLGA nanoparticles. *Eur. J. Pharm. Biopharm.* **2012**, *80*, 247–256. [CrossRef] [PubMed]

43. Poller, B.; Gutmann, H.; Krähenbühl, S.; Weksler, B.; Romero, I.; Couraud, P.O.; Tuffin, G.; Drewe, J.; Huwyler, J. The human brain endothelial cell line hCMEC/D3 as a human blood-brain barrier model for drug transport studies. *J. Neurochem.* **2008**, *107*, 1358–1368. [CrossRef] [PubMed]
44. Rajendran, L.; Knolker, H.J.; Simons, K. Subcellular targeting strategies for drug design and delivery. *Nat. Rev. Drug Discov.* **2010**, *9*, 29–42. [CrossRef] [PubMed]
45. Lin, K.H.; Hong, S.-T.; Wang, H.-T.; Lo, Y.-L.; Lin, A.M.-Y.; Yang, J.C.-H. Enhancing Anticancer Effect of Gefitinib across the Blood–Brain Barrier Model Using Liposomes Modified with One α-Helical Cell-Penetrating Peptide or Glutathione and Tween 80. *Int. J. Mol. Sci.* **2016**, *17*, 1998. [CrossRef] [PubMed]
46. Takeuchi, H.; Makhlof, A.; Fujimoto, S.; Tozuka, Y. In vitro and in vivo evaluation of WGA-carbopol modified liposomes as carriers for oral peptide delivery. *Eur. J. Pharm. Biopharm.* **2011**, *77*, 216–224. [CrossRef]
47. Huth, U.S.; Schubert, R.; Peschka-Suss, R. Investigating the uptake and intracellular fate of pH-sensitive liposomes by flow cytometry and spectral bio-imaging. *J. Control. Release* **2006**, *110*, 490–504. [CrossRef] [PubMed]

6

Intracellular Delivery of Natural Antioxidants via Hyaluronan Nanohydrogels

Elita Montanari [1], Chiara Di Meo [1,*], Tommasina Coviello [1], Virginie Gueguen [2], Graciela Pavon-Djavid [2,*] and Pietro Matricardi [1]

1 Department of Drug Chemistry and Technologies, Sapienza University of Rome, P.le Aldo Moro 5, 00185 Rome, Italy; elita.montanari@uniroma1.it (E.M.); tommasina.coviello@uniroma1.it (T.C.); pietro.matricardi@uniroma1.it (P.M.)

2 INSERM U1148, Laboratory for Vascular Translational Science, Cardiovascular Bioengineering, Paris 13 University, Sorbonne Paris Cite 99, Av. Jean-Baptiste Clément, 93430 Villetaneuse, France; virginie.gueguen@univ-paris13.fr

* Correspondence: chiara.dimeo@uniroma1.it (C.D.M.); graciela.pavon@univ-paris13.fr (G.P.-D.)

Abstract: Natural antioxidants, such as astaxanthin (AX), resveratrol (RV) and curcumin (CU), are bioactive molecules that show a number of therapeutic effects. However, their applications are remarkably limited by their poor water solubility, physico-chemical instability and low bioavailability. In the present work, it is shown that self-assembled hyaluronan (HA)-based nanohydrogels (NHs) are taken up by endothelial cells (Human Umbilical Vein Endothelial Cells, HUVECs), preferentially accumulating in the perinuclear area of oxidatively stressed HUVECs, as evidenced by flow cytometry and confocal microscopy analyses. Furthermore, NHs are able to physically entrap and to significantly enhance the apparent water solubility of AX, RV and CU in aqueous media. AX/NHs, RV/NHs and CU/NHs systems showed good hydrodynamic diameters (287, 214 and 267 nm, respectively), suitable ζ-potential values (−45, −43 and −37 mV, respectively) and the capability to neutralise reactive oxygen species (ROS) in tube. AX/NHs system was also able to neutralise ROS *in vitro* and did not show any toxicity against HUVECs. This research suggests that HA-based NHs can represent a kind of nano-carrier suitable for the intracellular delivery of antioxidant agents, for the treatment of oxidative stress in endothelial cells.

Keywords: drug delivery; astaxanthin; resveratrol; curcumin; hyaluronan; nanohydrogels; oxidative stress; intracellular therapy

---

1. Introduction

Reactive oxygen species (ROS) are highly reactive molecules derived from the molecular oxygen [1], which are produced as normal by-products of aerobic respiration in eukaryotic cells. Although physiological concentrations of ROS are crucial for ensuring the cell survival, the loss of redox equilibrium by over-production of ROS or by failed control systems is detrimental to cells and leads to oxidative stress (OS) [2]. Many research lines evidenced that OS and inflammation processes are key-factors for the development of several diseases, such as neurodegenerative diseases, cardiovascular disorders and cancer [3]. Epidemiological studies suggest that low levels of antioxidants are associated with an increased risk of disease, whilst an increased consumption seems to be protective. Targeting the reestablishment of redox homeostasis by stimulation/blocking of endogenous systems or by administration of exogenous drugs is a strategy followed in several pathologies. In a recent clinical trial, the association of N-acetylcysteine with metformin revealed good perspectives in the treatment of non-alcoholic steatohepatitis [4]. The combination of anti-inflammatory drugs, such as sulphasalazine [5] with natural antioxidants (e.g. curcumin and quercetin) [6,7], showed significant antioxidant properties in animal models.

Among natural antioxidants, carotenoids (e.g., astaxanthin, AX) present interesting biological properties: AX is a potent quencher of oxygen singlets, superoxide anions and hydroxyl radicals [8]. In previous works we showed that natural AX can protect human umbilical vein endothelial cells (HUVECs) under OS [9]. However, AX is a highly unsaturated molecule and easily decomposes when exposed to heat, light and oxygen. In addition, the applications of AX and other widely used antioxidants molecules, such as resveratrol (RV) [10,11] and curcumin (CU) [12,13], are often limited by their low solubility in water, their physico-chemical instability and their low bioavailability. Therefore, the use of novel drug delivery systems for enhancing the apparent water-solubility, stability and release of antioxidant molecules in the site of interest is crucial for the *in vivo* delivery and the development of antioxidant-based therapies. In this respect, nanohydrogels (NHs) [14,15], which are nano three-dimensional networks, are capable to deliver a variety of bioactive molecules at the target site, such as hydrophobic [16] as well as hydrophilic drugs [17], polypeptides [18] and genetic materials [19]. In fact, the porosity of the NHs network provides a reservoir for loading molecular and macromolecular therapeutics as well as protecting them from the environmental degradation. NHs are usually soft, hydrophilic, biocompatible and are able to absorb a high amount of water and easily swell and de-swell in aqueous media [20]. NHs can be prepared from natural [21] and/or synthetic polymers [22] and, based on the type of linkages present in the polymer network, NHs are subdivided into groups based on either physical or chemical cross-linking. Among the natural polymers, hyaluronan (HA) [23] is a linear, non-sulfated glycosaminoglycan, a poly-anionic polysaccharide, which occurs in all living organisms. HA is highly hydrophilic and can interact with a number of molecules and receptors which are involved in cellular signal transductions [24]. The major HA receptor is CD44 [25], which is known to be involved in the binding, endocytosis and metabolism of HA. A considerable number of publications reported that CD44 is up-regulated and plays a crucial role in a variety of inflammatory diseases [26,27]. However, the real functions of CD44 in inflammation processes are rather complex and they are still under investigation.

The present study aims to investigate the capability of HA-based NHs to enter healthy or oxidatively stressed endothelial cells (HUVECs) and to physically encapsulate three different antioxidant molecules, such as AX, RV and CU. AX/NHs, RV/NHs and CU/NHs systems were characterised in terms of size, polydispersity, ζ-potential and loading efficiency, while their antioxidant activity was investigated in tube. Moreover, the cellular antioxidant activity of AX/NHs and its toxicity were studied in oxidatively stressed HUVECs.

2. Materials and Methods

2.1. Chemicals

Hyaluronan (HA, $M_w = 2.2 \times 10^5$) was purchased from Contipro (Dolní Dobrouc ̌, Czech Republic) and was modified in the tetrabutylammonium salt (HA^-TBA^+) by using a Dowex cation exchange resin (Merck, Milan, Italy). Natural curcumin (CU, purity > 97.0% HPLC) and resveratrol (RV, purity > 99.0% HPLC) were purchased from Tokyo Chemical Industry Co., Ltd. (Tokyo, Japan). Natural astaxanthin from Haematococcus pluvialis (AX, purity > 97.0% HPLC), cholesterol (CH), 4-bromobutyric acid, *N*-methyl-2-pyrrolidone (NMP), *N*-(3-dimethylaminopropyl)-*N*′-(ethylcarbodimide hydrochloride) (EDC·HCl), 4-(dimethylamino) pyridine (DMAP), dimethyl sulfoxide (DMSO, American Chemical Society (ACS) grade reagent ≥ 99.9%), rhodamine B isothiocyanate (Rhod), 2,2′-azino-di-(3-ethylbenzthiazoline sulfonic acid) (ABTS) solution and potassium persulfate ($K_2S_2O_8$) were purchased from Sigma-Aldrich (Milan, Italy).

Human umbilical vein endothelial cells (HUVECs, ATCC CRL 1730) were purchased from LGC Standards S.a.r.l. (Molsheim, France). Antimicyn A (Streptomyces sp., AM), phalloidin, 4′,6-diamidino-2-phenylindole (DAPI), Triton, paraformaldehyde (PFA), dihydroethidium dye (DHE),

N-acetyl cysteine (NAC) were purchased from Sigma-Aldrich (Sigma Aldrich Chemie S.a.r.l., L'Isle d'Abeau Chesnes, France). Phosphate buffer saline (PBS), trypsin, Hank's Balanced Salt Solution (HBSS) and all reagents for cell culture were purchased from Invitrogen, ThermoFisher Scientific (Villebon sur Yvette, France). Culture plates were from Costar (Fisher Scientific SAS, Illkirch Cedex, France). CellTiter 96®AQueous One Solution Cell Proliferation Assay (MTS) was purchased from Promega (Charbonnières-les-Bains, France).

2.2. *Methods*

2.2.1. Synthesis of Empty and Fluorescent NHs

The methods for the synthesis of hyaluronan-cholesterol (HA-CH) derivative and the preparation of empty nanohydrogels formed by the self-assembling of HA-CH molecules (NHs) were extensively described in previous works [18,20] and will be not explained in detail here.

To obtain fluorescent NHs, the Rhod dye was covalently linked to the hydroxyl groups of NHs as previously reported [17].

2.2.2. Cell Culture

Cells were grown to 70–80% confluence, according to each experimental setting. In all experiments, untreated cells (which received PBS) were used and processed in parallel for an appropriate comparison.

Healthy HUVECs

HUVECs were cultured in complete low glucose Dulbecco's Modified Eagle Medium (DMEM, 1X GlutamaxTM-I) supplemented with 10% Foetal Calf Serum and 1% (*v/v*) Penicillin-Streptomycin-Amphotericin (PSA) solution, at 37 °C in a humidified atmosphere with 5% CO_2.

Oxidatively Stressed HUVECs

HUVECs were seeded in well plates and incubated for 48 h in complete DMEM. Cells were washed with PBS and, after the addition of fresh complete DMEM, cells were incubated with a suitable volume of 150 μM AM to obtain the final AM concentration of 11 μM, for 1 h at 37 °C in the dark, thus obtaining oxidatively stressed HUVECs.

2.2.3. Cell Binding/Uptake of NHs in HUVECs

The cell binding/uptake kinetics of fluorescent and empty NHs (Rhod-NHs) was studied in healthy or oxidatively stressed HUVECs, with a BD Accuri C6, BD 254 Bioscences (Erembodegem, Belgium) flow cytometer equipped with a 488 nm excitation laser beam and a 585/40 nm bandpass filter (FL2 channel). For each sample 50,000 events were collected. 300,000 cells/well (1.5 mL of cell suspension in complete DMEM) were seeded in a six-well plate and incubated for 48 h. Cell monolayers were then washed with 1 mL PBS, added by 1.5 mL of fresh complete DMEM and incubated with 0.35 mL of Rhod-NHs in PBS, at the final concentration of 0.1 mg mL^{-1}, for 3, 6 or 24 h at 37 °C. As negative control, cells received 0.35 mL PBS. Medium was removed, HUVECs were washed three times with PBS, allowed to detach with 0.7 mL trypsin and finally added to 2 mL complete DMEM. Cell suspensions were centrifuged for 5 min at 1200 rpm at 25 °C. Supernatants were removed and pellets were washed with 1 mL HBSS solution and centrifuged again. Pellets were re-suspended in 0.5 mL HBSS and the red fluorescence (due to the presence of Rhod) was detected with the flow cytometer. For the study of the binding/uptake kinetics in oxidatively stressed HUVECs, prior to the incubation with 0.35 mL, Rhod-NHs cells were added by 0.11 mL of AM solution (150 μM), for 1 h at 37 °C in the dark (AM final concentration = 11 μM), washed with 1 mL PBS and added by 1.5 mL of fresh complete DMEM. For the negative control, HUVECs received 0.35 mL PBS. Results were expressed as median fluorescence intensity (MFI). The dot plot was reported by plotting forward scattering (FSC-H) versus side scattering (SSC-H) and the gate was defined excluding cell debris. Each experiment was performed in triplicate ($n = 3$).

2.2.4. Cell Imaging: Confocal Microscopy

Immunofluorescence signal of Rhod-NHs was analysed by recording stained images using the Carl Zeiss®LSM 780, objective ×10, confocal microscope. Digital images were processed with ZEN software or Fiji-win 32 (ImageJ). 20,000 cells/well (400 µL of cell suspension in complete DMEM) were seeded in a Lab-Tek (Thermo Fisher Scientific, Milan, Italy) and incubated for 48 h. Cell monolayers were then washed with 400 µL PBS, added by 400 µL of fresh complete DMEM and incubated with 29 µL of PBS (healthy HUVECs) or 29 µL of 150 µM AM (oxidatively stressed HUVECs) for 1 h at 37 °C in the dark. Cells were washed with 400 µL PBS, added by 400 µL of fresh complete DMEM and incubated with 100 µL of 500 µg mL^{-1} Rhod-NHs in PBS (corresponding to a final concentration of 100 µg mL^{-1}) for 3 h and 24 h. As negative control, cells received 100 µL PBS. HUVECs were then washed with 400 µL PBS, fixed with 200 µL 2% PFA for 10 min at 4 °C, washed twice with 400 µL PBS and added by 200 µL DAPI (dilution 1:50,000) for 5 min at 25 °C. Cells were finally washed twice with 400 µL PBS and slides were mounted with 10 µL Dako and checked with the confocal microscope.

2.2.5. Preparation and Characterisation of AX-Loaded NHs

For the preparation of AX-loaded NHs samples of HA-CH (1.5 mg mL^{-1}, degree of functionalisation (Df) = 15%, mols of CH/ mols of HA repeating units) were left under magnetic stirring in bi-distilled water overnight, at 25 °C. The suspensions were then placed in an autoclave (121 °C, 1.1 bar for 20 min) where NHs were formed. AX was solubilised in DMSO (concentration = 9 mg mL^{-1}) and then added to NHs suspension (24 µL for 1 mg of HA-CH), corresponding to a weight ratio of 0.216 (mg of AX/mg of NHs). The nano-suspensions of AX/NHs were left for 5 h at 25 °C in the dark, dialysed against water for 6 h (MW cut-off: 12,000–14,000) and then centrifuged at 4000 rpm for 20 min at 25 °C. Pellets (unloaded AX) were discarded and the supernatants (AX/NHs) were freeze-dried. Mean hydrodynamic diameter ($\overline{d}_h$), polydispersity index (PDI) and ζ-potential (ζ-pot) of AX/NHs were measured by Dynamic Light Scattering (DLS) at 25 °C by using a Zetasizer Nano ZS instrument (Model ZEN3690, Malvern Instruments) equipped with a solid state HeNe laser ($\lambda = 633$ nm) at a scattering angle of 173°. The electrophoretic mobility of the samples was converted in ζ-pot by using the Smoluchowski equation. Empty NHs were also tested for an appropriate comparison. Each experiment was performed in triplicate ($n = 3$).

2.2.6. Preparation and Characterisation of RV or CU-Loaded NHs

Samples of HA-CH (1.0 mg mL^{-1}, Df of 15%) were left under magnetic stirring in bi-distilled water overnight, at 25 °C. The suspensions were then placed in an autoclave (121 °C, 1.1 bar for 20 min) where NHs were formed. RV or CU were solubilised in acetone at the concentration of 2 mg mL^{-1}; 0.5 mL of each drug solution were allowed to evaporate with Heidolph Hei-VAP rotary evaporator (Buchi, Schwabach, Germany) and the drug film was then added by 3 mL of NHs, corresponding to a weight ratio of 0.33 (mg of RV or CU / mg of NHs). The mixtures were kept under magnetic stirring for 14 h at 25 °C in the dark and then centrifuged at 4000 rpm for 10 min at 20 °C. Pellets (unloaded RV or CU) were discarded and the supernatants (RV/NHs or CU/NHs) were analysed with DLS. Each experiment was performed in triplicate ($n = 3$).

2.2.7. Quantification of Entrapped AX into NHs

The amount of AX entrapped into NHs was estimated using a Perkin-Elmer double beam "Lambda 3A" model Ultraviolet-Visible (UV-Vis) spectrometer (Milan, Italy). Freeze-dried AX/NHs were previously dispersed in few µL of water and then solubilised in a large excess of DMSO, by vortexing for few minutes. Samples were analysed at 25 °C, using 1 mm quartz cuvettes (Hellma

Analytics, Milan, Italy). The AX calibration curve was evaluated at the concentration range of 6.25–100 μg mL^{-1} ($R^2 = 0.999$, $\lambda = 490$ nm, $n = 5$). Each experiment was performed in triplicate ($n = 3$).

2.2.8. Quantification of Entrapped RV or CU into NHs

RV or CU pellets (free drugs) were solubilised in EtOH and quantified in order to obtain, by difference, the amount of entrapped drug into NHs. Analyses were performed by HPLC using a KnauerAzura instrument equipped with a binary pump (Azura P 6.1L) and a UV-Vis detector (190–750 nm, Azura UVD 2.1L), controlled by Clarity software. Samples (20 μL) were injected into a KnauerEurospher II C18 column (5 μm, 4.6 × 250 mm); the samples were injected at 1 mL min^{-1} in mixtures of water: acetonitrile (gradient mode) from 70:30 to 0:100 for RV and in water (+ 0.1% *v*/*v* of TFA): acetonitrile (+ 0.1% *v*/*v* of TFA) from 50:50 to 0:100 for CU. The unloaded RV was quantified at $\lambda = 306$ nm using a calibration curve previously recorded with RV standard solutions in ethanol in the range 6.25–50 μg mL^{-1} ($R^2 = 0.999$, $n = 5$); CU was detected at $\lambda = 425$ nm using a calibration curve in ethanol (0.39–50 μg mL^{-1}, $R^2 = 0.999$, $n = 8$) by integrating the three signals related to CU (~79 %), demethoxycurcumin (~18%) and bisdemethoxycurcumin (~3%).

Encapsulation Efficiency (EE) and Drug Loading (DL) of AX/NHs, RV/NHs and CU/NHs were calculated using the Equations (1) and (2):

$$\%EE = \frac{concentration\ of\ loaded\ drug}{concentration\ of\ added\ drug} \times 100 \tag{1}$$

$$\%DL = \frac{concentration\ of\ loaded\ drug}{polymer\ concentration} \times 100 \tag{2}$$

2.2.9. Antioxidant Activity of AX/NHs, RV/NHs and CU/NHs in Tube

ABTS assay: 5 mL of 3.8 mg mL^{-1} ABTS solution in bi-distilled water were added to 88 μL of 38 mg mL^{-1} $K_2S_2O_8$ solution in bi-distilled water, corresponding to a molar ratio of 2.3 (mol of ABTS per mol of $K_2S_2O_{48}$). The mixture (containing $ABTS^{\bullet+}$) was left overnight at 25 °C in the dark and diluted ~1:80 with bi-distilled water. 2.9 mL of the diluted $ABTS^{\bullet+}$ solution were added by 0.1 mL of nano-suspensions in bi-distilled water (AX/NHs, RV/NHs or CU/NHs and their controls) and the absorbance (Abs) was detected at $\lambda = 730$ nm between 12 s and 10 min, at 25 °C. The final concentration of all the antioxidant drugs was 13 μM. For an appropriate comparison, the ABTS assay was also tested on the free drugs: 2.9 mL of the diluted $ABTS^{\bullet+}$ solution in bi-distilled water were added by 0.1 mL of AX, RV or CU solutions in DMSO and the Abs was detected at $\lambda = 730$ nm. The final concentration of the free antioxidant drugs was the same as the loaded ones (13 μM). The antioxidant activity (AA) was calculated at 6 min, by using the following equation:

$$\%\,AA = \frac{Abs\ ABTS - Abs\ sample}{Abs\ ABTS} \times 100$$

2.2.10. Cell Viability

MTS Test: 10,000 cells/well (175 μL of cell suspension in complete DMEM) were seeded in a 96-well plate and incubated for 48 h. HUVECs were then washed with 100 μL PBS, added by 175 μL of fresh complete DMEM and treated with 13 μL of PBS (healthy HUVECs) or 13 μL of 150 μM AM (oxidatively stressed HUVECs) for 1 h at 37 °C in the dark. Cells were washed with 100 μL PBS, added by 175 μL of fresh complete DMEM and incubated with 25 μL of samples (AX/NHs or NHs in PBS) at specific final concentrations (ranging from 31 to 500 μg mL^{-1}, dilution factor (df) = 1:2) and incubated for 24 h. The highest concentration of AX in AX/NHs was 10 μg mL^{-1} (corresponding to 16.5 μM, df = 1:2). For an appropriate comparison, cells received 25 μL of PBS. The medium was then removed, cells were gently washed with 100 μL PBS and added by 100 μL of complete DMEM. 20 μL MTS were added to each well and the number of viable cells was measured by reading the Abs at 490 nm with the TECAN Infinite 200PRO plate reader (Mannedorf, Switzerland). Results were processed by using i-Control 1.10 software. Each experiment was performed on 8 wells ($n = 3$).

2.2.11. Cell Morphology

10,000 cells/well (400 μL of cell suspension in complete DMEM) were seeded in a Lab-Tek and incubated for 48 h. HUVECs were then washed with 100 μL PBS, added by 175 μL of fresh complete DMEM and treated with 13 μL of PBS (healthy HUVECs) or 13 μL of 150 μM AM (oxidatively stressed HUVECs) for 1 h at 37 °C in the dark. Cells were washed with 100 μL PBS, added by 175 μL of fresh complete DMEM and incubated with 25 μL of samples (AX/NHs or NHs in PBS) at the final concentration of 250 μg mL^{-1} and incubated for 24 h. For an appropriate comparison, cells received 25 μL of PBS. HUVECs were washed with 400 μL PBS, fixed with 200 μL 4% PFA for 30 min at 4 °C, washed twice with 400 μL PBS and added by 200 μL of 0.1% Triton for 5 min at 25 °C. Cells were washed again twice with 400 μL PBS and then treated with 200 μL DAPI (dilution 1:1000) and phalloidin (dilution 1:200) solution for 30 min at 25 °C. Cells were finally washed twice with PBS (400 μL), slides were fixed and then digital images were obtained and analysed using Nanozoomer digital pathology software (Hamamatsu, Japan).

2.2.12. Cellular Antioxidant Activity of AX/NHs

Cellular antioxidant activity (CAA) test: 10,000 cells/well (175 μL of cell suspension in complete DMEM) were seeded in 96 well plates and incubated for 48 h. HUVECs were then washed with 100 μL PBS, added by 175 μL of fresh complete DMEM and treated with 25 μL of samples (AX/NHs or NHs in PBS) at the final concentrations of 250 and 500 μg mL^{-1}) and incubated for 6 h at 37 °C. The highest concentration of AX in AX/NHs was 10 μg mL^{-1}, corresponding to 16.5 μM. As negative control, cells received 25 μL of PBS, whilst as positive control cells received 15 μL of 300 mM NAC (corresponding to a final concentration of 22 μM). The medium was then removed, cells were carefully washed with 100 μL PBS and added by 130 μL of 5 μM DHE dye and incubated for 30 min in the dark at 37 °C. Then 10 μL of 150 μM AM were added and HUVECs were incubated for 1 h at 37 °C in the dark. Cells were washed with PBS, added by 100 μL PBS and fluorescence was red with the TECAN Infinite 200PRO plate reader, using an excitation wavelength at 500 nm and an emission wavelength at 600 nm. Results were processed by using i-Control 1.10 software. Each experiment was performed on 4 wells ($n = 3$).

2.2.13. Statistical Analysis

CAA of AX/NHs or NHs: viable cell counts were calculated using four biological replicate count data (each derived from three technical replicate data). All data are normalised to the negative control (untreated cells that received PBS) and are expressed as the mean value ± standard deviation. Statistical significance was determined using four biological replicate data ($n = 3$) with a Mann–Whitney test by using SPSS 20 Software. Values of $p < 0.05$ were considered significant. Asterisk denotes statistically significant differences ($^{*}p < 0.05$).

Cell Viability: viable HUVECs (MTS test) were calculated using three biological replicates (each derived from 8 wells). All data are normalised to the negative control (untreated cells that received PBS) and are expressed as the mean value ± standard deviation. Statistical significance was determined using 8 wells ($n = 3$) with One-way ANOVA analysis in Prism (GraphPad 5.0 Software, Inc., La Jolla, CA, USA). Differences between the two groups were determined by a Turkey's multiple comparison test. Asterisks denote statistically significant differences ($^{*}p < 0.05$; $^{**}p < 0.01$; $^{***}p < 0.005$).

3. Results

3.1. Cell Binding/Uptake Kinetics of NHs in Healthy or Oxidatively Stressed HUVECs

Rhod dye was covalently linked to the hydroxyl groups of NHs [17] and the obtained fluorescent NHs were used for the binding/internalization kinetics study in healthy or oxidatively stressed HUVECs by flow cytometry (Figure 1A) and confocal microscopy (Figure 1B). Flow cytometry analysis evidenced that both, healthy and oxidatively stressed HUVECs, incubated for 3 h with Rhod-NHs, showed a significant increase in fluorescence intensity, indicating an evident binding/uptake of NHs within the cells, followed by a plateau up to 6 h; after 24 h the fluorescence intensity of HUVECs increased again (Figure 1A). Interestingly, the fluorescent intensity of oxidatively stressed HUVECs was almost two-fold higher than that of healthy HUVECs, at all the tested time points, suggesting that HUVECs are able to bind/take up more NHs in stress conditions. According to confocal microscopy analysis, NHs are located into vesicle-like structures in the perinuclear area, suggesting an intracellular location of NHs (Figure 1B). A similar outcome was already obtained, by incubating human keratinocytes (HaCaT) with Rhod-NHs [17]. Moreover, micro-graphs of oxidatively stressed cells showed a higher red fluorescence than that observed for healthy cells, confirming that HUVECs take up more NHs in stress conditions.

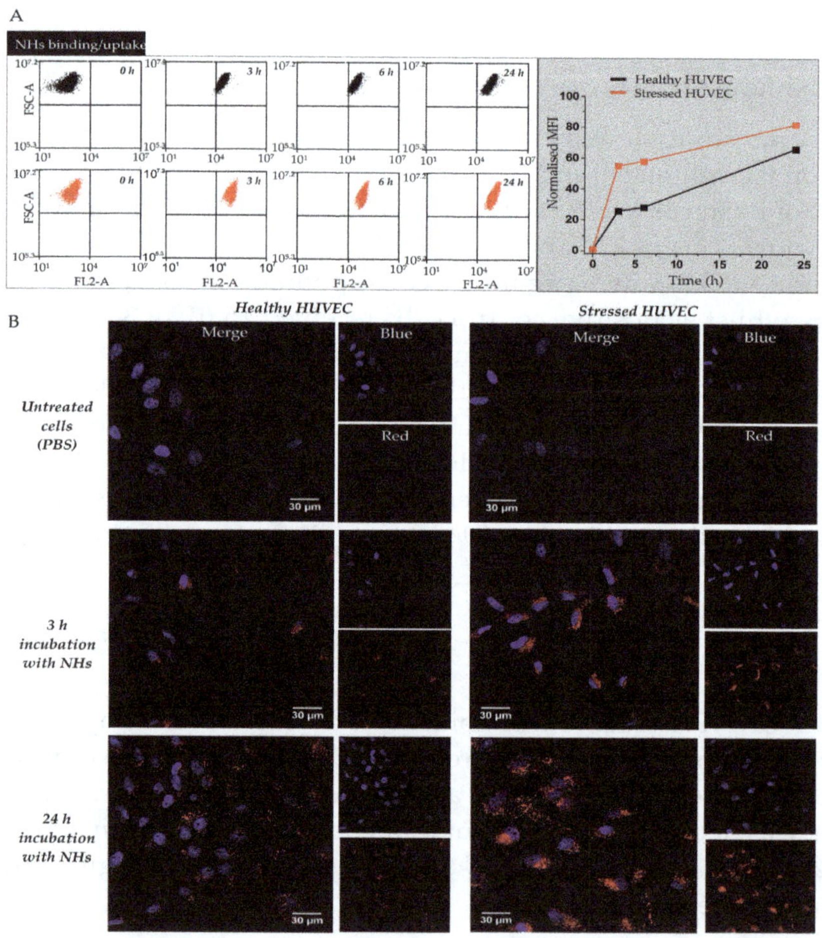

Figure 1. (**A**) Flow cytometry analysis of healthy or oxidatively stressed Human Umbilical Vein Endothelial Cells (HUVECs) incubated with rhodamine B isothiocyanate-nanohydrogels (Rhod-NHs). Cells were cultured in complete Dulbecco's Modified Eagle Medium (DMEM) for 48 h and then incubated from 3 to 24 h with 100 μg mL^{-1} Rhod-NHs. (**B**) Confocal micro-graphs (scale bars: 30 μm) of healthy (left) or oxidatively stressed (right) HUVECs, incubated with 100 μg mL^{-1} Rhod-NHs for 3 or 24 h. Blue colour refers to nuclei incubated with 4′,6-diamidino-2-phenylindole (DAPI), whilst red colour refers to Rhod-NHs. Untreated cells received PBS.

3.2. Preparation and Characterisation of AX/NHs, RV/NHs and CU/NHs Systems

AX, RV and CU, which are three natural antioxidant molecules poorly soluble in water, were loaded into NHs with the aim to enhance their solubilisation in aqueous environments, their intracellular accumulation as well as their therapeutic efficacy. NHs aqueous suspensions, obtained by autoclaving [28], were added by AX, RV or CU (according to the experimental procedures described in Sections 2.2.5 and 2.2.6), for drug encapsulation. The obtained AX/NHs, RV/NHs and CU/NHs (Figure 2A) were purified from the free antioxidant drugs by centrifugation (4000 rpm for 10 or 20 min) and the EE% and the DL% were evaluated with HPLC (RV/NHs and CU/NHs) or with a UV-Vis spectrometer (AX/NHs). The amounts of entrapped drugs are reported in Figure 2D: RV loading (%EE, 32.6 ± 1.1) was similar to that of CU (%EE, 27.0 ± 5.0) and higher than that of AX (%EE, 12.3 ± 0.6). This may be due to the lower MW (smaller size) of RV or CU compared to AX. AX/NHs, RV/NHs and CU/NHs were characterised in terms of $\overline{d}_h$, PDI and ζ-pot, as summarised in Figure 2B–D, showing average sizes of 287 nm (AX/NHs), 214 nm (RV/NHs) and 267 nm (CU/NHs), which appear to be dependent on the MW of the drugs (AX > CU > RV). The ζ-pot net values of loaded-NHs (ranging from ≈ |45| to |37| mV) were lower than those of unloaded NHs (≈ |49| mV), but high enough to ensure a good stability of the nano-formulations.

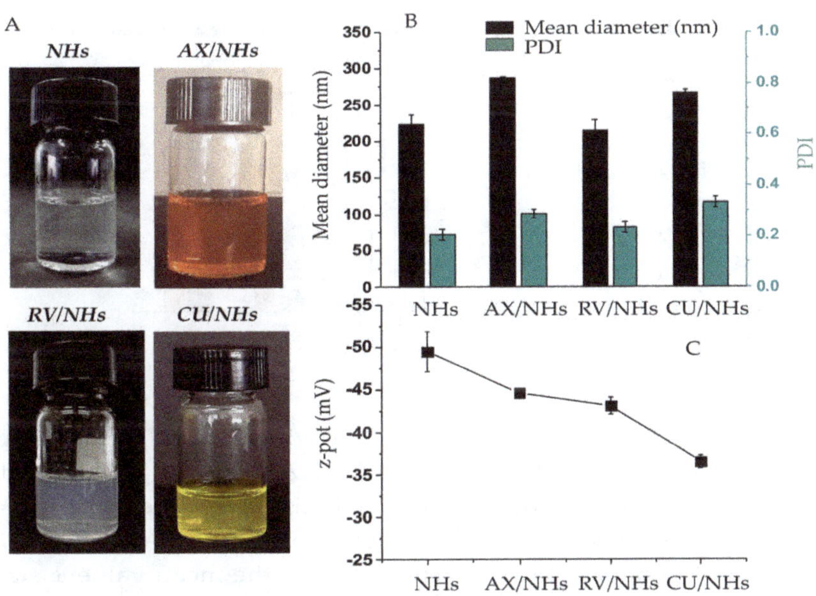

D

	$\overline{d}_h$ (nm)	PDI	z-pot (mV)	%EE	%DL
NHs	224 ± 13	0.21 ± 0.02	- 49.5 ± 2.4		
AX/NHs	287 ± 2	0.29 ± 0.01	- 44.6 ± 0.6	12.3 ± 0.6	4.1 ± 0.2
RV/NHs	214 ± 16	0.23 ± 0.02	- 43.1 ± 1.0	32.6 ± 1.1	11 ± 1
CU/NHs	267 ± 5	0.33 ± 0.02	- 36.5 ± 0.7	27.0. ± 5.0	9 ± 2

Figure 2. (**A**) Pictures of NHs, astaxanthin/nanohydrogels (AX/NHs), resveratrol/nanohydrogels (RV/NHs) and curcumin/nanohydrogels (CU/NHs) samples. (**B**) mean hydrodynamic diameter ($\overline{d}_h$) and polydispersity index (PDI) and (**C**) ζ-potential (ζ-pot) of free NHs, AX/NHs, RV/NHs and CU/NHs. Samples were characterised with dynamic light scattering (DLS) (**D**) Table summarising the physico-chemical properties ($\overline{d}_h$, PDI and ζ-pot), the encapsulation efficiency (EE%) and the drug loading (DL%) of AX/NHs, RV/NHs and CU/NHs.

3.3. Antioxidant Activity of AX/NHs, RV/NHs and CU/NHs Samples in Tube and in Vitro

Once loaded into NHs, the AA of AX, RV and CU were checked with the ABTS test [29] and compared to that of the free drugs. ABTS assay measures the ability of the antioxidant molecules to scavenge the $ABTS^{\bullet+}$, which is generated by the reaction of ABTS salt with a strong oxidising agent, such as potassium persulfate. The reduction of the blue-green $ABTS^{\bullet+}$ coloured solution (due to the presence of hydrogen-donating antioxidant molecules) is due to the suppression of its characteristic absorption spectrum at λ = 730 nm. Results evidenced that free NHs do not show any AA, whilst RV has the highest AA, followed by CU and finally by AX. The AA of AX molecules did not change when they were loaded into NHs (Figure 3A,B); conversely, loaded molecules of RV and CU lost 23 and 27% of AA, respectively, compared to those of the starting drugs. This result may be due to the longer encapsulation process (14 h for RV and CU and 5 h for AX), needed to obtain stable nano-formulations with suitable physico-chemical properties. The highest AA was evidenced by RV/NHs (60%), whilst AX/NHs and CU/NHs showed similar AA (38 and 40%, respectively).

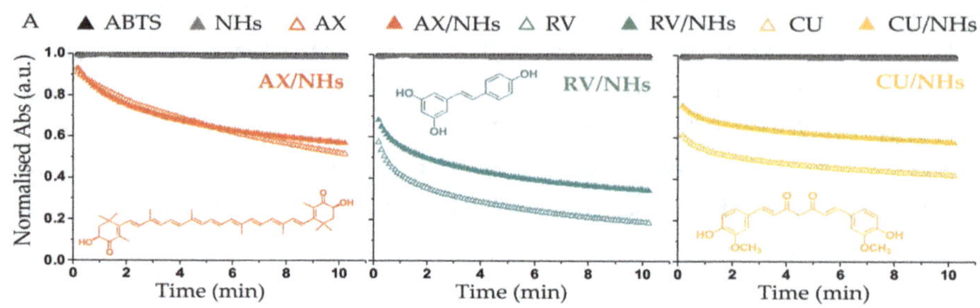

B

	Normalised AA (%) in tube
NHs	0
AX	39 ± 2
AX/NHs	38 ± 1
RV	78 ± 4
RV/NHs	60 ± 1
CU	55 ± 3
CU/NHs	40 ± 8

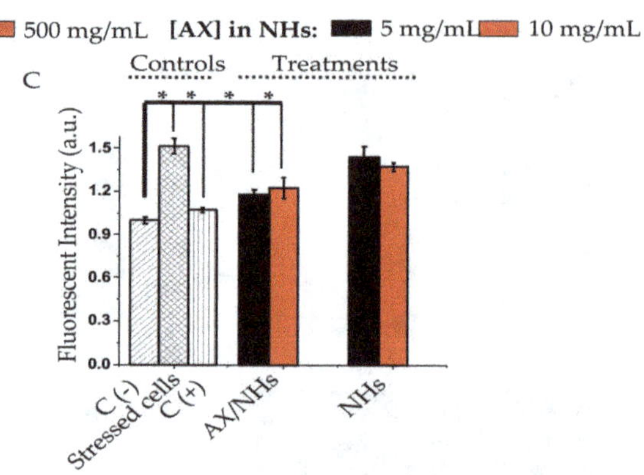

Figure 3. (**A**) Normalised Abs (λ = 730 nm) of AX/NHs, RV/NHs, CU/NHs and their controls versus 2,2′-azino-di-(3-ethylbenzthiazoline sulfonic acid) (ABTS). AX, RV and CU (loaded into NHs) were studied at the final concentration of 13 µM, respectively. Their absorbance (Abs) was compared to that of the free drugs at the same concentration. (**B**) Antioxidant activity (AA, %) of AX/NHs, RV/NHs, CU/NHs and their controls at 6 min. Data are expressed as the mean value ± standard deviation; experiments were performed in triplicate (n = 3). (**C**) Cell antioxidant activity (CAA) of AX/NHs and free NHs in oxidatively stressed HUVECs at two different concentrations (corresponding to NHs concentration of 500 and 250 µg mL^{-1} and AX concentration of 5 µg mL^{-1} (8 µM) and 10 µg mL^{-1} (16 µM). Experiments were performed on 4 wells (n = 3). Statistical significance was determined with Mann-Whitney test and asterisk denotes statistically significant differences ($^*p < 0.05$).

According to the obtained results, AX/NHs sample was chosen for the *in vitro* test. In HUVECs, ROS were generated with AM, which is a molecule able to inhibit succinate oxidase, NADH oxidase and the mitochondrial electron transport between cytochrome b and c [30]. The inhibition of electron transport causes both the collapse of the proton gradient across the mitochondrial inner membrane and the production of ROS. DHE dye was employed for monitoring the ROS production. Results show the OS occurs when HUVECs are incubated with AM (final concentration 11 µM), such ROS production is reduced by NAC, which is the antioxidant typically employed as a positive control. When HUVECs were incubated with AX/NHs, the nano-formulation showed a similar CAA as NAC, thus confirming the capability of AX/NHs to inhibit the ROS production in oxidatively stressed HUVECs, at all tested concentrations (Figure 3C). In contrast, unloaded NHs did not show any CAA in these conditions (Figure 3C).

3.4. Cell Viability and Morphology

To determine the effects of AX/NHs and free NHs on cell viability, healthy or oxidatively stressed HUVECs (Figure 4A) were incubated with AX/NHs or free NHs over 24 h, at several concentrations (ranging from 31 to 500 μg mL^{-1} (NHs) and from 1 to 16 μM (AX)). Both cell morphology (Figure 4B) and MTS (Figure 4C) showed that nano-formulations were not toxic to healthy or oxidatively stressed HUVECs, as neither HUVECs morphology nor metabolism was significantly affected by any of the tested concentrations after 24 h (Figure 4B,C). However, stressed HUVECs appear to be slightly smaller and a bit less metabolically active (18%) than healthy HUVECs.

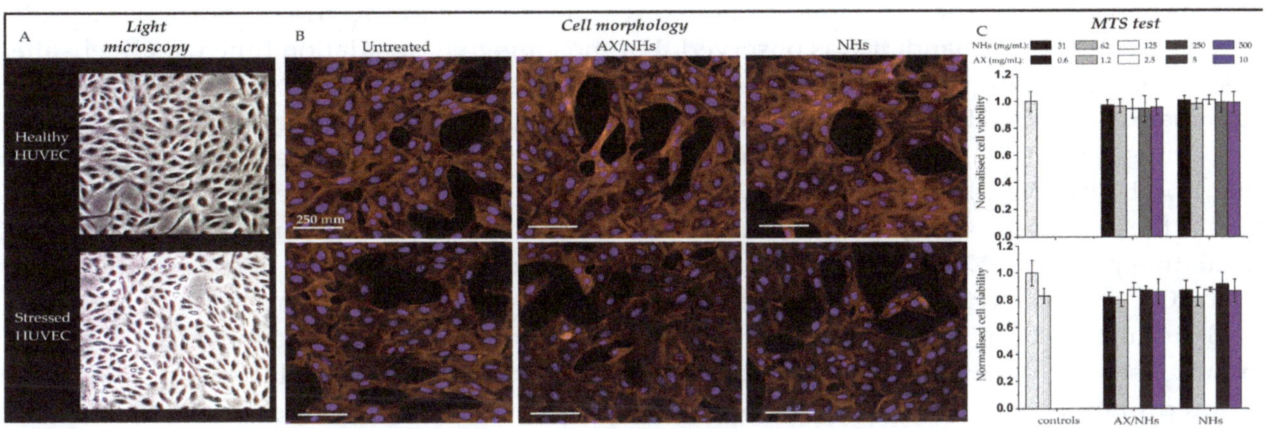

Figure 4. (**A**) Light microscopy micro-graphs of healthy or oxidatively stressed HUVECs. (**B**) Fluorescence microscopy micro-graphs (cell morphology) of healthy or oxidatively stressed HUVECs incubated with AX/NHs or free NHs at the concentration of 250 μg mL^{-1} (NHs) and 8 μM (AX) for 24 h. Nuclei were stained with DAPI (blue), whilst actin filaments were stained with phalloidin (red). (**C**) Cell metabolism (MTS test) of healthy or oxidatively stressed HUVECs. Cells were incubated with AX/NHs or free NHs over 24 h, at several concentrations (ranging from 31 to 500 μg mL^{-1} (NHs) and from 1 to 16 μM (AX)). Data were normalised to the negative control (HUVECs that received PBS). Statistical significance was determined with Mann-Whitney test and asterisk denote statistically significant differences ($^*p < 0.05$). Statistical significance was determined with One-way ANOVA analysis and differences between the two groups were not detected. Results are expressed as the mean value ± standard deviation and experiments were performed on 8 wells ($n = 3$).

4. Discussion

In order to prepare NHs, the carboxyl groups of HA were covalently linked to the functionalised cholesterol (CH-Br), leading to the amphiphilic HA-CH polymer (Df = 15, mol%) [18]. HA-CH macromolecules are able to self-assemble into nano-sized structures (NHs) after a suitable treatment (i.e., autoclaving at 121 °C for 20 min) [28]. Such nanoparticles are formed by internal hydrophobic domains and by external hydrophilic layers.

A detailed characterisation of NHs systems, their dimensions and spherical shape, their soft nature and their swelling capability, was already reported in previous works [18,20].

Furthermore, the ability of NHs to entrap hydrophilic antibiotics (e.g., gentamicin and levofloxacin) and to enhance their antimicrobial activity against intracellular pathogens was evidenced in keratinocytes (HaCaT) [17] and HeLa cells [31].

In the present work, NHs were physically loaded with natural and poorly water-soluble antioxidant compounds. The NHs capability to accumulate into healthy or oxidatively stressed endothelial cells (HUVECs) and to entrap AX, RV and CU molecules, as well as to retain/enhance their antioxidant activity, both in tube and *in vitro*, was investigated. Flow cytometry and confocal microscopy data (Figure 1) showed that NHs enter HUVECs and accumulate in their perinuclear area; a similar result was obtained in keratinocytes and reported in a previous work [17]. Moreover, the experiments clearly show that NHs were taken up by oxidatively stressed HUVECs more than by the healthy ones (~ two-fold). Such results suggest NHs may deliver antioxidants inside the cells and preferentially to endothelial cells that are under oxidative stress. However, additional studies are necessary to elucidate the internalisation mechanism with which NHs bind/enter HUVECs.

AX, RV and CU molecules were successfully loaded into NHs, leading to nano-formulations with suitable size, PDI and ζ-pot values (Figure 2) for biomedical applications. Furthermore, as expected, the apparent water solubility of AX, RV and CU was significantly enhanced when loaded into NHs, offering the opportunity to improve the administration, bioavailability and therapeutic efficacy of these compounds. The encapsulation time of RV and CU (14 h) was longer than that of AX (5 h), as RV/NHs and CU/NHs did not show suitable physico-chemical properties at shorter encapsulation time points. On the other hand, it was observed that the longer encapsulation time negatively affected the AA of the molecules. In fact, once loaded into NHs, the AA of AX (AX/NHs) was fully retained, whereas the AA of RV/NHs and CU/NHs decreased of 23 and 27%, respectively, when compared to the starting drugs (Figure 3A). Hence, the shortest encapsulation time was chosen for each nano-system, to obtain both suitable physico-chemical and antioxidant properties. Since RV and CU evidenced the loss of the AA after loading (possibly due to the partial oxidation of the molecules after the long encapsulation process), AX/NHs was selected as the best nano-system for the *in vitro* studies. In order to test the CAA of AX/NHs, HUVECs were oxidatively stressed with AM, a molecule able to enhance the ROS production at the mitochondrial level. The ROS increase can be studied by DHE, a compound commonly used for detecting cytosolic superoxide [32]. Upon reaction with the ROS species, DHE forms a red fluorescent product with maximum excitation and emission peaks at 500 and 580 nm, respectively. After incubation with AM, HUVECs showed a significant increase in fluorescence (~ 1.5-fold), thus confirming the oxidative stress (Figure 3B) occurred. The stressed HUVECs were incubated with AX/NHs or free NHs in order to investigate their CAA capability; NAC was tested as a positive control. Results show AX/NHs were able to inhibit the oxidative stress in HUVECs as much as NAC, at all the tested concentrations suggesting that I) NHs can effectively deliver AX into HUVECs; II) AX retains its antioxidant activity after encapsulation. Free NHs did not show any AA inside the cells. Promising results were also obtained by loading AX into cyclodextrins and lipid nanoparticles as reported by other researchers [9,33,34]. Cyclodextrins/AX complexes were found to be efficient in delivering AX from the PVA cardiac patches [35] as well as from the pullulan-dextran natural matrix, in an ischemia reperfusion rat model [33]. Both AX/NHs and free NHs did not evidence any significant toxicity against healthy or oxidatively stressed HUVECs, at all tested concentrations (Figure 4), as shown by cell metabolism data (MTS test) and morphology micro-graphs.

These results suggest self-assembled HA-based NHs may represent a suitable candidate for the delivery of natural antioxidants. Furthermore, it is worth noting that HA is among the most widely used biopolymers in cosmetics. Hence, formulations based on antioxidants-loaded HA NHs may be developed and tested both in pharmaceutical and cosmetic fields [36].

5. Conclusions

HA-based NHs are capable to entrap natural and poorly water-soluble antioxidants, such as AX, RV and CU and to significantly enhance their apparent water solubility in aqueous media. The nano-formulations are able to neutralise ROS species, as evidenced by in tube and *in vitro* (AX/NHs only) studies and do not show any toxicity against HUVECs cells. Since previous results suggest NHs are highly taken up by oxidatively stressed HUVECs, they may represent a suitable nano-carrier for delivering antioxidant molecules intracellularly. *In vivo* studies will help to evaluate the potential use of these systems for the medical treatment of OS pathologies, particularly in cardiovascular diseases such as ischemia/reperfusion (I/R) injuries.

Author Contributions: Data curation, T.C. and V.G.; Funding acquisition, G.P.-D. and P.M.; Investigation, E.M. and C.D.M.; Methodology, E.M. and G.P.-D.; Project administration, C.D.M., G.P.-D. and P.M.; Supervision, C.D.M. and G.P.-D.; Writing—original draft, E.M.; Writing—review and editing, T.C. and V.G.

Acknowledgments: The authors are grateful to Valeria Rocchi, Madalina Nistorescu and Marisole Zuluaga, Pauline Di Luise and Marialuisa Di Bari for their contribution to the work. Our thanks to Teresa Simon-yarza, Marie Noelle Labour and Marie Le Borgne for their technical support.

References

1. Halliwell, B. Reactive oxygen species in living systems: Source, biochemistry, and role in human disease. *Oxid. Antioxid. Pathophysiol. Determ. Ther. Agents* **1991**, *91*, S14–S22. [CrossRef]
2. Schieber, M.; Chandel, N.S. ROS function in redox signaling and oxidative stress. *Curr. Biol. CB* **2014**, *24*, R453–R462. [CrossRef] [PubMed]
3. Sies, H.; Berndt, C.; Jones, D.P. Oxidative Stress. *Annu. Rev. Biochem.* **2017**, *86*, 715–748. [CrossRef] [PubMed]
4. Oliveira, C.P.; Cotrim, H.P.; Stefano, J.T.; Siqueira, A.C.G.; Salgado, A.L.A.; Parise, E.R. N-acetylcysteine and/or ursodeoxycholic acid associated with metformin. *Arq. Gastroenterol.* **2019**, *56*, 184–190. [CrossRef]
5. Soliman, N.A.; Keshk, W.A.; Rizk, F.H.; Ibrahim, M.A. The possible ameliorative effect of simvastatin versus sulfasalazine on acetic acid induced ulcerative colitis in adult rats. *Chem. Biol. Interact.* **2019**, *298*, 57–65. [CrossRef]
6. Kusuhara, H.; Furuie, H.; Inano, A.; Sunagawa, A.; Yamada, S.; Wu, C.; Fukizawa, S.; Morimoto, N.; Ieiri, I.; Morishita, M.; et al. Pharmacokinetic interaction study of sulphasalazine in healthy subjects and the impact of curcumin as an in vivo inhibitor of BCRP. *Br. J. Pharmacol.* **2012**, *166*, 1793–1803. [CrossRef]
7. Osawe, S.O.; Farombi, E.O. Quercetin and rutin ameliorates sulphasalazine-induced spermiotoxicity, alterations in reproductive hormones and steroidogenic enzyme imbalance in rats. *Andrologia* **2018**, *50*, e12981. [CrossRef]
8. Xue, X.-L.; Han, X.-D.; Li, Y.; Chu, X.-F.; Miao, W.-M.; Zhang, J.-L.; Fan, S.-J. Astaxanthin attenuates total body irradiation-induced hematopoietic system injury in mice via inhibition of oxidative stress and apoptosis. *Stem Cell Res. Ther.* **2017**, *8*, 7. [CrossRef]
9. Zuluaga, M.; Barzegari, A.; Letourneur, D.; Gueguen, V.; Pavon-Djavid, G. Oxidative Stress Regulation on Endothelial Cells by Hydrophilic Astaxanthin Complex: Chemical, Biological, and Molecular Antioxidant Activity Evaluation. *Oxid. Med. Cell. Longev.* **2017**, *2017*, 8073798. [CrossRef]
10. Francioso, A.; Mastromarino, P.; Masci, a.; d'Erme, M.; Mosca, L. Chemistry, Stability and Bioavailability of Resveratrol. *Med. Chem.* **2014**, *10*, 237–245. [CrossRef]
11. Gokce, E.H.; Korkmaz, E.; Dellera, E.; Sandri, G.; Bonferoni, M.C.; Ozer, O. Resveratrol-loaded solid lipid nanoparticles versus nanostructured lipid carriers: Evaluation of antioxidant potential for dermal applications. *Int. J. Nanomed.* **2012**, *7*, 1841–1850. [CrossRef] [PubMed]
12. Nagpal, M.; Sood, S. Role of curcumin in systemic and oral health: An overview. *J. Nat. Sci. Biol. Med.* **2013**, *4*, 3–7.
13. Fan, Y.; Yi, J.; Zhang, Y.; Yokoyama, W. Fabrication of curcumin-loaded bovine serum albumin (BSA)-dextran nanoparticles and the cellular antioxidant activity. *Food Chem.* **2018**, *239*, 1210–1218. [CrossRef] [PubMed]
14. Kabanov, A.V.; Vinogradov, S.V. Nanogels as Pharmaceutical Carriers: Finite Networks of Infinite Capabilities. *Angew. Chem.* **2009**, *48*, 5418–5429. [CrossRef] [PubMed]
15. Soni, K.S.; Desale, S.S.; Bronich, T.K. Nanogels: An overview of properties, biomedical applications and obstacles to clinical translation. *J. Control. Release* **2016**, *240*, 109–126. [CrossRef] [PubMed]
16. Choi, K.Y.; Min, K.H.; Na, J.H.; Choi, K.; Kim, K.; Park, J.H.; Kwon, I.C.; Jeong, S.Y. Self-assembled hyaluronic acid nanoparticles as a potential drug carrier for cancer therapy: Synthesis, characterization, and in vivo biodistribution. *J. Mat. Chem.* **2009**, *19*, 4029–4280. [CrossRef]
17. Montanari, E.; Oates, A.; Di Meo, C.; Meade, J.; Cerrone, R.; Francioso, A.; Devine, D.; Coviello, T.; Mancini, P.; Mosca, L.; et al. Hyaluronan-Based Nanohydrogels for Targeting Intracellular S. Aureus in Human Keratinocytes. *Adv. Healthcare Mater.* **2018**, *7*, e1701483. [CrossRef]
18. Montanari, E.; Capece, S.; Di Meo, C.; Meringolo, M.; Coviello, T.; Agostinelli, E.; Matricardi, P. Hyaluronic Acid Nanohydrogels as a Useful Tool for BSAO Immobilization in the Treatment of Melanoma Cancer Cells. *Macromol. Biosci.* **2013**, *13*, 1185–1194. [CrossRef]

19. Ganguly, K.; Chaturvedi, K.; More, U.A.; Nadagouda, M.N.; Aminabhavi, T.M. Polysaccharide-based micro/nanohydrogels for delivering macromolecular therapeutics. *J. Control. Release* **2014**, *193*, 162–173. [CrossRef]
20. Montanari, E.; Di Meo, C.; Sennato, S.; Francioso, A.; Marinelli, A.L.; Ranzo, F.; Schippa, S.; Coviello, T.; Bordi, F.; Matricardi, P. Hyaluronan-cholesterol nanohydrogels: Characterisation and effectiveness in carrying alginate lyase. *New Biotechnol.* **2017**, *37*, 80–89. [CrossRef]
21. Akiyoshi, K.; Deguchi, S.; Moriguchi, N.; Yamaguchi, S.; Sunamoto, J. Self-aggregates of hydrophobized polysaccharides in water. Formation and characteristics of nanoparticles. *Macromolecules* **1993**, *26*, 3062–3068. [CrossRef]
22. Vinogradov, S.V.; Batrakova, E.; Kabanov, A.V. Poly(ethylene glycol)–polyethyleneimine NanoGel™ particles: Novel drug delivery systems for antisense oligonucleotides. *Colloid Surf. B-Biointerfaces* **1999**, *16*, 291–304. [CrossRef]
23. Laurent, T.C.; Fraser, J.R. Hyaluronan. *FASEB J.* **1992**, *99*, 2397–2404. [CrossRef]
24. Day, A.J.; Prestwich, G.D. Hyaluronan-binding Proteins "Tying up the Giant". *J. Biol. Chem.* **2002**, *277*, 4585–4588. [CrossRef] [PubMed]
25. Ponta, H.; Sherman, L.; Herrlich, P.A. CD44: From adhesion molecules to signalling regulators. *Nat. Rev. Mol. Cel. Biol.* **2003**, *4*, 33–45. [CrossRef] [PubMed]
26. Pure, E.; Cuff, C.A. A crucial role for CD44 in inflammation. *Trends Mol. Med.* **2001**, *7*, 213–221. [CrossRef]
27. Rafi-Janajreh, A.Q.; Chen, D.; Schmits, R.; Mak, T.W.; Grayson, R.L.; Sponenberg, D.P.; Nagarkatti, M.; Nagarkatti, P.S. Evidence for the involvement of CD44 in endothelial cell injury and induction of vascular leak syndrome by IL-2. *J. Immunol.* **1999**, *163*, 1619–1627.
28. Montanari, E.; De Rugeriis, M.C.; Di Meo, C.; Censi, R.; Coviello, T.; Alhaique, F.; Matricardi, P. One-step formation and sterilization of gellan and hyaluronan nanohydrogels using autoclave. *J. Mater. Sci. Mater. Med.* **2015**, *26*, 32–37. [CrossRef]
29. Miller, N.J.; Rice-Evans, C.A. Factors influencing the antioxidant activity determined by the ABTS+ radical cation assay. *Free Radic. Res.* **1997**, *26*, 195–199. [CrossRef]
30. Campo, M.L.; Kinnally, K.W.; Tedeschi, H. The effect of antimycin A on mouse liver inner mitochondrial membrane channel activity. *J. Biol. Chem.* **1992**, *267*, 8123–8127.
31. Montanari, E.; D'Arrigo, G.; Di Meo, C.; Virga, A.; Coviello, T.; Passariello, C.; Matricardi, P. Chasing bacteria within the cells using levofloxacin-loaded hyaluronic acid nanohydrogels. *Eur. J. Pharm. Biopharm.* **2014**, *87*, 518–523. [CrossRef] [PubMed]
32. Gomes, A.; Fernandes, E.; Lima, J.L. Fluorescence probes used for detection of reactive oxygen species. *J. Biochem. Biophys. Methods* **2005**, *65*, 45–80. [CrossRef] [PubMed]
33. Zuluaga Tamayo, M.; Choudat, L.; Aid-Launais, R.; Thibaudeau, O.; Louedec, L.; Letourneur, D.; Gueguen, V.; Meddahi-Pellé, A.; Couvelard, A.; Pavon-Djavid, G. Astaxanthin Complexes to Attenuate Muscle Damage after In Vivo Femoral Ischemia-Reperfusion. *Mar. Drugs* **2019**, *17*, 354. [CrossRef] [PubMed]
34. Rodriguez-Ruiz, V.; Salatti-Dorado, J.Á.; Barzegari, A.; Nicolas-Boluda, A.; Houaoui, A.; Caballo, C.; Caballero-Casero, N.; Sicilia, D.; Bastias Venegas, J.; Pauthe, E.; et al. Astaxanthin-Loaded Nanostructured Lipid Carriers for Preservation of Antioxidant Activity. *Molecules* **2018**, *23*, 2601. [CrossRef] [PubMed]
35. Zuluaga, M.; Gregnanin, G.; Cencetti, C.; Di Meo, C.; Gueguen, V.; Letourneur, D.; Meddahi-Pelle, A.; Pavon-Djavid, G.; Matricardi, P. PVA/Dextran hydrogel patches as delivery system of antioxidant astaxanthin: A cardiovascular approach. *Biomed. Mater. Bristol Engl.* **2017**, *13*, 015020. [CrossRef]
36. Montanari, E.; Zoratto, N.; Mosca, L.; Cervoni, L.; Lallana, E.; Angelini, R.; Matassa, R.; Coviello, T.; Di Meo, C.; Matricardi, P. Halting hyaluronidase activity with hyaluronan-based nanohydrogels: Development of versatile injectable formulations. *Carbohydr. Polym.* **2019**, *221*, 209–220. [CrossRef]

7

Enhanced Delivery of Therapeutic siRNA into Glioblastoma Cells Using Dendrimer-Entrapped Gold Nanoparticles Conjugated with β-Cyclodextrin

Jieru Qiu [1,2], Lingdan Kong [2], Xueyan Cao [2], Aijun Li [2], Ping Wei [2], Lu Wang [2], Serge Mignani [3,4,*], Anne-Marie Caminade [5,6], Jean-Pierre Majoral [5,6,*] and Xiangyang Shi [1,2,4,*]

1 Department of Radiology, Shanghai Tenth People's Hospital, Tongji University School of Medicine, Shanghai 200072, China; jieruq@outlook.com
2 College of Chemistry, Chemical Engineering and Biotechnology, Donghua University, Shanghai 201620, China; lingdankong@hotmail.com (L.K.); caoxy_116@dhu.edu.cn (X.C.); andrewaijun.lee@gmail.com (A.L.); weiping876@hotmail.com (P.W.); wanglu2013@dhu.edu.cn (L.W.)
3 Université Paris Descartes, PRES Sorbonne Paris Cité, CNRS UMR 860, Laboratoire de Chimie et de Biochimie Pharmacologiques et Toxicologique, 45, rue des Saints Peres, 75006 Paris, France
4 CQM—Centro de Química da Madeira, MMRG, Universidade da Madeira, Campus da Penteada, 9020-105 Funchal, Portugal
5 Laboratoire de Chimie de Coordination du CNRS, 205 Route de Narbonne, BP 44099, 31077 Toulouse CEDEX 4, France; anne-marie.caminade@lcc-toulouse.fr
6 Université de Toulouse, UPS, INPT, 31077 Toulouse CEDEX 4, France
* Correspondence: serge_mignani@orange.fr (S.M.); majoral@lcc-toulouse.fr (J.-P.M.); xshi@dhu.edu.cn (X.S.);

Abstract: We describe a safe and highly effective non-viral vector system based on β-cyclodextrin (β-CD)-modified dendrimer-entrapped gold nanoparticles (Au DENPs) for improved delivery small interfering RNA (siRNA) to glioblastoma cells. In our approach, we utilized amine-terminated generation 5 poly(amidoamine) dendrimers partially grafted with β-CD as a nanoreactor to entrap Au NPs. The acquired β-CD-modified Au DENPs (Au DENPs-β-CD) were complexed with two different types of therapeutic siRNA (B-cell lymphoma/leukemia-2 (Bcl-2) siRNA and vascular endothelial growth factor (VEGF) siRNA). The siRNA compression ability of the Au DENPs-β-CD was evaluated by various methods. The cytocompatibility of the vector/siRNA polyplexes was assessed by viability assay of cells. The siRNA transfection capability of the formed Au DENPs-β-CD vector was evaluated by flow cytometric assay of the cellular uptake of the polyplexes and Western blot assays of the Bcl-2 and VEGF protein expression. Our data reveals that the formed Au DENPs-β-CD carrier enables efficiently delivery of siRNA to glioma cells, has good cytocompatibility once complexed with the siRNA, and enables enhanced gene silencing to inhibit the expression of Bcl-2 and VEGF proteins. The developed Au DENPs-β-CD vector may be used for efficient siRNA delivery to different biosystems for therapeutic purposes.

Keywords: PAMAM dendrimers; β-CD; gold nanoparticles; gene silencing; siRNA

---

1. Introduction

Gene therapy is becoming a promising strategy for cancer therapy by transfecting genetic materials (such as DNA [1–3], RNA [4,5] and antisense oligonucleotides [6,7]) into target cancer cells to achieve the therapeutic purposes. Among that, RNA interference has been considered as one of the most potential strategies for cancer therapy through silencing the specific genes up-regulated in cancer cells or involved in cell division [8,9]. Small interfering RNA (siRNA) has played a central role for RNA interference.

For efficient siRNA delivery, one has to consider to use a carrier system owing to the electrostatic repulsion of the negatively-charged cell membrane and the negatively-charged siRNA backbone [10,11]. For gene delivery, non-viral vectors are increasingly employed considering their better bio-safety profile than viral ones, relative ease to be synthesized, targeting specificity to cell/tissue after surface modification [12–14], structural diversity, and capacity to transfect plasmid of varying sizes [15,16]. The currently used non-viral vectors such as cationic lipids [17,18], polymers [12,19,20], polypeptides [21,22], and inorganic nanoparticles (NPs) [23,24] can be used to form vector/DNA polyplexes at the nanoscale [10,11,25]. In any case, development of novel vector systems for safe and effective transfection of siRNA still remains a critical research area [26–32].

Poly(amidoamine) (PAMAM) dendrimers are a class of monodispersed macromolecules [33–35] with branched interior and well-fixed molecular conformation and controlled surface functionalities [36–39]. These properties of PAMAM dendrimers make them act as desired carrier systems for non-viral siRNA delivery [13,40–42]. In this direction, several studies have reported that by functional modifications of generation 5 (G5) PAMAM dendrimers via dendrimer periphery modification of polyethylene glycol chains [43] or entrapment of gold (Au) NPs within dendrimer internal cavities [44], the cytotoxicity of the vector has been significantly reduced, while the gene transfection efficiency has been prominently enhanced [14,44–47]. Previously, we have shown that the Au NP entrapment within G5 PAMAM dendrimers to form dendrimer-entrapped Au NPs (Au DENPs) is beneficial to reduce the cytotoxicity of dendrimers and simultaneously enhance the gene delivery efficiency [44]. On one hand, the entrapped Au NPs are able to compensate the dendrimer terminal amine cytotoxicity by reducing the density of amine groups, thus improving the cytocompatibility of the dendrimers; on the other hand, the Au NPs entrapped helps to maintain the globular conformation of the dendrimer, thereby enhancing the compaction capacity of DNA.

Recently, we have used β-cyclodextrin (β-CD) to modify the surface of G5 PAMAM dendrimers and used the β-CD-modified G5 dendrimers for the synthesis of Au NPs within the dendrimers [48]. The prepared β-CD-modified Au DENPs (Au DENPs-β-CD) displayed weakened cytotoxicity and enhanced DNA compression capability, and enabled the enhanced transfection of plasmid DNA (pDNA) encoding either luciferase gene or enhanced the green fluorescent protein gene into 293T cells. The enhanced gene delivery efficiency could be resulted from the entrapped Au NPs. Meanwhile, the attached β-CD moieties might facilitate the release of pDNA or the siRNA complex from endosomes after endocytic uptake [49]. These promising results strongly stimulate us to further explore the performance of the Au DENPs-β-CD to deliver siRNA to silence genes in cancer cells.

In this work, we prepared the Au DENPs-β-CD vector according to the procedure previously reported [48]. The prepared Au DENPs-β-CD were employed as a vector to compact two different types of siRNA including B-cell lymphoma 2 (Bcl-2) siRNA and vascular endothelial growth factor (VEGF) siRNA under the appropriate N/P (dendrimer terminal amine/siRNA phosphate) ratios for oncogene silencing (Scheme 1). The siRNA compaction ability of the vector was explored by gel electrophoresis, dynamic light scattering, and zeta potential measurements. The cytocompatibility of the prepared vector/siRNA polyplexes was also analyzed by cell viability assay. Furthermore, flow cytometry assay and confocal microscopic observations of cells were used to assess the efficiency of gene transfection of the vector/siRNA polyplexes. Finally, we used Western blot assay to prove the oncogene silencing efficiency of the Au DENPs-β-CD/siRNA polyplexes in glioblastoma cancer cells.

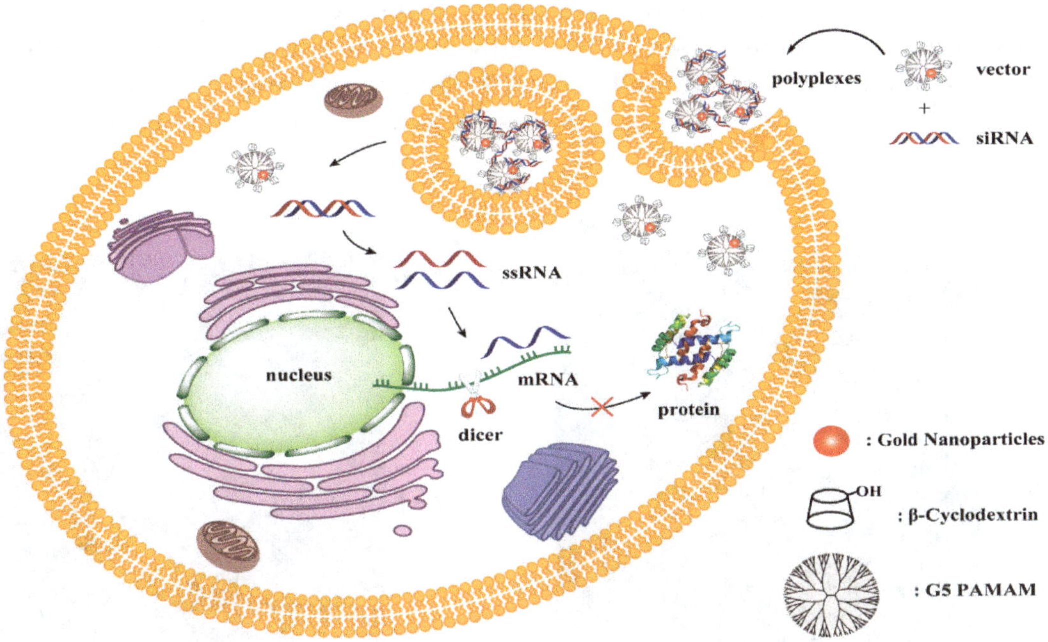

Scheme 1. Schematic illustration of the gene delivery process.

2. Results and Discussion

2.1. Characterization of Vector/siRNA Polyplexes

Herein, we aimed to explore the enhanced delivery efficiency of siRNA using the Au DENPs-β-CD (Q2) vector. Au DENPs without β-CD modification (Q1) and pristine G5.NH_2 dendrimers (Q0) were used for comparison. We first checked the siRNA compaction capability of the vectors. Agarose gel retardation assay was used to analyze the obtained vector/siRNA polyplexes (Figure 1). Apparently, the migration of both siRNAs is able to be blocked at higher N/P ratios. For Bcl-2 siRNA, all vectors fully inhibit the siRNA migration at the N/P ratio of 2:1 or above (Figure 1a). For VEGF siRNA, Q0 and Q1 retard the siRNA migration at the N/P ratio of 2:1 or above (Figure 1b), similar to Bcl-2 siRNA. It seems that Q2 displays a better compaction capacity of VEGF siRNA than Q0 and Q1, and the siRNA migration can be completely retarded at the N/P ratio above 1:1. Clearly, the conjugation of β-CD onto G5 dendrimers is beneficial for enhanced siRNA compaction, in accordance with our previous study [48]. These results demonstrated that both Bcl-2 siRNA and VEGF siRNA could be efficiently compressed by the vectors at N/P ratios greater than 2:1.

DLS and zeta potential measurements were utilized to characterize the vector/siRNA polyplexes (Figure 2 and Table S1, Supporting Information). Apparently, the hydrodynamic particle size of the vector/siRNA polyplexes decreases with the N/P ratio. This may be attributed to the situation that at a higher N/P ratio, more vector materials are present and the siRNA can be more compacted to have a smaller size. It appears that polyplexes composed of the vectors with Au NPs entrapped have a slightly larger size than those gained using dendrimers without the entrapment of Au NPs, which is different from the vector/pDNA in our earlier work [44]. This difference is probably owing to the much smaller molecular weight of siRNA, and the size of the polyplexes could be mainly derived from that of the vectors.

We determined the surface potentials of the vector/siRNA polyplexes under the given N/P ratios (Figure 3). Clearly, at the same N/P ratios, the surface potential of the polyplexes obeys the order of Q0/siRNA > Q1/siRNA > Q2/siRNA for both Bcl-2 siRNA (Figure 3a) and VEGF siRNA (Figure 3b). These data suggest that the modification of β-CD on the dendrimer periphery and the entrapment of Au NPs within the dendrimer internal cavity reduce the density of dendrimer surface amines, thus decreasing the surface potentials of the formed polyplexes. This is beneficial for them to have an improved cytocompatibility (see below). However, the surface potentials of the Q1/siRNA and Q2/siRNA are still positively charged. Overall, the positive surface potential along with the appropriate hydrodynamic sizes of the polyplexes may allow them to be used for effective gene delivery [48].

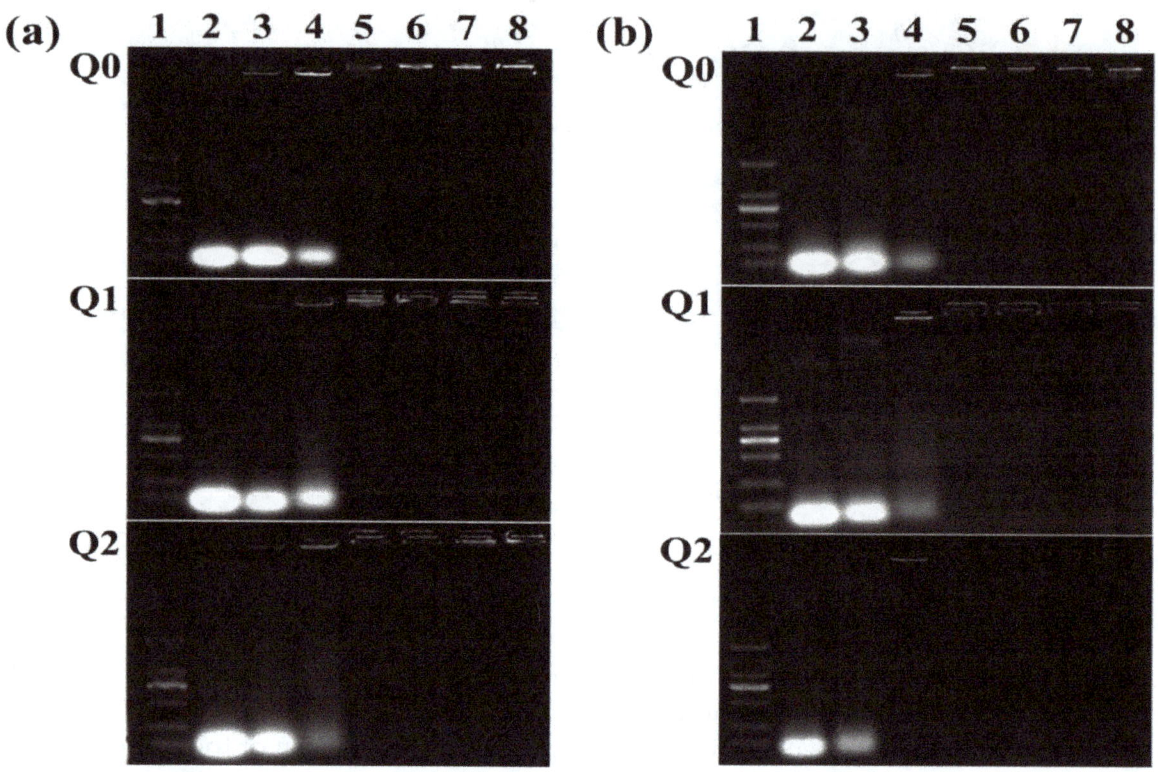

Figure 1. Gel retardation assay of B-cell lymphoma/leukemia-2 (Bcl-2) siRNA (**a**) and vascular endothelial growth factor (VEGF) siRNA (**b**) complexed with Q0, Q1 and Q2 at various N/P ratios, respectively. Lane 1: DNA marker; lane 2: N/P = 0.25:1; lane 3: N/P = 0.5:1; lane 4: N/P = 1:1; lane 5: N/P = 2:1; lane 6: N/P = 3:1; lane 7: N/P = 4:1; and lane 8: N/P = 5:1.

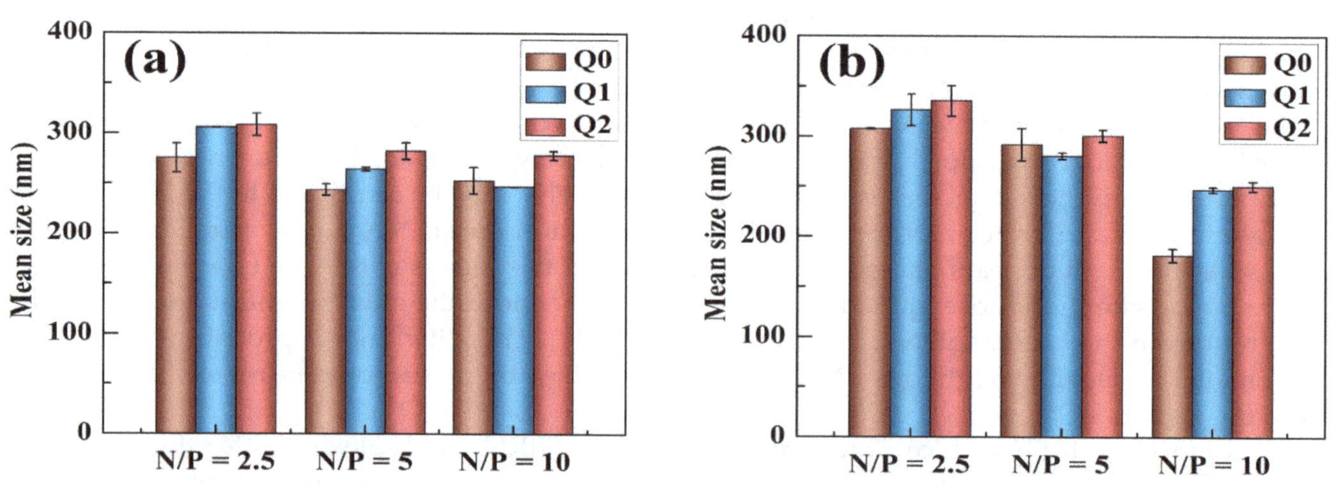

Figure 2. Mean hydrodynamic size of Bcl-2 siRNA (**a**) and VEGF siRNA (**b**) complexed with Q0, Q1, and Q2 at N/P ratios of 2.5:1, 5:1, or 10:1, respectively (mean ± SD, $n = 3$).

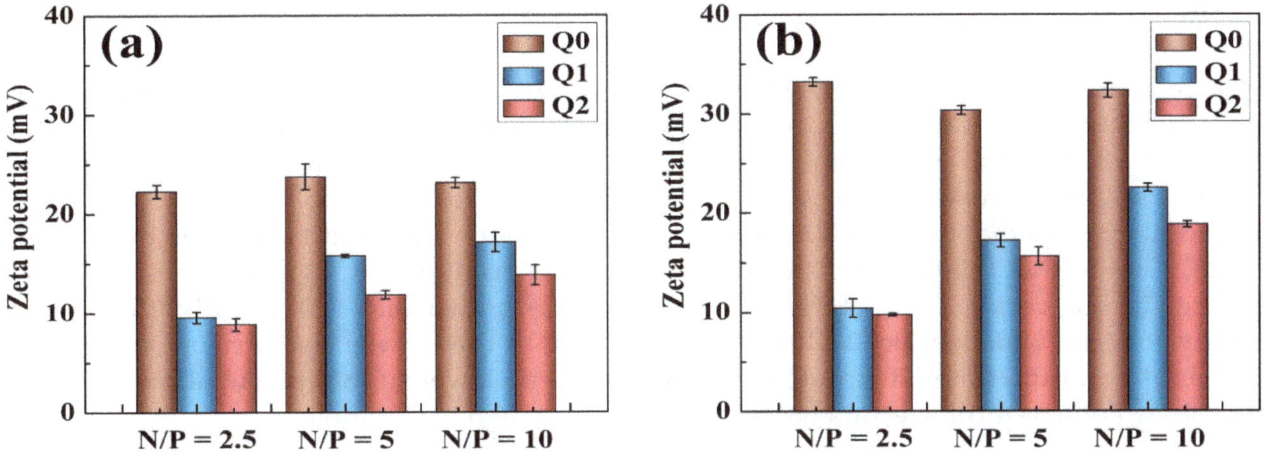

Figure 3. Surface potentials of Bcl-2 siRNA (**a**) and VEGF siRNA (**b**) complexed with Q0, Q1, and Q2 at N/P ratios of 2.5:1, 5:1 or 10:1, respectively (mean ± SD, $n = 3$).

2.2. *Cytotoxicity Assay*

MTT assay of cell viability was next carried out to test the cytotoxicity of vector/siRNA polyplexes (Figure 4). The cell viability is reduced with the vector concentration. The cytotoxicity of the vector/siRNA polyplexes obeys the order of Q2/siRNA < Q1/siRNA < Q0/siRNA at the same vector concentration for either Bcl2 siRNA (Figure 4a) or VEGF siRNA (Figure 4b). Even at the highest vector concentration of 2000 nM, the cells incubated with the Q2/siRNA polyplexes still display a viability higher than 80%, while the cells co-cultured with the Q0/siRNA polyplexes show a viability lower than 60%. Our results suggest that Q2 could be adopted as a relatively 'safe' gene delivery vector when compared with Q0 and Q1. Our data emphasize that the dendrimer periphery modification with β-CD and the internal loading of Au NPs are beneficial to compromise the cytotoxicity of G5 PAMAM dendrimers.

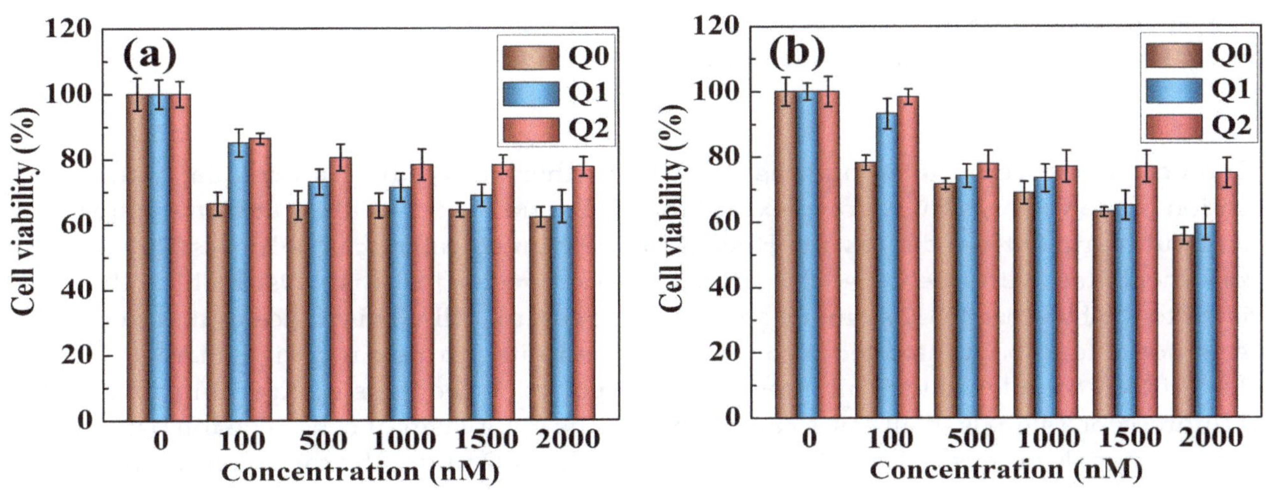

Figure 4. MTT viability assay of Uppsala 87 Malignant Glioma (U87MG) cells treated with the vector/Bcl-2 siRNA (**a**) and vector/VEGF siRNA; and (**b**) polyplexes under distinct vector concentrations (mean ± SD, $n = 6$).

2.3. Uptake of Vector/siRNA Polyplexes by Cancer Cells

The cellular uptake of the vector/siRNA polyplexes was investigated by flow cytometry analysis (Figure S1, Supporting Information). As shown in Figure 5, for both vector/Cy3-Bcl-2 siRNA and vector/Cy3-VEGF siRNA polyplexes, the percentages of fluorescent cells associated with the Cy3-labeled siRNA are relatively higher at the higher N/P ratios of the polyplexes. Under the same conditions, it appears that Bcl-2 siRNA (Figure 5a) can be more significantly uptaken by the U87MG cells than VEGF siRNA (Figure 5b). The percentage of cells having the Cy3 fluorescence signals after transfection by the vector/Cy3-Bcl-2 siRNA polyplexes is higher than 80% for all different vectors. The ability of vector to deliver Bcl-2 siRNA and VEGF siRNA follows the tendency of Q0 < Q1 < Q2 at N/P ratios of 5 and 10. It should be noted that Q2 possesses a lower surface potential, thus being more liable to show enhanced transfection efficiency of genes at high N/P ratios.

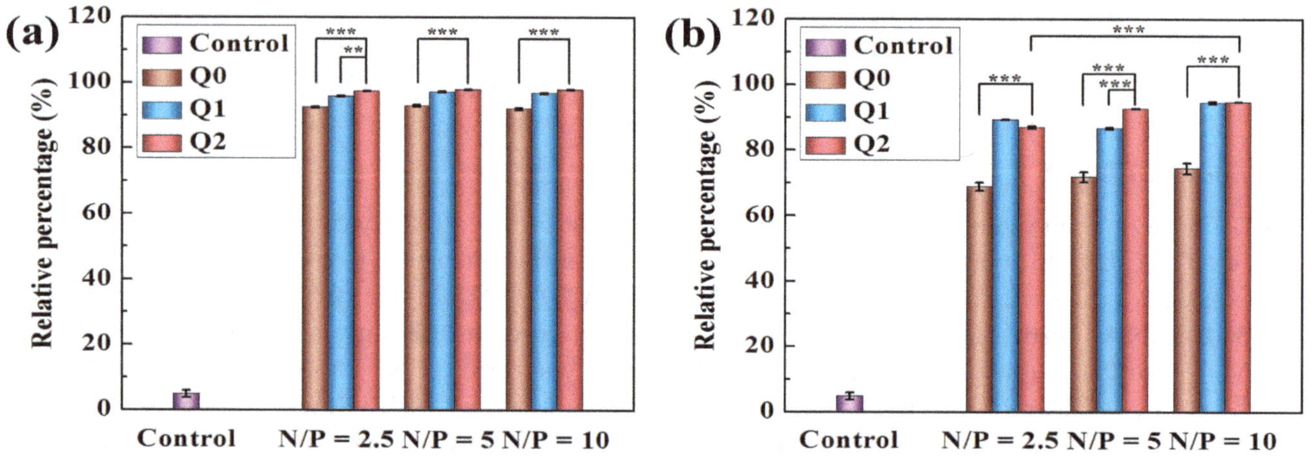

Figure 5. Flow cytometry analysis of U87MG cells transfected using vector/Cy3-Bcl-2 siRNA (**a**) and vector/Cy3-VEGF siRNA (**b**) polyplexes at the N/P ratios of 2.5:1, 5:1, and 10:1, respectively. Cells without treatment were used as control. Data are shown with mean ± SD (n = 3). For (**a**,**b**), ** and *** mean that the p values of statistical analyses are <0.01 and <0.001, respectively.

Confocal microscopic imaging was used to further study the transcellular pathways and localization of the vector/siRNA polyplexes at the N/P ratio of 5:1. As illustrated in Figure 6, control cells without treatment just display the Hoechst 33342-stained cell nuclei, which is blue fluorescent. The cells incubated with free Cy3-Bcl-2 siRNA without vector just displays the blue fluorescence associated to the Hoechst 33342 staining, similar to the control cells. This indicates that free Cy3-Bcl-2 siRNA is not able to be transfected into the cells due to its intrinsic negative charge. In contrast, Cy3-Bcl-2 siRNA complexed with all three different vectors can be transfected within the cancer cells, as red fluorescence signals in all cases can be seen in the cytoplasm of cells. The intensity of the red fluorescence signals of cells follows the order of Q0 < Q1 < Q2 under the same condition, suggesting that the siRNA delivery efficiency follows the same order, in agreement with the flow cytometry assay data. For the Cy3-VEGF siRNA delivery (Figure S2, Supporting Information), the same trend of cellular uptake of the polyplexes can be seen.

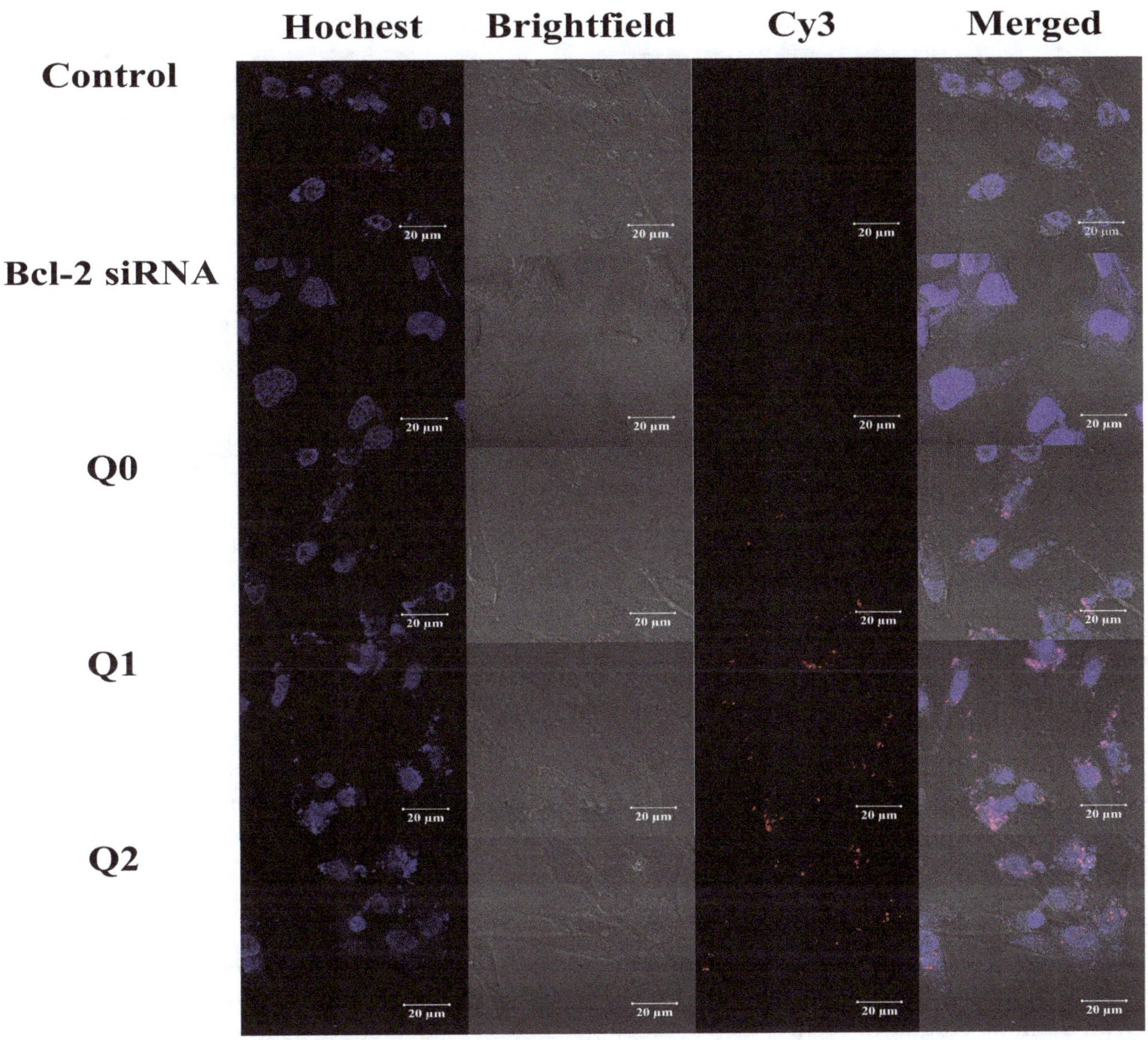

Figure 6. Confocal microscopic images (63×) of U87MG cells showing the intracellular localization of the vectors/Cy3-Bcl-2 siRNA polyplexes that were prepared with an N/P of 5:1 (red: Cy3-labeled siRNA; blue: Hoechst 33342 stained cell nuclei).

2.4. Gene Silencing with VEGF and Bcl-2 siRNAs

With the goal to study the effective siRNA delivery using the designed vector systems, Western blot analysis was undertaken to explore the gene silencing capabilities of vector/siRNA polyplexes at the N/P ratio of 5:1. We used naked siRNA without any protection as a control and GAPDH protein was adopted as the reference protein. As shown in Figure 7a, the Bcl-2 gene is not able to be silenced by naked Bcl-2 siRNA, which is similar to the control cells. In contrast, decreased expression of Bcl-2 protein can be seen in cells treated with all vector/siRNA polyplexes, and the gene silencing efficacy follows the order of Q2 > Q1 > Q0. Similarly, VEGF siRNA is also able to be transfected after complexation with the vectors of Q0, Q1, and Q2 to lower the expression of VEGF protein (Figure 7b), and the gene silencing trend follows the same order. These results prove that the Au DENPs-β-CD (Q2) possess excellent siRNA transfection ability and the formed polyplexes are able to silence the genes in cancer cells for effective gene therapy applications.

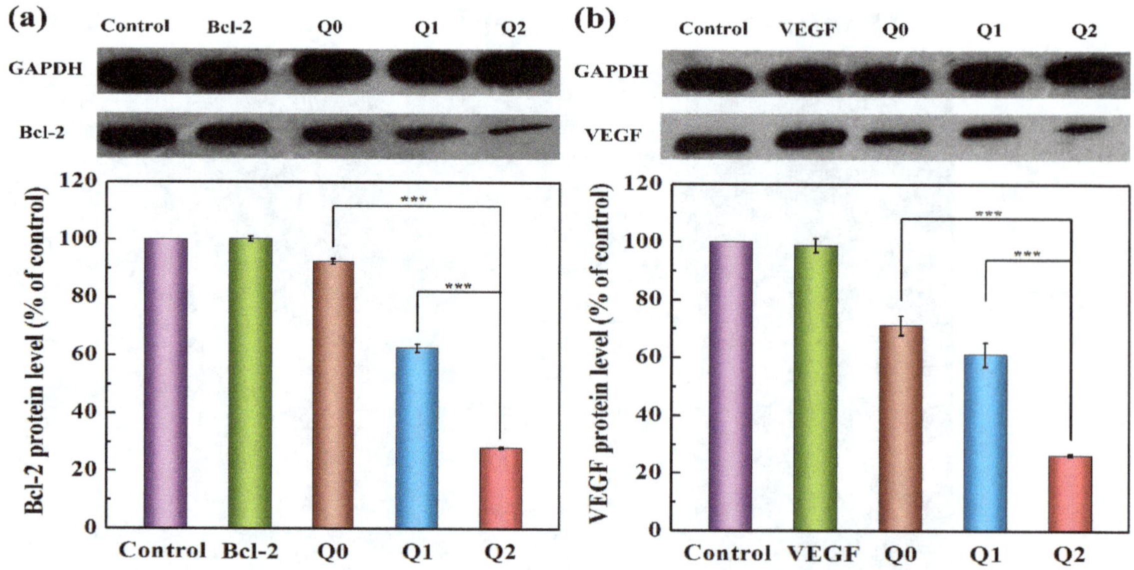

Figure 7. Relative Bcl-2 (**a**) and VEGF (**b**) protein expression levels in U87MG cells transfected with vector/siRNA polyplexes at an N/P ratio of 5:1. The GAPDH protein was used as a reference for the Western blot data. For (**a**,**b**), *** means that the p values of statistical analyses are <0.001.

3. Experimental Section

3.1. *Synthesis of Au DENPs-β-CD*

G5.NH_2, Au DENPs, and Au DENPs-β-CD were obtained using the same procedures described in our previous work [48]. For clarity, the structure of G5.NH_2 PAMAM dendrimer and β-CD can be seen in Figure S3 (Supporting Information). Besides, for simplicity, the above materials were referred to as Q0, Q1, and Q2, respectively.

3.2. *Preparation of Vectors/siRNA Polyplexes*

Bcl-2 and VEGF siRNAs were respectively complexed with vectors with various N/P ratios. Both vectors and siRNA (1 μg) were dissolved in phosphate buffered saline (PBS, 0.01 mol/L, pH 7.4) to reach an ultimate volume of 100 μL, then blended gently and incubated for 20 min at room temperature.

3.3. *Gene Silencing with VEGF and Bcl-2 siRNAs*

U87MG cells were incubated into 12-well flat-bottomed plates at a density of 1×10^5 cells/well as described above. When the cells were brought to a 60–70% confluence, the medium in each well was substituted with 1 mL of fresh DMEM containing 100 μL of vector/siRNA polyplexes prepared using 1 μg of siRNA at the N/P ratio of 5:1. After incubation for 4 h, the cell medium was exchanged to fresh DMEM supplemented with 10% FBS and the cells were then cultivated for additional 48 h. Then, the cells were treated with pre-chilled PBS and digested with lysis buffer (400 μL/well) for 30 min under ice bath. The lysates were centrifuged at 12,000 rpm for 5 min at 4 °C. Thereafter, the supernatants were collected for Western-blot assay according to protocols in our previous work [13]. Both the Bcl-2 and VEGF proteins were detected using a Western Lightning® Plus-ECL (Enhanced Chemiluminescence) Kit (PerkinElmer, Inc., Boston, MA, USA). More detailed information of experimental can be seen in Supporting Information.

4. Conclusions

To summarize, we used the synthesized Au DENPs-β-CD as a carrier for highly efficient delivery of siRNA to glioblastoma cells. The Au DENPs-β-CD are much more efficient to compact siRNA under appropriate N/P ratios, and exhibit lower cytotoxicity and better siRNA delivery efficiency than the pristine G5.NH_2 dendrimers and the Au DENPs without β-CD modification. These results are related to the dendrimer surface modification of β-CD and dendrimer internal cavity entrapment of Au NPs. In addition, with the assistance of the Au DENPs-β-CD vector, both Bcl-2 and VEGF siRNAs are able to be transfected to silence of glioblastoma cancer cells by downregulation of the respective proteins. Strongly, our study suggests that Au DENPs-β-CD may be employed as a prospective carrier for safe and effective transfection of siRNA to treat a variety of cancer cells based on specific siRNAs.

Acknowledgments: This research is financially supported by the Science and Technology Commission of Shanghai Municipality (17540712000), the National Natural Science Foundation of China (81761148028 and 21773026, and 31400816), and the Fundamental Research Funds for the Central Universities (for Lu Wang, Xueyan Cao and Xiangyang Shi). Xiangyang Shi also thanks the support of the Sino-French Cai Yuanpei Programme, as well as the support by FCT-Fundaca õ para a Ciência e a Tecnologia (project No. PEst-OE/QUI/UI0674/2013, CQM, Portuguese Government funds) and by ARDITI-Agência Regional para o Desenvolvimento da Investigaca õ Tecnologia e Inovaca õ through the project No. M1420-01-0145-FEDER-000005-Centro de Quim ica da Madeira-CQM+ (Madeira 14-20).

Author Contributions: Xiangyang Shi designed the whole experiments; Jieru Qiu carried out the primary parts of the experiments, analyzed the data, and wrote the paper; Lingdan Kong performed some of the experiments of cell culture and edited the manuscript; Aijun Li, Ping Wei, Xueyan Cao, and Lu Wang contributed to some in vitro experiments; and Serge Mignani, Anne-Marie Caminade, Jean-Pierre Majoral, and Xiangyang Shi revised and proofread the whole manuscript.

References

1. Sonawane, N.D.; Szoka, F.C.; Verkman, A.S. Chloride accumulation and swelling in endosomes enhances DNA transfer by polyamine-DNA polyplexes. *J. Biol. Chem.* **2003**, *278*, 44826–44831. [CrossRef] [PubMed]
2. Pantarotto, D.; Singh, R.; McCarthy, D.; Erhardt, M.; Briand, J.P.; Prato, M.; Kostarelos, K.; Bianco, A. Functionalized carbon nanotubes for plasmid DNA gene delivery. *Angew. Chem. Int. Edit.* **2004**, *43*, 5242–5246. [CrossRef] [PubMed]
3. Farmer, H.; McCabe, N.; Lord, C.J.; Tutt, A.N.J.; Johnson, D.A.; Richardson, T.B.; Santarosa, M.; Dillon, K.J.; Hickson, I.; Knights, C.; et al. Targeting the DNA repair defect in BRCA mutant cells as a therapeutic strategy. *Nature* **2005**, *434*, 917–921. [CrossRef] [PubMed]
4. Borgheti-Cardoso, L.N.; Depieri, L.V.; Diniz, H.; Calzzani, R.A.J.; Fantini, M.C.D.; Iyomasa, M.M.; Vicentini, F.; Bentley, M. Self-assembling gelling formulation based on a crystalline-phase liquid as a non-viral vector for siRNA delivery. *Eur. J. Pharm. Sci.* **2014**, *58*, 72–82. [CrossRef] [PubMed]
5. Liu, H.M.; Li, Y.; Mozhi, A.; Zhang, L.; Liu, Y.L.; Xu, X.; Xing, J.M.; Liang, X.J.; Ma, G.H.; Yang, J.; et al. SiRNA-phospholipid conjugates for gene and drug delivery in cancer treatment. *Biomaterials* **2014**, *35*, 6519–6533. [CrossRef] [PubMed]
6. Van Hauwermeiren, F.; Vandenbroucke, R.E.; Grine, L.; Puimege, L.; Van Wonterghem, E.; Zhang, H.; Libert, C. Antisense oligonucleotides against TNFR1 prevent toxicity of TNF/IFN gamma treatment in mouse tumor models. *Int. J. Cancer* **2014**, *135*, 742–750. [CrossRef] [PubMed]
7. Itoh, M.; Nakaura, M.; Imanishi, T.; Obika, S. Target gene knockdown by 2′,4′-BNA/LNA antisense oligonucleotides in zebrafish. *Nucleic Acid Ther.* **2014**, *24*, 186–191. [CrossRef] [PubMed]
8. Putral, L.N.; Gu, W.Y.; McMillan, N.A.J. RNA interference for the treatment of cancer. *Drug News Perspect.* **2006**, *19*, 317–324. [CrossRef] [PubMed]
9. Izquierdo, M. Short interfering RNAs as a tool for cancer gene therapy. *Cancer Gene Ther.* **2005**, *12*, 217–227. [CrossRef] [PubMed]
10. Aagaard, L.; Rossi, J.J. RNAi therapeutics: Principles, prospects and challenges. *Adv. Drug Deliv. Rev.* **2007**, *59*, 75–86. [CrossRef] [PubMed]

11. Castano, S.; Delord, B.; Fevrier, A.; Lehn, J.M.; Lehn, P.; Desbat, B. Brewster angle microscopy and PMIRRAS study of DNA interactions with BGTC, a cationic lipid used for gene transfer. *Langmuir* **2008**, *24*, 9598–9606. [CrossRef] [PubMed]
12. Kong, L.D.; Qiu, J.R.; Sun, W.J.; Yang, J.; Shen, M.W.; Wang, L.; Shi, X.Y. Multifunctional PEI-entrapped gold nanoparticles enable efficient delivery of therapeutic siRNA into glioblastoma cells. *Biomater. Sci.* **2017**, *5*, 258–266. [CrossRef] [PubMed]
13. Kong, L.D.; Wu, Y.L.; Alves, C.S.; Shi, X.Y. Efficient delivery of therapeutic siRNA into glioblastoma cells using multifunctional dendrimer-entrapped gold nanoparticles. *Nanomedicine* **2016**, *11*, 3103–3115. [CrossRef] [PubMed]
14. Xiao, T.Y.; Hou, W.X.; Cao, X.Y.; Wen, S.H.; Shen, M.W.; Shi, X.Y. Dendrimer-entrapped gold nanoparticles modified with folic acid for targeted gene delivery applications. *Biomater. Sci.* **2013**, *1*, 1172–1180. [CrossRef]
15. Paleos, C.M.; Tziveleka, L.A.; Sideratou, Z.; Tsiourvas, D. Gene delivery using functional dendritic polymers. *Expert Opin. Drug Deliv.* **2009**, *6*, 27–38. [CrossRef] [PubMed]
16. Wu, J.; Yamanouchi, D.; Liu, B.; Chu, C.C. Biodegradable arginine-based poly(ether ester amide)s as a non-viral DNA delivery vector and their structure-function study. *J. Mater. Chem.* **2012**, *22*, 18983–18991. [CrossRef]
17. Stamatatos, L.; Leventis, R.; Zuckermann, M.J.; Silvius, J.R. Interactions of cationic lipid vesicles with negatively charged phospholipid-vesicles and biological-membranes. *Biochemistry* **1988**, *27*, 3917–3925. [CrossRef] [PubMed]
18. Behr, J.P.; Demeneix, B.; Loeffler, J.P.; Mutul, J.P. Efficient gene-transfer into mammalian primary endocrine-cells with lipopolyamine-coated DNA. *Proc. Natl. Acad. Sci. USA* **1989**, *86*, 6982–6986. [CrossRef] [PubMed]
19. Boussif, O.; Lezoualch, F.; Zanta, M.A.; Mergny, M.D.; Scherman, D.; Demeneix, B.; Behr, J.P. A versatile vector for gene and oligonucleotide transfer into cells in culture and in-vivo-polyethylenimine. *Proc. Natl. Acad. Sci. USA* **1995**, *92*, 7297–7301. [CrossRef] [PubMed]
20. Pack, D.W.; Hoffman, A.S.; Pun, S.; Stayton, P.S. Design and development of polymers for gene delivery. *Nat. Rev. Drug Discov.* **2005**, *4*, 581–593. [CrossRef] [PubMed]
21. Haralambidis, J.; Duncan, L.; Tregear, G.W. The solid-phase synthesis of oligonucleotides containing a 3′-peptide moiety. *Tetrahedron Lett.* **1987**, *28*, 5199–5202. [CrossRef]
22. Derossi, D.; Joliot, A.H.; Chassaing, G.; Prochiantz, A. The 3rd helix of the antennapedia homeodomain translocates through biological-membranes. *J. Biol. Chem.* **1994**, *269*, 10444–10450. [PubMed]
23. Kuriyama, S.; Mitoro, A.; Tsujinoue, H.; Nakatani, T.; Yoshiji, H.; Tsujimoto, T.; Yamazaki, M.; Fukui, T. Particle-mediated gene transfer into murine livers using a newly developed gene gun. *Gene Ther.* **2000**, *7*, 1132–1136. [CrossRef] [PubMed]
24. Srinivasan, C.; Lee, J.; Papadimitrakopoulos, F.; Silbart, L.K.; Zhao, M.H.; Burgess, D.J. Labeling and intracellular tracking of functionally active plasmid DNA with semiconductor quantum dots. *Mol. Ther.* **2006**, *14*, 192–201. [CrossRef] [PubMed]
25. Mintzer, M.A.; Simanek, E.E. Nonviral vectors for gene delivery. *Chem. Rev.* **2009**, *109*, 259–302. [CrossRef] [PubMed]
26. Guillot-Nieckowski, M.; Eisler, S.; Diederich, F. Dendritic vectors for gene transfection. *New J. Chem.* **2007**, *31*, 1111–1127. [CrossRef]
27. Li, S.; Huang, L. Nonviral gene therapy: Promises and challenges. *Gene Ther.* **2000**, *7*, 31–34. [CrossRef] [PubMed]
28. Itaka, K.; Kanayama, N.; Nishiyama, N.; Jang, W.D.; Yamasaki, Y.; Nakamura, K.; Kawaguchi, H.; Kataoka, K. Supramolecular nanocarrier of siRNA from peg-based block catiomer carrying diamine side chain with distinctive pk(a) directed to enhance intracellular gene silencing. *J. Am. Chem. Soc.* **2004**, *126*, 13612–13613. [CrossRef] [PubMed]
29. Minakuchi, Y.; Takeshita, F.; Kosaka, N.; Sasaki, H.; Yamamoto, Y.; Kouno, M.; Honma, K.; Nagahara, S.; Hanai, K.; Sano, A.; et al. Atelocollagen-mediated synthetic small interfering RNA delivery for effective gene silencing in vitro and in vivo. *Nucleic Acids Res.* **2004**, *32*, e109. [CrossRef] [PubMed]
30. Spagnou, S.; Miller, A.D.; Keller, M. Lipidic carriers of siRNA: Differences in the formulation, cellular uptake, and delivery with plasmid DNA. *Biochemistry* **2004**, *43*, 13348–13356. [CrossRef] [PubMed]

31. Dalby, B.; Cates, S.; Harris, A.; Ohki, E.C.; Tilkins, M.L.; Price, P.J.; Ciccarone, V.C. Advanced transfection with lipofectamine 2000 reagent: Primary neurons, siRNA, and high-throughput applications. *Methods* **2004**, *33*, 95–103. [CrossRef] [PubMed]
32. Unnamalai, N.; Kang, B.G.; Lee, W.S. Cationic oligopeptide-mediated delivery of dsRNA for post-transcriptional gene silencing in plant cells. *FEBS Lett.* **2004**, *566*, 307–310. [CrossRef] [PubMed]
33. Tomalia, D.A.; Baker, H.; Dewald, J.; Hall, M.; Kallos, G.; Martin, S.; Roeck, J.; Ryder, J.; Smith, P. A new class of polymers-starburst-dendritic macromolecules. *Polym. J.* **1985**, *17*, 117–132. [CrossRef]
34. Tomalia, D.A.; Baker, H.; Dewald, J.; Hall, M.; Kallos, G.; Martin, S.; Roeck, J.; Ryder, J.; Smith, P. Dendritic macromolecules-synthesis of starburst dendrimers. *Macromolecules* **1986**, *19*, 2466–2468. [CrossRef]
35. Bielinska, A.U.; Chen, C.L.; Johnson, J.; Baker, J.R. DNA complexing with polyamidoamine dendrimers: Implications for transfection. *Bioconjug. Chem.* **1999**, *10*, 843–850. [CrossRef] [PubMed]
36. He, H.; Li, Y.; Jia, X.R.; Du, J.; Ying, X.; Lu, W.L.; Lou, J.N.; Wei, Y. PEGylated poly(amidoamine) dendrimer-based dual-targeting carrier for treating brain tumors. *Biomaterials* **2011**, *32*, 478–487. [CrossRef] [PubMed]
37. Shakhbazau, A.; Isayenka, I.; Kartel, N.; Goncharova, N.; Seviaryn, I.; Kosmacheva, S.; Potapnev, M.; Shcharbin, D.; Bryszewska, M. Transfection efficiencies of PAMAM dendrimers correlate inversely with their hydrophobicity. *Int. J. Pharm.* **2010**, *383*, 228–235. [CrossRef] [PubMed]
38. Zeng, F.W.; Zimmerman, S.C. Dendrimers in supramolecular chemistry: From molecular recognition to self-assembly. *Chem. Rev.* **1997**, *97*, 1681–1712. [CrossRef] [PubMed]
39. Bosman, A.W.; Janssen, H.M.; Meijer, E.W. About dendrimers: Structure, physical properties, and applications. *Chem. Rev.* **1999**, *99*, 1665–1688. [CrossRef] [PubMed]
40. Zhou, J.H.; Wu, J.Y.; Hafdi, N.; Behr, J.P.; Erbacher, P.; Peng, L. PAMAM dendrimers for efficient siRNA delivery and potent gene silencing. *Chem. Commun.* **2006**, *22*, 2362–2364. [CrossRef] [PubMed]
41. Nam, H.Y.; Nam, K.; Hahn, H.J.; Kim, B.H.; Lim, H.J.; Kim, H.J.; Choi, J.S.; Park, J.S. Biodegradable PAMAM ester for enhanced transfection efficiency with low cytotoxicity. *Biomaterials* **2009**, *30*, 665–673. [CrossRef] [PubMed]
42. Navarro, G.; de Ilarduya, C.T. Activated and non-activated PAMAM dendrimers for gene delivery in vitro and in vivo. *Nanomed. Nanotechnol. Biol. Med.* **2009**, *5*, 287–297. [CrossRef] [PubMed]
43. Hou, W.X.; Wei, P.; Kong, L.D.; Guo, R.; Wang, S.G.; Shi, X.Y. Partially PEGylated dendrimer-entrapped gold nanoparticles: A promising nanoplatform for highly efficient DNA and siRNA delivery. *J. Mater. Chem. B* **2016**, *4*, 2933–2943. [CrossRef]
44. Shan, Y.B.; Luo, T.; Peng, C.; Sheng, R.L.; Cao, A.M.; Cao, X.Y.; Shen, M.W.; Guo, R.; Tomas, H.; Shi, X.Y. Gene delivery using dendrimer-entrapped gold nanoparticles as nonviral vectors. *Biomaterials* **2012**, *33*, 3025–3035. [CrossRef] [PubMed]
45. Qi, R.; Gao, Y.; Tang, Y.; He, R.R.; Liu, T.L.; He, Y.; Sun, S.; Li, B.Y.; Li, Y.B.; Liu, G. PEG-conjugated PAMAM dendrimers mediate efficient intramuscular gene expression. *AAPS J.* **2009**, *11*, 395–405. [CrossRef] [PubMed]
46. Xiao, T.Y.; Cao, X.Y.; Hou, W.X.; Peng, C.; Qiu, J.R.; Shi, X.Y. Poly(amidoamine) dendrimers modified with 1,2-epoxyhexane or 1,2-epoxydodecane for enhanced gene delivery applications. *J. Nanosci. Nanotechnol.* **2015**, *15*, 10134–10140. [CrossRef] [PubMed]
47. Hou, W.X.; Wen, S.H.; Guo, R.; Wang, S.G.; Shi, X.Y. Partially acetylated dendrimer-entrapped gold nanoparticles with reduced cytotoxicity for gene delivery applications. *J. Nanosci. Nanotechnol.* **2015**, *15*, 4094–4105. [CrossRef] [PubMed]
48. Qiu, J.R.; Kong, L.D.; Cao, X.Y.; Li, A.J.; Tan, H.R.; Shi, X.Y. Dendrimer-entrapped gold nanoparticles modified with β-cyclodextrin for enhanced gene delivery applications. *RSC Adv.* **2016**, *6*, 25633–25640. [CrossRef]
49. Kihara, F.; Arima, H.; Tsutsumi, T.; Hirayama, F.; Uekama, K. In vitro and in vivo gene transfer by an optimized alpha-cyclodextrin conjugate with polyamidoamine dendrimer. *Bioconjug. Chem.* **2003**, *14*, 342–350. [CrossRef] [PubMed]

8

SPC Liposomes as Possible Delivery Systems for Improving Bioavailability of the Natural Sesquiterpene β-Caryophyllene: Lamellarity and Drug-Loading as Key Features for a Rational Drug Delivery Design

Antonella Di Sotto [1,*], Patrizia Paolicelli [2,*], Martina Nardoni [2], Lorena Abete [1], Stefania Garzoli [2], Silvia Di Giacomo [1], Gabriela Mazzanti [1], Maria Antonietta Casadei [2] and Stefania Petralito [2,*]

1 Department of Physiology and Pharmacology "V. Erspamer", Sapienza University of Rome, P.le Aldo Moro 5, 00185 Rome, Italy; lorena.abete@uniroma1.it (L.A.); silvia.digiacomo@uniroma1.it (S.D.G.); gabriela.mazzanti@uniroma1.it (G.M.)

2 Department of Chemistry and Technology of Drugs, Sapienza University of Rome, P.le Aldo Moro 5, 00185 Rome, Italy; martina.nardoni@uniroma1.it (M.N.); stefania.garzoli@uniroma1.it (S.G.); mariaantonietta.casadei@uniroma1.it (M.A.C.)

* Correspondence: antonella.disotto@uniroma1.it (A.D.S.); patrizia.paolicelli@uniroma1.it (P.P.); stefania.petralito@uniroma1.it (S.P.)

Abstract: The natural sesquiterpene β-caryophyllene (CRY) has been highlighted to possess interesting pharmacological potentials, particularly due to its chemopreventive and analgesic properties. However, the poor solubility of this sesquiterpene in aqueous fluids can hinder its uptake into cells, resulting in inconstant responses of biological systems, thus limiting its application. Therefore, identifying a suitable pharmaceutical form for increasing CRY bioavailability represents an important requirement for exploiting its pharmacological potential. In the present study, the ability of soybean phosphatidylcholine (SPC) liposomes to improve bioavailability and absorption of CRY in cancer cells has been evaluated. Liposomal formulations of CRY, differing for lamellarity (i.e., unilamellar and multilamellar vesicles or ULV and MLV) and for the drug loading (i.e., 1:0.1, 1:0.3 and 1:0.5 mol/mol between SPC and CRY) were designed with the aim of maximizing CRY amount in the liposome bilayer, while avoiding its leakage during storage. The low-loaded formulations significantly potentiated the antiproliferative activity of CRY in both HepG2 and MDA-MB-468 cells, reaching a maximum IC_{50} lowering (from two to five folds) with 1:0.3 and 1:0.1 SPC/CRY MLV. Conversely, increasing liposome drug-loading reduced the ability for CRY release, likely due to a possible interaction between SPC and CRY that affects the membrane properties, as confirmed by physical measures.

Keywords: lipophilic compound; caryophyllene sesquiterpene; antiproliferative activity; liposomes; lamellarity; drug loading

1. Introduction

β-caryophyllene or *trans*-caryophyllene (CRY), a bicyclic sesquiterpene with a rare cyclobutane ring (Figure 1), is a volatile compound found in large amounts in the essential oil of many different spice and food plants, particularly *Eugenia caryophyllata* L., *Copaifera multijuga* (copaiba) and *Cannabis sativa* L [1].

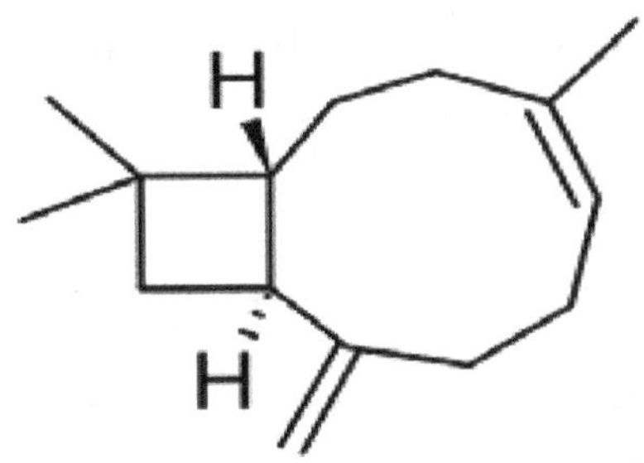

Figure 1. Chemical structure of β-caryophyllene (CRY).

In nature, β-caryophyllene is usually found together with small amount of its isomers α-caryophyllene and γ-caryophyllene or in a mixture with its oxidation product, β-caryophyllene oxide. Several biological activities have been reported for β-caryophyllene, including antimicrobial, antileishmanial, antimalarial, local anesthetic, spasmolytic and anticonvulsivant activities [2]. It has been reported to partly act as an agonist of the CB2 receptor, which represents a therapeutic target for the treatment of inflammation, pain, atherosclerosis, and inflammatory-based diseases, including colitis, cerebral ischemia and brain inflammation [3–7]. Also, it has been recently shown to possess chemopreventive properties [1,8–11] and displayed a chemosensitizing power when administered in combination with anticancer drugs, thus resensitizing chemoresistant cancer cells [12]. It was found to be able to interfere with targeted signalling pathways involved in inflammation and cancer, including HMGB1/TLR4 signalling and STAT3 [10,13,14].

Despite these promising biological activities, β-caryophyllene is characterized by high lipophilicity and poor stability in hydrophilic media (such as biological fluids), which limit its bioavailability and absorption into cells. Bioavailability depends on the nature and chemical-physical properties of a molecule and is mainly due to water solubility (or dissolution rate) and membrane permeability [15]. Low bioavailability is a common feature of different natural substances, defined as "poorly water-soluble drugs", and can hinder their administration, clinical application and market entry. In this context, improving bioavailability represents an important requirement for exploiting the pharmacological potential of such natural substances and meeting the need for suitable pharmaceutical formulations.

To this end, various strategies, including formulation in complex forms as micelles, liposomes, polymeric nanoparticles and lipid nanoparticles, have been approached. Among them, liposomes have been extensively applied in the years as biomembrane models and as drug carriers in the pharmaceutical and medical fields, owing to their excellent biocompatibility and biodegradability, low toxicity and lack of immunogenicity [16,17]. They have also been adopted as efficient systems for incorporating natural compounds, such as essential oil components, and improving their solubility and chemical stability [18].

Liposome structure allows the incorporation of different types of drugs: hydrophilic substances are encapsulated in the inner aqueous compartments, while lipophilic drugs are mainly entrapped within the lipid bilayer [19]. According to lamellarity and size, they are usually classified as multilamellar vesicles (MLV; greater than 0.5 μm), small unilamellar vesicles (SUV; between 20 and 100 nm) and large unilamellar vesicles (LUV; greater than 100 nm) [20].

Taking into account the strong lipophilicity of CRY and its low dissolution rate in biological fluids, in the present study we propose a rational design of soy phosphatidylcholine (SPC) liposomal formulations for improving cellular uptake of CRY and then its antiproliferative activity in cancer cells, focusing on lamellarity and drug-loading as major key features to develop optimized delivery systems. SPC is commonly used in different types of drug delivery formulations, due to its structural similarity with biomembrane phospholipids, and seems to represent an interesting molecule to be used for designing liposomal chemotherapy formulations, since it could enhance the antiproliferative activity of anticancer drugs by affecting the cholesterol-induced stiffening of cancer cell biomembrane, thus favoring drug permeability. It is well accepted that cancer cells, respect to normal cells, are characterized by changes in biomembrane phospholipid composition and a constitutive activation of the fatty acid biosynthesis seems to support the increased cell proliferation [21]. Particularly, higher accumulation of cholesterol leads to a more rigid and low-permeable membrane, with increased resistance to cancer chemotherapy.

In order to characterize the best features of SPC liposomes in improving the dissolution of CRY in biological fluids and its cellular uptake, both unilamellar (ULV) and multilamellar (MLV) formulations were studied. In fact, due to the physico-chemical properties of CRY, it is expected that the drug is incorporated within the phospholipid bilayer of liposomes. Therefore, liposomal formulations of CRY have been rationally designed taking into account that the loading of CRY in the bilayer of liposomes, while avoiding its leakage during storage, requires special consideration in product development and represents a key feature for optimizing the formulation. The lipid composition, lamellarity, the manufacturing process and drug incorporation can all influence the physicochemical properties of a liposomal formulation, including the drug release performance. Therefore, when liposomes are investigated as drug delivery vehicles of hydrophobic drugs, the influence of the drug–lipid ratio on the arrangement of the nonpolar region of the vesicles membrane should be considered to design a delivery vehicle that is at the same time able to catch and release the encapsulated payload in order to achieve the therapeutic purpose [22].

In line with this evidence, in the present study different formulations at three loading degrees, characterized by SPC phospholipid and CRY molar ratio of 1:0.1, 1:0.3 and 1:0.5 as well as different lamellarity were prepared. A physicochemical characterization by dynamic light scattering, fluorescence anisotropy and entrapment efficiency of CRY were performed. The increased bioavailability was evaluated on the basis of the cytotoxicity potency of the formulations encapsulating CRY with respect to the substance alone. In specific, the antiproliferative activity of CRY-loaded SPC ULV and MLV with respect to that of CRY alone was studied in liver cancer HepG2cells. Also, triple negative MDA-MB-468 breast cancer cells were used being high-responsive to CRY cytotoxicity respect to HepG2 cells.

2. Materials and Methods

2.1. Chemicals

β-Caryophyllene (CRY; >98.5% purity), soybean phosphatidylcholine (Phospholipon90; SPC), HEPES [4-(2-hydroxyethyl) piperazine-1-ethane-sulfonic acid], thiocyanatoiron (III), 1,6-diphenyl-1,3,5-hexatriene (DPH) and (4,5-dimethyl-2-thiazolyl)-2,5-diphenyl-2H-tetrazolium bromide (MTT; ≥97.5% purity) and cholesterol (Chol) were purchased from Sigma-Aldrich Co (St. Louis, MO, USA). Dulbecco's Modified Eagle's medium (DMEM) was from Aurogene (Rome, Italy). Chloroform, dimethyl sulfoxide, ethanol, 1,2-dicloroethane and hydrochloric acid were supplied by Carlo Erba Reagents (Arese, Italy) and were of analytical grade. All solutions were prepared in the better solvent, sterilized by filtration and stored for a just conservation time at recommended temperature, i.e., room temperature (RT) or refrigerated conditions (from 4 °C to −20 °C).

For the cytotoxicity assay, the sesquiterpene was dissolved in absolute EtOH (100% v/v): at the tested concentrations, and the percentage of ethanol was less than 1% v/v in the final mixture, in order to exclude a potential toxicity due to the solvent. Conversely, both the CRY-loaded and plain SPC liposomes were directly dispersed in the culture medium at different concentrations.

2.2. Liposome Preparation

Liposomes were prepared by the thin-film hydration method followed by extrusion [23]. Specifically, 250 mg of SPC and different amount of CRY (7, 20 or 33 mg) were dissolved in a 50 mL round-bottom flask in the minimum volume of chloroform to give lipid-to-drug molar ratio of 1:0.1, 1:0.3 and 1:0.5.

The solvent was removed by rotary evaporation under reduced pressure to form a thin layer on the flask wall. The resultant thin film was further dried with a high vacuum oil pump for at least 2 h.

Dried film was hydrated in 5 mL of a 10 mM HEPES buffer solution (pH 7.4) at 25 °C and the dispersion was shaken vigorously with a vortex mixer to form multi-lamellar vesicles (MLV).

The generated multilamellar vesicles were repeatedly extruded at 25 °C through polycarbonate membranes of decreasing pore size using a thermobarrel Extruder, (Lipex Biomembrane, Vancouver, BC, Canada) until a defined size distribution was achieved (2 times through 400 nm membranes and finally 6 times through 200 nm membranes). All liposome formulations were flushed with nitrogen gas, stored at 4 °C and used within two weeks.

2.3. *Gas Chromatographic/Mass Spectrometric (GC/MS)*

Purity of CRY and its concentration obtained in the liposomal dispersion was determined by the gas chromatographic/mass spectrometric (GC/MS) technique. The GC/MS analyses were performed on a Clarus 500 series from Perkin Elmer instruments (Waltham, MA, USA) operating in the electron impact mode (70 eV) and equipped with NIST (National Institute of Standards and Technology) libraries. A Stabilwax fused-silica capillary column (Restek, Bellefonte, PA, USA) (60 m × 0.25 mm, 0.25 mm film thickness) was used with helium as carrier gas (1.0 mL/min). 1 μL of sample was injected into the GC injector at the temperature of 280 °C and in splitless mode. The oven of GC was programmed to rise from 90 °C to 200 °C at 3 °C/min and then held at 200 °C for 2 min. All analyses were performed at constant flow. A calibration curve was generated by running various solutions containing graded amounts of the CRY and injecting a constant volume of each standard solution exactly measured. The calibration curve was obtained by plotting the peaks area (automatically calculated by the computer) on the ordinate and the amounts on the abscissa.

2.4. *Physicochemical Characterization of Liposomes*

2.4.1. Dynamic Light Scattering (DLS) and Zeta-Potential Measurements

Particle size distribution and zeta-potential were measured with a Zetasizer Nano ZS90 (Malvern Panalytical, Malvern, UK). Hydrodynamic diameter and polydispersity index were evaluated by dynamic light scattering (DLS) experiments, whereas zeta-potential was measured by electrophoretic light scattering (ELS) experiments. The DLS and ELS techniques used a photon correlator spectrometer equipped with a 4 mW He/Ne laser source operating at 633 nm. All measurements were performed at a scattering angle of 90° and were thermostatically controlled at 25 °C. The samples were opportunely diluted with 10 mM HEPES (pH 7.4) before analysis. Size, polydispersity index and zeta-potential values of the liposome formulations are the mean of three different preparation batches ± standard deviation.

2.4.2. Assay of Phospholipids

Phospholipid content in liposomes was quantified as reported in literature [24]. Briefly, 0.4 mL of sample (20–200 nmol) was mixed with 0.2 mL of ethanol, 1 mL of thiocyanatoiron (III) and 0.6 mL of 0.17 N hydrochloric acid. 3 mL of 1,2-dichloroethane were added to extract the thiocyanatoiron–phospholipid complex formed after shaking for 2 min. The sample was then centrifuged for 5 min at 12,000 rpm. The absorbance of the organic phase was read at a wavelength of 470 nm in a Lambda 25 spectrophotometer (Perkin Elmer, Waltham, USA). The calibration curve was obtained with several solutions of known SPC concentration.

2.4.3. Evaluation of Total Amount of β-Caryophyllene (CRY) in Liposomal Suspensions

Phospholipids and drug molecules dissolved in the organic phase may be get lost during solvent removal under vacuum and high-pressure extrusion steps. Considering that CRY is a liquid with an initial boiling point of 129 °C, to evaluate the amount of the sequiterpene actually present in the different liposomal formulations, it was first extracted from vesicles and then its concentration was determined by the GC/MS technique reported in Section 2.3. In particular, 5 mL of CRY-loaded SPC

ULV were diluted with 10 mL of 10 mM HEPES (pH 7.4) and extracted with $CHCl_3$ (5 mL). To promote the separation of the two phases, $CaCl_2$ (460 mg) was added to the biphasic system and the organic phase then collected. The extraction procedure was repeated three times, all the organic phases were mixed and made up to known volume before GC/MS analysis.

2.4.4. Steady-State and Time-Resolved Fluorescence Measurements

Steady state anisotropy of DPH in liposomes was measured to assess the effect of CRY and its concentration on the fluidity of SPC liposome membranes. To this end, DPH-loaded SPC liposomes were prepared by the thin-film hydration method reported in Section 2.2, dissolving SPC (250 mg) and DPH (0.15 mg; 6.46×10^{-4} mmol) in a 50 mL round-bottom flask in the minimum volume of chloroform to give a lipid-to-DPH molar ratio of 1:0.002.

The solvent was removed as previously described and the resultant thin film was hydrated in 5 mL of a 10 mM HEPES buffer solution (pH 7.4) at 25 °C. The generated multilamellar vesicles were repeatedly extruded at 25 °C through polycarbonate membranes of decreasing pore size.

DPH normally is located within the hydrophobic region of the bilayer membrane. DPH responds to changes in physical properties of the acyl chain region of the membrane that affect its ability to rotate. Probe movement is quantified by measuring the degree to which DPH fluorescence emission is depolarized following excitation by polarized light. These fluorescence anisotropy measurements respond to changes in the order degree of the DPH surrounding environment: changes in the liquid–crystalline state organization of the liposome membrane alter the rate of probe movement; in particular, the more disordered the membrane environment, the greater is the motional freedom of the fluorophore and hence the lower the observed anisotropy. An increase in steady state anisotropy of DPH in membranes may imply a reduction in mobility of lipids.

Steady-state fluorescence anisotropy measurements, for DPH-loaded liposomes, were carried out at room temperature with a Perkin-Elmer LS50B spectrofluorometer. The excitation and emission wavelengths were 350 and 450 nm, respectively, and all slits were set to a width of 2.5/2.5 nm.

Samples, opportunely diluted with 10 mM HEPES buffer pH 7.4, were illuminated by vertically (V) or horizontally (H) polarized monochromatic light at $\lambda = 350$ nm and the emitted fluorescence intensities (I) parallel or perpendicular to the direction of the excitation beam were recorded at $\lambda = 450$ nm. Total fluorescence intensity $[I_f = (I_{/\!/})V + 2G(I_{\perp})H]$ is obtained by addition of the respectively horizontally $[I_{\perp}]$ and vertically $[I_{/\!/}]$ intensities polarised light emission. The stationary fluorescence anisotropy (r) was determined using the typical calculation:

$$r = \frac{(I_{/\!/})V - G(I_{\perp})H}{I_f}$$

Total fluorescence intensity and anisotropy measurements required correction for the gain of photomultipler detector $[G = (I_{/\!/})H/(I_{\perp})H]$.

The effect of CRY incorporation on the phospholipid bilayer of SPC liposomes was evaluated by comparison with the well-known effect produced by cholesterol (Chol) on the membrane behavior.

Anisotropy data are represented as the mean $\pm$ standard deviation (SD).

2.5. Cytotoxicity Studies

2.5.1. Human Cancer Cell Lines

Liver cancer HepG2 cells were a kind gift of Prof. Eufemi (Sapienza University of Rome, Italy), while triple negative MDA-MB-468 breast cancer cells were purchased from IRCCS AOU San Martino -IST (Genoa, Italy). The cells were grown under standard conditions (37 °C and 5% CO_2) in DMEM-F12 medium containing L-glutamine (1% v/v) and HEPES (15 mM) and supplemented with 10% heat-inactivated FBS, 100 U/mL penicillin and 100 µg/mL streptomycin in 75 cm^2 flasks.

Subcultures were prepared every 4 days, renewing growth medium every 2–3 days. All experiments were performed when cells reached the logarithmic growth phase.

2.5.2. Cytotoxicity Assay

The cultured cells were seeded into 96-well microplates (20,000 cells/well), allowed to grow for 24 h, then treated with CRY (1–75 μg/mL in EtOH 1% *v*/*v*) or CRY loaded SPC liposomes. The concentrations of pure CRY were prepared by progressive dilution in EtOH 100% *v*/*v*, then added to cells at 1% *v*/*v* in the final mixture, at which ethanol was nontoxic. A vehicle control (EtOH 1% *v*/*v* in the final mixture for CRY and 10 mM HEPES for SPC ULV and MLV), corresponding to 100% cell viability and a standard cytotoxic agent (i.e., doxorubicin, 10 μg/mL in the final mixture) were also included in the experiments.

After 24 h incubation, the cytotoxicity of the treatment was measured by the 3-[4,5-dimethylthiazol-2-yl]-2,5-diphenyl tetrazolium bromide (MTT) assay according to previous published methods [25]. The assay was carried out at least in three biological replicates, and in each experiment each concentration was tested in six technical triplicates. The treatment was considered cytotoxic when the cell viability was lower than 70% with respect to vehicle treated cells [26].

The results were expressed as percentage of cell viability (about three experiments including 8-10 replicates for each treatment) with respect to the vehicle.

Results of cytotoxicity studies are expressed as mean ± standard error (SE). The concentration–response curves were constructed using the Hill equation:

$$E = \frac{E_{max}}{[1 + (10logIC_{50} - A)Hill\ Slope]}$$

where E is the effect at a given concentration of the substance, E_{max} is the maximum activity, IC_{50} is the concentration that produces a 50% of the inhibitory response, A is the substance molar concentration, *HillSlope* is the curve slope.

2.6. Statistical Analysis

Statistical analysis was performed by GraphPad Prism™ (Version 4.00) software (GraphPad Software, Inc., San Diego, CA, USA). The one-way analysis of variance (one-way ANOVA), followed by Dunnett's multiple comparison post-test, was used to analyze the difference among different treatments, while the Student's *t*-test was applied to determine the statistical significance between two different experimental conditions. The values of $p < 0.05$ were considered significant.

3. Results

3.1. Physicochemical Characterization of Soybean Phosphatidylcholine (SPC) Unilamellar and Multilamellar Vesicles (ULV and MLV)

Results obtained by DLS measurements highlighted that high pure CRY did not alter the vesicles formation, since no significant changes in physicochemical features (i.e., mean diameter, zeta-potential and size distribution) of CRY-loaded SPC ULV and MLV, compared to conventional liposomes, were found even at the highest molar ratio tested (1:0.5 mol/mol) (Tables 1 and 2). Moreover, no loss of CRY was observed during the preparation process. In fact, GC/MS analysis performed after the extraction of CRY from liposomes evidenced a perfect overlap of the actual recovered amount with the theoretical one, thus indicating that no losses of sesquiterpene occurred. When the physicochemical features of liposomes were evaluated in the presence of cell medium, no interference with the dimensional analysis was highlighted, thus suggesting a suitable stability of the formulation in cell culture environment (data not shown). The amount of structured phospholipids in the liposomal suspensions, with and without CRY, resulted in not being affected by the presence of the sesquiterpene, thus suggesting their compatibility.

Table 1. Physicochemical features of soybean phosphatidylcholine (SPC) unilamellar vesicles (ULV) liposomes.

Sample	Hydrodynamic Diameter (nm)	PdI	ζ-Potential (mV)	SPC Recovery (%)
Unloaded SPC vesicles	180.6 ± 4.7	0.079 ± 0.015	−15.3 ± 0.4	92.2 ± 1.7
SPC/CRY vesicles (mol/mol)				
1:0.1	185.5 ± 4.2	0.076 ± 0.006	−14.1 ± 0.2	89.5 ± 1.2
1:0.3	176.7 ± 7.5	0.075 ± 0.005	−14.3 ± 0.5	88.5 ± 0.5
1:0.5	181.4 ± 2.1	0.085 ± 0.012	−13.5 ± 0.6	85.2 ± 2.2

Hydrodynamic diameter (Z-Average, nm); polydispersity index (PdI); ζ-potential (mV) and % of SPC recovery.

Table 2. Physicochemical features of SPC multilamellar vesicles (MLV) liposomes.

Sample	Hydrodynamic Diameter (nm)	PdI
Unloaded SPC vesicles	699.7 ± 6.6	0.359 ± 0.069
SPC/CRY vesicles (mol/mol)		
1:0.1	643.9 ± 13.6	0.339 ± 0.045
1:0.3	631.5 ± 21.1	0.371 ± 0.005
1:0.5	497.1 ± 7.9	0.387 ± 0.025

Hydrodynamic diameter (Z-Average, nm); polydispersity index (PdI).

3.2. Cytotoxicity of CRY and Plain SPC-Based Liposomes

Under our experimental conditions, CRY did not affect the cell viability of HepG2 cells up to 10 µg/mL, although a slight cell viability reduction (about 10%) was found starting from 5 µg/mL. A significant decrease of cell viability (about 45% reduction respect to control) was found at 25 µg/mL, reaching a greatest inhibition of about 90% at 75 µg/mL (Figure 2). In MDA-MB-468 cells, CRY produced early toxicity signs (inhibition of 10%) at 2.5 µg/mL, with a biologically significant effect at 15, 25 and 50 µg/mL (inhibition of 38%, 84% and 98% respectively) (Figure 2). The IC_{50} values were 44.7 (C.L. 19.5–96.8) and 19.2 (C. L. 15.4–23.8) µg/mL in HepG2 and MDA-MB-468 cells, respectively.

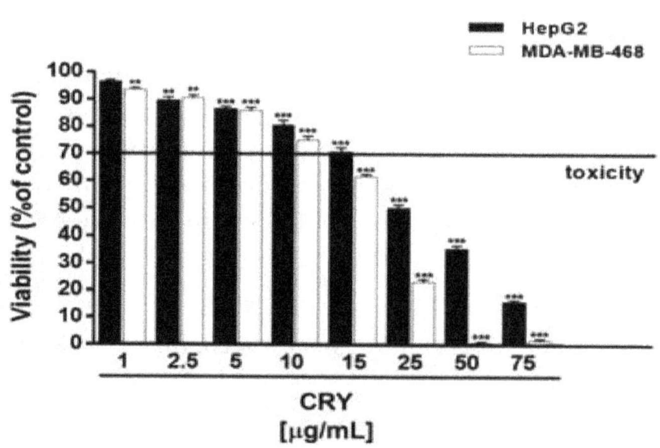

Figure 2. Effect of CRY on the viability of HepG2 and MDA-MB-468 cells. ** $p < 0.01$ and *** $p < 0.001$ (analysis of variance (ANOVA) + multiple Dunnett's comparison post-test); denotes a statistically significant reduction of cell viability compared to control (i.e., vehicle-treated cells). A cell viability lower than 70% respect to control was considered as cytotoxic [26].

The cytotoxicity of plain SPC ULV and MLV (1–1000 µg/mL) in HepG2 and MDA-MB-468 cells was preliminarily evaluated, in order to define the maximum concentration at which liposomal formulations did not affect cell viability. Plain SPC ULV were nontoxic up to the concentration of 100 µg/mL in both HepG2 and MDA-MB-468 cells, with biologically significant cytotoxic effects (from 40% to 56% inhibition of cell viability) starting from 200 µg/mL (Figure 3). Conversely, plain SPC MLV produced biologically significant cytotoxic effects (from 40% to 50% inhibition of cell viability) at

1000 μg/mL in both HepG2 and MDA-MB-468 cells, with early toxicity signs (about 25% inhibition of cell viability) at 500 μg/mL (Figure 3).

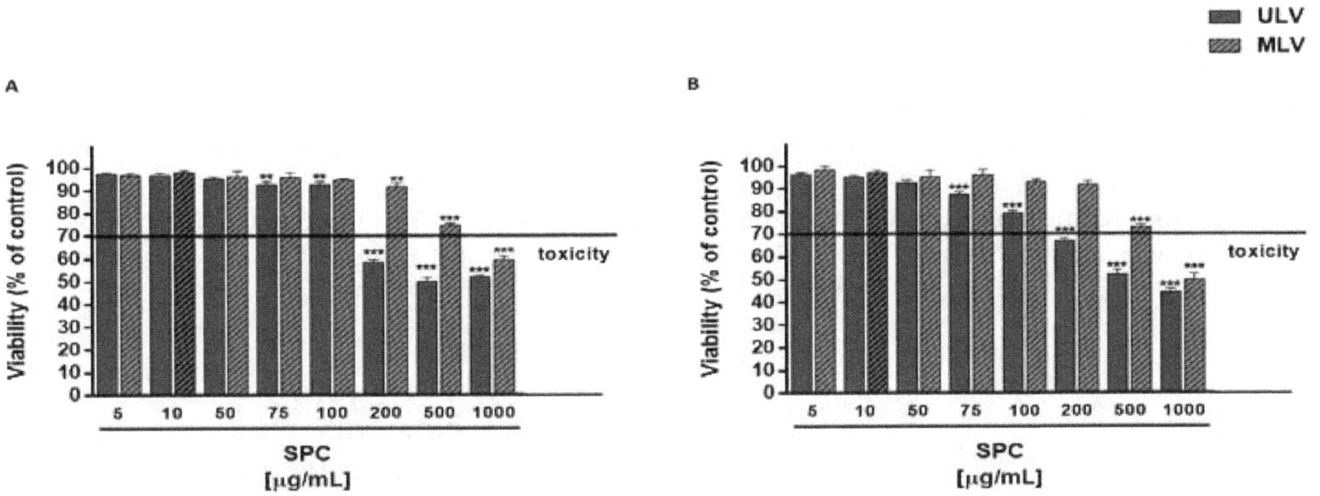

Figure 3. Effect of SPC ULV and MLV on the viability of HepG2 (**A**) and MDA-MB-468 (**B**) cells. ** $p < 0.01$ and *** $p < 0.001$ vs. control (i.e., vehicle-treated cells), denotes a statistically significant reduction of cell viability compared to control (ANOVA + multiple Dunnett's comparison post-test). A cell viability lower than 70% respect to control was considered as cytotoxic [26].

3.3. *Cytotoxicity of CRY-Loaded SPC ULV at Different Molar Ratio*

When assessed in HepG2 cells, different behaviour was found for CRY-loaded SPC ULV respect to pure CRY, as a function of their molar ratio (Figure 4). In particular, the 1:0.1 molar ratio between SPC and CRY produced about a 40% cytotoxicity increase of CRY at low concentrations of 0.1, 1, 5 and 10 μg/mL, which were non-effective when CRY was administered as pure compound. Conversely, a progressive loss of the cytotoxic effect of CRY was found at highest concentrations of 25, 50 and 75 μg/mL of 1:0.1 SPC/CRY ULV, reaching a maximum 40% inhibition (Figure 4). In spite of a biologically significant cytotoxicity of low-dose 1:0.1 SPC/CRY ULV, the 1:0.3 and 1:0.5 unilamellar formulations produced non-biologically relevant cytotoxic effects and progressively reduced the antiproliferative activity of pure CRY at all the tested concentrations, reaching a maximum of 63% inhibition (Figure 4).

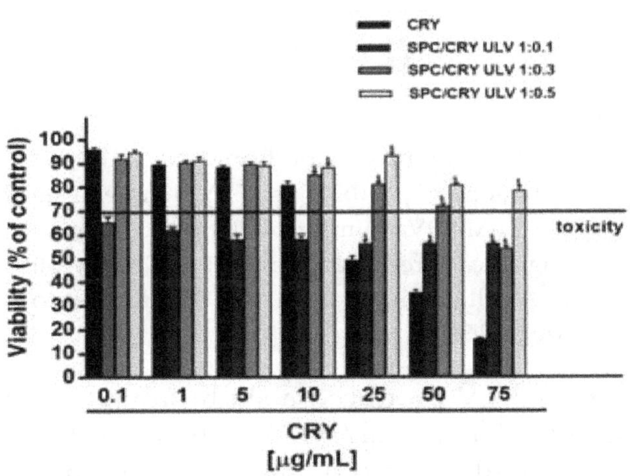

Figure 4. Cytotoxicity of SPC ULV differently loaded with CRY (1:0.1, 1:0.3 and 1:0.5 mol/mol) in HepG2 cells after 24 h incubation. *** $p < 0.001$ vs CRY; denotes a statistically significant increase of cytotoxicity respect to pure CRY (ANOVA + multiple Dunnett's comparison post-test). § $p < 0.001$ vs. CRY, denotes a statistically significant reduction respect to CRY cytotoxicity (ANOVA + multiple Dunnett's comparison post-test). A cell viability lower than 70% respect to control (i.e., vehicle-treated cells) was considered as cytotoxic [26].

Furthermore, the highest doses of loaded liposomes (starting from 25 μg/mL of 1:0.1 and 1:0.3 SPC/CRY ULV) significantly reduced the cytotoxicity of plain SPC ULV, at the corresponding concentrations (Figure 4). This evidence suggested that increasing molar ratio between SPC and CRY in ULV formulations can hinder CRY release and retain the molecule into liposomes; also, some interactions between SPC and CRY could be expected, so explaining the reduced toxicity of plain SPC ULV. A similar behaviour was observed in MDA-MB-468 cells for 1:0.5 SPC/CRY ULV, which did not potentiate CRY cytotoxicity in all the experimental conditions, while inhibiting the antiproliferative activity of pure CRY by about 20%, at concentrations of 25 and 50 μg/mL (Figure 5). Conversely, the 1:0.1 loaded formulation induced a significant potentiation of CRY cytotoxicity (from about 20 to 30%) at concentrations of 2.5 and 5 μg/mL, which disappeared at the highest tested concentrations.

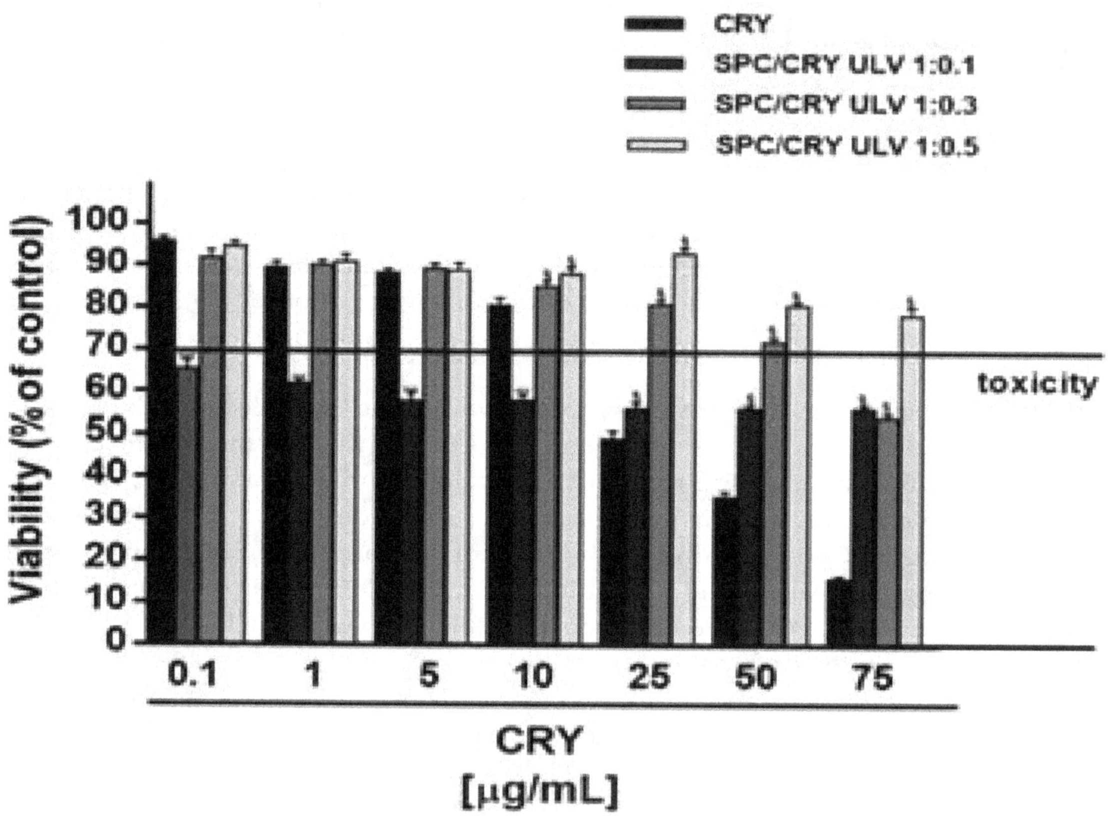

Figure 5. Cytotoxicity of SPC ULV differently loaded with CRY (1:0.1, 1:0.3 and 1:0.5 mol/mol) in MDA-MB-468 cells after 24 h incubation. *** $p < 0.001$ vs. CRY, denotes a statistically significant increase of cytotoxicity respect to pure CRY (ANOVA + multiple Dunnett's comparison post-test). § $p < 0.001$ vs. CRY, denotes a statistically significant reduction respect to CRY cytotoxicity (ANOVA + multiple Dunnett's comparison post-test). A cell viability lower than 70% respect to control (i.e., vehicle-treated cells) was considered as cytotoxic [26].

Similarly, the 1:0.3 SPC/CRY ULV produced a slight (about 10%) but significant increase of CRY toxicity at concentrations of 2.5 and 5 μg/mL. It is noteworthy that potentiation occurred at non-effective concentrations of CRY administered as a pure compound. For all loaded formulations, the highest concentrations of 25 and 50 μg/mL induced a significant inhibition (from about 10 to 28%) of CRY antiproliferative activity, thus suggesting a possible loss of activity of the drug or the loss of the carrier's ability to deliver the incorporated substance (Figure 5). When CRY was administered as 1:0.1 SPC ULV, the IC_{50} values were not evaluable in HepG2 cells, while a slight reduction (about 1.5 folds) was obtained in MDA-MB-468 cells (Table 3).

Table 3. IC_{50} values of CRY administered as pure compound or as ULV and MLV formulations in HepG2 and MDA-MB-468 cells.

	HepG2	**MDA-MB-468**
	IC_{50} (CL) μg/mL *RR*	
CRY	44.7 (19.5–96.8)	19.2 (15.4–23.8)
	SPC/CRY ULV (mol/mol)	
1:0.1	ne	12.4 (6.4–109.9) *1.5*
1:0.3	ne	ne
1:0.5	ne	ne
	SPC/CRY MLV (mol/mol)	
1:0.1	ne	4.9 (2.4–9.9) *3.9*
1:0.3	9.1 (2.6–32.0) *4.9*	8.3 (6.1–11.2) *2.3*
1:0.5	ne	ne

CL, confidential limits; RR, reversal ratio (ratio between the IC_{50} values of CRY alone and CRY-loaded SPC liposomes); ne, not evaluable as a lower than 80% inhibition of cell viability was reached.

3.4. Cytotoxicity of CRY-Loaded SPC MLV at Different Molar Ratio

Under our experimental conditions, multilamellar liposomes produced different cytotoxic effects as a function of drug loading. In HepG2 cells, 1:0.1 SPC/CRY MLV did not affect the cell viability up to 1 μg/mL, while it produced a marked potentiation of CRY cytotoxicity, at concentrations from 5 to 25 μg/mL, reaching the greatest effect of about 45% at 5 μg/mL (Figure 6). A significant and progressive increase of CRY antiproliferative activity, with a maximum potentiation of about 40%, was also produced by 1:0.3 loaded multilamellar formulation (Figure 6) within the concentrations of 1 and 50 μg/mL: the IC_{50} value of CRY was reduced about five-fold (Table 3). Conversely, the 1:0.5 molar ratio between SPC and CRY increased the biological activity of CRY at concentrations of 5 and 10 μg/mL, with a maximum potentiation of 30% at 5 μg/mL (Figure 6). At the highest concentration of 75 μg/mL, all the CRY-loaded multilamellar formulations markedly reduced the antiproliferative activity of pure CRY, reaching a maximum 26% inhibition (Figure 6).

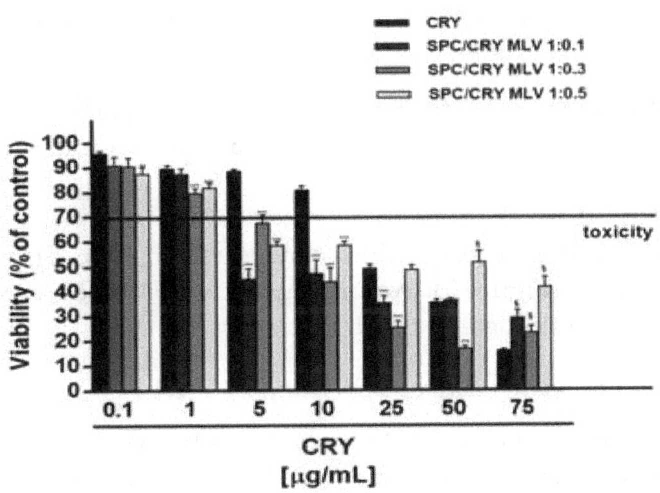

Figure 6. Cytotoxicity of SPC MLV differently loaded with CRY (1:0.1, 1:0.3 and 1:0.5 mol/mol) in HepG2 cells after 24 h incubation. ** $p < 0.01$ and *** $p < 0.001$ vs CRY; denotes a statistically significant increase of cytotoxicity respect to pure CRY (ANOVA + multiple Dunnett's comparison post-test). § $p < 0.001$ vs. CRY, denotes a statistically significant reduction respect to CRY cytotoxicity (ANOVA + multiple Dunnett's comparison post-test). A cell viability lower than 70% respect to control (i.e., vehicle-treated cells) was considered as cytotoxic [26].

Analogously, in MDA-MB-468 cells, the 1:0.1 SPC/CRY MLV induced a significant potentiation of CRY cytotoxicity from 0.1 to 10 µg/mL, with a maximum increase of about 30% at 5 and 10 µg/mL (Figure 7). The 1:0.3 and 1:0.5 loaded formulations produced lower potentiation of CRY activity (about 10–25%) from 0.1 to 10 µg/mL. Conversely, the highest concentrations of 25 and 50 µg/mL reduced the antiproliferative activity of pure CRY, reaching a maximum 30% inhibition (Figure 7).

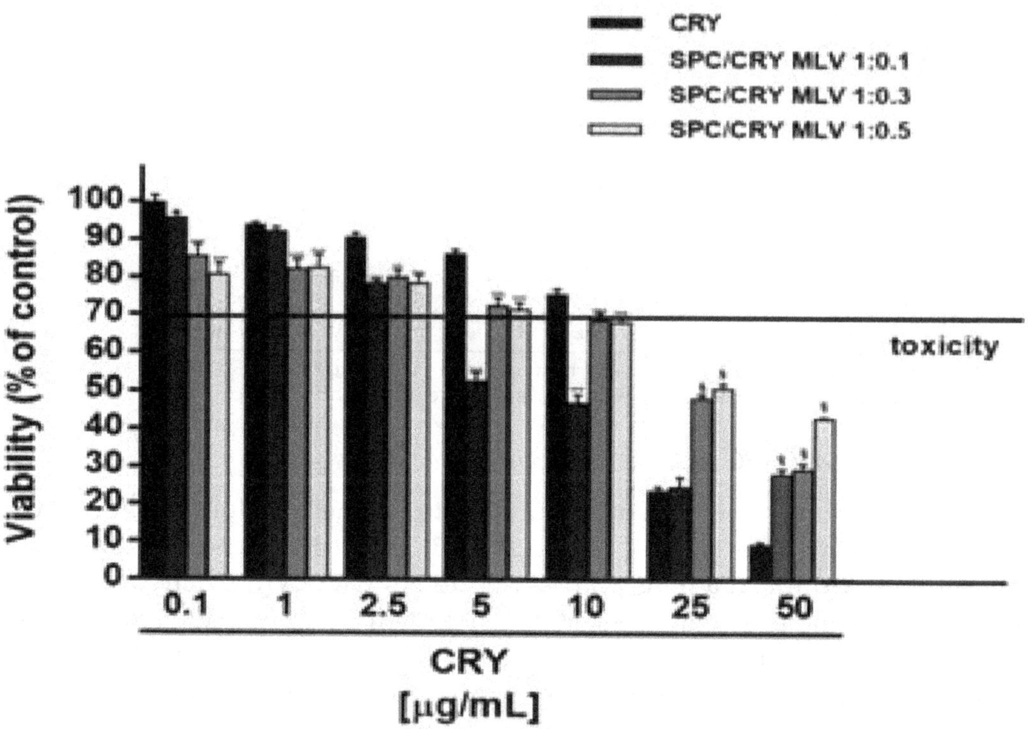

Figure 7. Cytotoxicity of SPC MLV differently loaded with CRY (1:0.1, 1:0.3 and 1:0.5 mol/mol) in MDA-MB-468 cells after 24 h incubation. ** $p < 0.01$ and *** $p < 0.001$ vs. CRY, denotes a statistically significant increase of cytotoxicity respect to pure CRY (ANOVA + multiple Dunnett's comparison post-test). § $p < 0.001$ vs. CRY, denotes a statistically significant reduction respect to CRY cytotoxicity (ANOVA + multiple Dunnett's comparison post-test). A cell viability lower than 70% respect to control (i.e., vehicle-treated cells) was considered as cytotoxic [26].

Within the concentrations from 0.1 to 25 µg/mL, the IC_{50} value of CRY was reduced about four-fold when CRY was administered as 1:0.1 MLV, while about two-fold when CRY was administered as 1:0.3 MLV (Table 3).

Furthermore, the highest dose (75 µg/mL) of 1:0.5 SPC/CRY MLV significantly reduced the cytotoxicity of plain SPC MLV at the corresponding concentration, thus displaying a behaviour similar to that found for CRY-loaded ULV (Figure 7). Accordingly, a possible segregation of CRY into liposome due to its interaction with SPC could be expected.

3.5. Evaluation of the Potential Interaction between CRY and SPC ULV

In order to better characterize the possible interaction between CRY and SPC ULV, additional experiments in which the two separate components were co-administered to cells, at the same concentrations found in liposome formulations, were performed in HepG2 cells.

When administered in the presence of SPC ULV, CRY exhibited a lower cytotoxic behaviour with respect to the pure compound. Despite a biologically relevant toxicity of the pure compound alone, the presence of SPC ULV induced a significant loss of CRY bioactivity. About a 30% reduction of its antiproliferative effect is observed (Figure 8) probably due to the high hydrophobic nature of CRY, which is therefore carried off by liposomes.

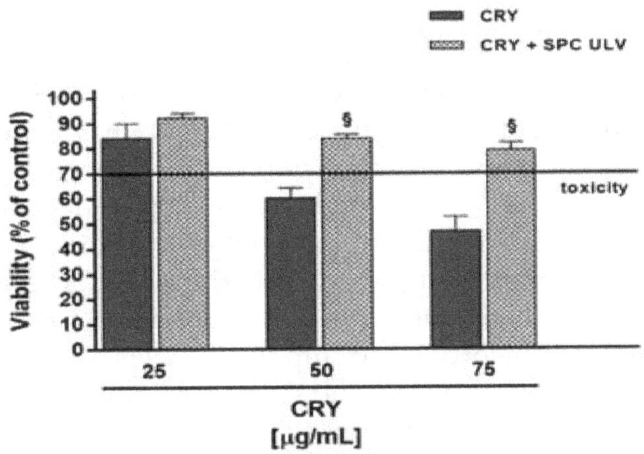

Figure 8. Cytotoxicity of CRY and the combination of SPC/CRY ULV (1:0.5 mol/mol) in HepG2 cells after 24 h incubation. § $p < 0.001$ vs. CRY, denotes a statistically significant reduction respect to CRY cytotoxicity (ANOVA + multiple Dunnett's comparison post-test). A cell viability lower than 70% respect to control (i.e., vehicle-treated cells) was considered as cytotoxic [26].

Similar results were reported by Botré et al. [27], who observed that the addition of empty liposomes to urine samples containing free steroids interfere with the recovery of the drugs, with consequent important implication on doping analysis. These results support our hypothesis that the reduced bioactivity of CRY, when administered as SPC ULV with low molar ratio or at high concentration of the drug, could be due to a close interaction of the substance with phospholipid components as a consequence of its high-grade lipophilicity.

To test this hypothesis, fluorescence anisotropy studies were carried out in order to evaluate the effect of CRY and its concentration on the fluidity of the SPC bilayer membrane of liposomes. The results obtained were compared with that produced by cholesterol (Chol) on the membrane behavior (Figure 9). Fluorescence anisotropy studies have found that lipophilic molecules, such as cholesterol and caryophyllene sesquiterpene, can affect the typical fluidity of SPC-based vesicles and reduce the mobility of the hydrocarbon chains of membrane fatty acids. In order to determine how CRY affects membrane structure, we analyze the extent to which this molecule mimics the behavior of cholesterol in L_d liposomes. Liposomes made of SPC, SPC/Chol and SPC/CRY respectively were tested.

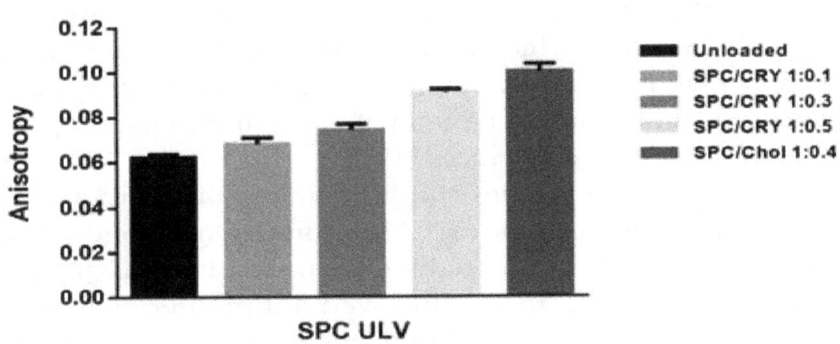

Figure 9. Anisotropy measures obtained by DPH-probe fluorescence for 1:0.1, 1:0.3 and 1:0.5 SPC/CRY ULV and 1:0.4 SPC/cholesterol (Chol) ULV.

As shown in Figure 9, conventional SPC ULV liposomes produced an average anisotropy value of 0.062. SPC bilayer was expected to be in a homogenous liquid disordered (L_d) state; the low anisotropy value obtained reflects the freedom of movement of the DPH fluorophore in the fluid disordered state of plain SPC liposome.

The thickening effect obtained as a result of cholesterol addition to a fluid bilayer is well documented [27] and the results reported in Figure 9 are in good agreement with previous published data. When cholesterol 40% mol/mol was incorporated in L_d SPC/Chol bilayer, in fact, the DPH fluorescence anisotropy increases, thus indicating that at this cholesterol amount, a greater order level exists for the phospholipid acyl chain packing. According to Marsh [28], cholesterol in the liposomal fluid bilayer promotes the formation of a phase that coexists with the L_d phase. In SPC/Chol liposomes the close contact between the sterol and adjacent phospholipids results in the formation of the so called liquid-ordered (L_o) phase. This new intermediate fluid phase exhibits translational degrees of freedom of the lipid molecules that are similar to those in a conventional fluid bilayer state, while the conformational degrees of freedom of the lipid hydrocarbon chains resemble those of the gel state. In contrast, a progressive increase of the anisotropy value appeared for CRY-loaded liposomes that is proportional to the amount of drug incorporated into the vesicles bilayer.

Increasing the mixing ratios between SPC and CRY, the fluorescence anisotropies of DPH were increased almost linearly, suggesting that rotational motion of DPH in SPC liposomes was restricted by CRY entrapment. Comparing the behaviour of SPC/CRY ULV with a 1:0.5 molar ratio and that of SPC/Chol ULV, very similar anisotropy values were found (Figure 9).

In line with these results, our hypothesis is that liposome formulations with a higher than 1:0.1 molar ratio between SPC and CRY can modify the phospholipid bilayer organization, thus hindering drug release.

4. Discussion

Low solubility of the natural sesquiterpene β-caryophyllene (CRY) in aqueous fluids and the subsequent poor bioavailability represent key aspects limiting its use in therapy. CRY also exhibited sensitivity to light, oxygen, humidity, and high temperatures [29]: these conditions decrease its stability and limit its biological effectiveness. A possible strategy to overcome these problems is the use of drug delivery systems, which may provide much higher bioavailability of this compound and ensure obtaining desired biological effects. Previous studies proposed cyclodextrin complexation to improve the bioavailability of CRY [30–32]. Recently, oil/water microemulsions have been also reported to possess suitable properties for effective topical delivery of β-caryophyllene [33].

Many synthetic and herbal drugs possess the problem of poor oral bioavailability, due to their very low water solubility or poor permeation through the biological membranes, thus leading to a limited dissolution profile in biological fluids and inefficacy in therapy. Increased reports highlighted the promising role of phospholipid-based formulations as effective drug delivery systems for natural bioactive constituents [34]. Being the main components of cellular membrane, phospholipids are characterized by an excellent biocompatibility; also, they possess amphiphilic structures and surface-active wetting characteristics, which allow enhancing the hydrophilicity of hydrophobic compounds. In water, phospholipids self-assemble into supramolecular aggregates, among which liposomes displayed high cell affinity and tissue compatibility, improving drug stability and ability to deliver both hydrophilic and lipophilic substances [34].

In line with this evidence, in the present study the internalization of CRY into the cells was increased using soybean phosphatidylcholine (SPC) liposomes Our hypothesis was that CRY, when administered as liposomal formulations, rationally designed in term of drug to lipid ratio, can be easily uptaken from cells, thus leading to an improved antiproliferative activity. SPC has been used as phospholipid molecule forming the lipid bilayer not only for its structural similarity with cell biomembrane constituents, but also for its ability to affect the cholesterol-induced stiffening of cancer cell biomembrane, which has been found responsible for reduced drug permeability and chemoresistance development in cancer cells [21].

In our cancer cell models, high concentrations of SPC exhibited early cytotoxicity signs, likely due to its ability to increase the permeability of cancer cell biomembrane, through the interference with cholesterol accumulation. In line with this evidence and considering that previous studies highlighted the ability of phosphatidylcholine to induce cholesterol depletion and to be inversely related to cholesterol amount [35,36], we hypothesize that the cytotoxicity found at higher concentrations of plain SPC liposomes can be, at least in part, due to a cholesterol transfer between liposomes and cells. Liposomes could reduce the cholesterol/phospholipid ratio and increase lipid disorder in cell membrane. Depletion of cholesterol in cell thus, could make cell more vulnerable, also to physical stress [37]; similarly, methyl-beta-cyclodextrin has been used for cholesterol removal, although the effect was incomplete [38].

Under our experimental conditions, the encapsulation of CRY within SPC liposomes highlighted that the cellular uptake of CRY can be improved or reduced as a function of the molar ratio between SPC and CRY.

Characterizing the optimal concentration of CRY in liposomal formulations represents a key point for the increase of its antiproliferative effectiveness. Both ULV and MLV liposomes loaded with the highest molar ratio between SPC and CRY (i.e., 1:0.5) induced a progressive loss of the antiproliferative potential of the sesquiterpene. The results obtained highlighted that, despite a possible improvement of low-dose CRY cytotoxicity, increased molar ratio between SPC and CRY markedly interfere with the biological activity of pure compound. This phenomenon suggests that the substance can be greatly retained and become stuck into liposomes, likely due to a stable interaction between CRY and phosphatidylcholine and a stiffening of the membrane structure, which hinders the sesquiterpene release by vesicles and its uptake into cells. Accordingly, Sarpietro et al. [39] showed that CRY possessed a great capacity to interact with membrane phospholipids and to spread through the lipophilic matrix, determining an alteration of the cooperativity. This hypothesis is also in agreement with the more accepted ordering effect induced by cholesterol in biomembrane bilayer and SPC ULV [28]. Therefore, we hypothesize that incorporating high concentrations of CRY in the ULV bilayer can alter membrane packing of SPC liposomes by inducing conformational phospholipid ordering, thus leading to a decreased fluidity and permeability of the bilayer of the phospholipid carrier.

The enhanced rigidity of the membrane, that could be generated by the inclusion of hydrophobic CRY, might seal the system and reduce the drug release. Moreover, the release of high CRY concentrations embedded within the lipid bilayers could be compromised due to strong hydrophobic interactions that might develop between the drug and the phospholipid acyl chains.

The trend displayed by SPC multilamellar vesicles support the hypothesis of the reduced bioactivity of CRY due to a condensing effect of this molecule on the bilayer. In fact, the results observed with the MLV system were partly similar to SPC ULV only at the highest CRY concentrations. We reasonable speculate that CRY reduces the fluidity of the SPC MLV bilayer to a lesser extent with respect to SPC ULV. In fact, for a fixed SPC/CRY ratio, the number of CRY molecules included in each of the lamella of the multilamellar carrier was smaller with respect to ULV, thus leading to a reduced extent of the stiffness effect.

5. Conclusions

In the present study, SPC liposomes have been developed as potential effective delivery systems to increase the in vitro bioavailability and stability of the natural sesquiterpene CRY. According to widely accepted evidence that release is governed by molecule lipophilicity and liposome features, our results allow us to hypothesize that CRY release by SPC liposomes is strictly dependent on lamellarity and drug-to-lipid ratio. Lipid-to-drug ratio is a critical parameter as it may influence the therapeutic efficacy of the drug, in particular with lipophilic drugs. The increase of drug encapsulation could be not a valid strategy in liposomal formulation, as the drug release properties of the liposomal product could be negatively affected by the molar concentration of drug in liposomes. In fact, as SPC liposome loading increases, a condensing effect of the loaded molecule on the fluid bilayer occurs. As a consequence, the substance can be greatly retained, and its release restrained. In the case of CRY, this feature can negatively affect and hinder its anticancer effectiveness. Therefore, the SPC to CRY ratio seems to represent a key tool for the development of optimized liposomal formulation to control membrane fluidity and permeability of SPC liposomes, and thus predict the release abilities. In fact, low-loaded MLV appears to induce the maximum increase of CRY antiproliferative activity in both HepG2 and

MDA-MB-468 cells, thus suggesting the ability of these formulations to better carry the lipophilic cargo inside cells. However, further in vitro studies are necessary to measure the CRY release by SPC vesicles and the achieved intracellular levels effectively.

In conclusion, our results highlight the importance of rationally designing formulations to develop the optimal liposomal composition, taking into account not only the chemical nature of the payload but also that the high drug loading in liposomes could be critical for the maximum usefulness of its therapeutic potential.

Author Contributions: Conceptualization, A.D.S., P.P. and S.P.; Formal analysis, A.D.S., P.P. and M.N.; Funding acquisition, A.D.S.; Investigation, A.D.S., P.P., M.N., L.A., S.G., S.D.G. and S.P.; Methodology, A.D.S., P.P., S.D.G., M.A.C. and S.P.; Project administration, A.D.S., P.P. and S.P.; Supervision, G.M. and M.A.C.; Visualization, A.D.S. and M.N.; Writing–original draft, A.D.S., P.P., G.M., M.A.C. and S.P.

References

1. Di Sotto, A.; Evandri, M.G.; Mazzanti, G. Antimutagenic and mutagenic activities of some terpenes in the bacterial reverse mutation assay. *Mutat. Res.* **2008**, *653*, 130–133. [CrossRef]
2. Fidyt, K.; Fiedorowicz, A.; Strządała, L.; Szumny, A. β-caryophyllene and β-caryophyllene oxide-natural compounds of anticancer and analgesic properties. *Cancer Med.* **2016**, *5*, 3007–3017. [CrossRef] [PubMed]
3. Gertsch, J. Antiinflammatory cannabinoids in diet—Towards a better understanding of CB2 receptor action? *Commun. Integr. Biol.* **2008**, *1*, 26–28. [CrossRef] [PubMed]
4. Bento, A.F.; Marcon, R.; Dutra, R.C.; Claudino, R.F.; Cola, M.; Leite, D.F.; Calixto, J.B. β-Caryophyllene inhibits dextran sulfate sodium-induced colitis in mice through CB2 receptor activation and PPARγ pathway. *Am. J. Pathol.* **2011**, *178*, 1153–1166. [CrossRef] [PubMed]
5. Chang, H.J.; Kim, J.M.; Lee, J.C.; Kim, W.K.; Chun, H.S. Protective effect of betacaryophyllene; a natural bicyclic sesquiterpene; against cerebral ischemic injury. *J. Med. Food* **2013**, *16*, 471–480. [CrossRef] [PubMed]
6. Liu, H.; Song, Z.; Liao, D.; Zhang, T.; Liu, F.; Zhuang, K.; Luo, K.; Yang, L. Neuroprotective effects of trans-caryophyllene against kainic acid induced seizure activity and oxidative stress in mice. *Neurochem. Res.* **2015**, *40*, 118–123. [CrossRef]
7. Viveros-Paredes, J.M.; González-Castañeda, R.E.; Gertsch, J.; Chaparro-Huerta, V.; López-Roa, R.I.; Vázquez-Valls, E.; Beas-Zarate, C.; Camins-Espuny, A.; Flores-Soto, M.E. Neuroprotective Effects of β-Caryophyllene against Dopaminergic Neuron Injury in a Murine Model of Parkinson's Disease Induced by MPTP. *Pharmaceuticals* **2017**, *10*, 60. [CrossRef]
8. Di Sotto, A.; Mazzanti, G.; Carbone, F.; Hrelia, P.; Maffei, F.; Mazzanti, G. Inhibition by beta-caryophyllene of ethyl methanesulfonate-induced clastogenicity in cultured human lymphocytes. *Mutat. Res.* **2010**, *699*, 23–28. [CrossRef]
9. Di Giacomo, S.; Mazzanti, G.; Di Sotto, A. Mutagenicity of cigarette butt waste in the bacterial reverse mutation assay: The protective effects of β-caryophyllene and β-caryophyllene oxide. *Environ. Toxicol.* **2016**, *31*, 1319–1328. [CrossRef]
10. Di Giacomo, S.; Abete, L.; Cocchiola, R.; Mazzanti, G.; Eufemi, M.; Di Sotto, A. Caryophyllane sesquiterpenes inhibit DNA-damage by tobacco smoke in bacterial and mammalian cells. *Food Chem. Toxicol.* **2018**, *111*, 393–404. [CrossRef]
11. Hanušová, V.; Caltová, K.; Svobodová, H.; Ambrož, M.; Skarka, A.; Murínová, N.; Králová, V.; Tomšík, P.; Skálová, L. The effects of β-caryophyllene oxide and trans-nerolidol on the efficacy of doxorubicin in breast cancer cells and breast tumor-bearing mice. *Biomed. Pharmacother.* **2017**, *95*, 828–836. [CrossRef]
12. Di Giacomo, S.; Di Sotto, A.; El-Readi, M.Z.; Mazzanti, G.; Wink, M. Chemosensitizing Properties of β-Caryophyllene and β-Caryophyllene Oxide in Combination with Doxorubicin in Human Cancer Cells. *Anticancer Res.* **2017**, *37*, 1191–1196. [PubMed]

13. Fontes, L.B.A.; Dias, D.D.S.; Aarestrup, B.J.V.; Aarestrup, F.M.; Da Silva Filho, A.A.; Corrêa, J.O.D.A. β-Caryophyllene ameliorates the development of experimental autoimmune encephalomyelitis in C57BL/6 mice. *Biomed. Pharmacother.* **2017**, *91*, 257–264. [CrossRef] [PubMed]
14. Zhou, L.; Zhan, M.L.; Tang, Y.; Xiao, M.; Li, M.; Li, Q.S.; Yang, L.; Li, X.; Chen, W.W.; Wang, Y.L. Effects of β-caryophyllene on arginine ADP-ribosyltransferase 1-mediated regulation of glycolysis in colorectal cancer under high-glucose conditions. *Int. J. Oncol.* **2018**, *53*, 1613–1624. [CrossRef]
15. Kawabata, Y.; Wada, K.; Nakatani, M.; Yamada, S.; Onoue, S. Formulation design for poorly water-soluble drugs based on biopharmaceutics classification system: Basic approaches and practical applications. *Int. J. Pharm.* **2011**, *420*, 1–10. [CrossRef] [PubMed]
16. Sarfraz, M.; Afzal, A.; Raza, S.M.; Bashir, S.; Madni, A.; Khan, M.W.; Ma, X.; Xiang, G. Liposomal co-delivered oleanolic acid attenuates doxorubicin-induced multi-organ toxicity in hepatocellular carcinoma. *Oncotarget* **2017**, *8*, 47136–47153. [CrossRef]
17. Yang, G.; Yang, T.; Zhang, W.; Lu, M.; Ma, X.; Xiang, G. In vitro and in vivo antitumor effects of folatetargeted ursolic acid stealth liposome. *J. Agric. Food Chem.* **2014**, *62*, 2207–2215. [CrossRef]
18. Coimbra, M.; Isacchi, B.; van Bloois, L.; Torano, J.S.; Ket, A.; Wu, X.; Broere, F.; Metselaar, J.M.; Rijcken, C.J.; Storm, G.; et al. Improving solubility and chemical stability of natural compounds for medicinal use by incorporation into liposomes. *Int. J. Pharm.* **2011**, *416*, 433–442. [CrossRef]
19. Rodríguez, J.; Martín, M.J.; Ruiz, M.A.; Clares, B. Current encapsulation strategies for bioactive oils: From alimentary to pharmaceuical perspectives. *Food Res. Int.* **2016**, *83*, 41–59. [CrossRef]
20. Mishra, G.P.; Bagui, M.; Tamboli, V.; Mitra, A.K. Recent applications of liposomes in ophthalmic drug delivery. *J. Drug Deliv.* **2011**, *2011*, 863734. [CrossRef] [PubMed]
21. Lladó, V.; López, D.J.; Ibarguren, M.; Alonso, M.; Soriano, J.B.; Escribá, P.V.; Busquets, X. Regulation of the cancer cell membrane lipid composition by NaCHOleate: Effects on cell signaling and therapeutical relevance in glioma. *Biochim. Biophys. Acta* **2014**, *1838*, 1619–1627. [CrossRef] [PubMed]
22. Kannan, V.; Balabathula, P.; Divi, M.K.; Thoma, L.A.; Wood, G.C. Optimization of drug loading to improve physical stability of paclitaxel-loaded long-circulating liposomes. *J. Liposome Res.* **2015**, *25*, 308–315. [CrossRef] [PubMed]
23. Bangham, A.D. Properties and uses of lipid vesicles: An overview. *Ann. N. Y. Acad. Sci.* **1978**, *308*, 2–7. [CrossRef] [PubMed]
24. Yoshida, Y.; Furuya, E.; Tagawa, K. A direct colorimetric method for the determination of phospholipids with dithiocyanatoiron reagent. *J. Biochem.* **1980**, *88*, 463–468. [CrossRef] [PubMed]
25. Di Sotto, A.; Mazzanti, G.; Savickiene, N.; Staršelskyte, R.; Baksenskaite, V.; Di Giacomo, S.; Vitalone, A. Antimutagenic and antioxidant activity of a protein fraction from aerial parts of Urtica dioica. *Pharm. Biol.* **2014**, *53*, 935–938. [CrossRef] [PubMed]
26. International Organization for Standardization. *Biological Evaluation of Medical Devices—Part 5: Tests for In Vitro Cytotoxicity (ISO 10993-5)*; International Organization for Standardization: Geneva, Switzerland, 2009.
27. Botrè, F.; Esposito, S.; de la Torre, X. How we risk: Liposomes and steroids. In *Recent Advances in Doping Analysis*; Schanzer, W., Geyer, H., Gotzmann, A., Mareck, U., Eds.; Sport und Buch Strauß: Koln, Germany, 2011; Volume 19, pp. 24–33.
28. Marsh, D. Liquid-ordered phases induced by cholesterol: A compendium of binary phase diagrams. *Biochim. Biophys. Acta* **2010**, *1798*, 688–699. [CrossRef] [PubMed]
29. Sköld, M.; Karlberg, A.T.; Matura, M.; Börje, A. The fragrance chemical β-caryophyllene-air oxidation and skin sensitization. *Food Chem. Toxicol.* **2006**, *44*, 538–545. [CrossRef] [PubMed]
30. Liu, H.; Yang, G.; Tang, Y.; Cao, D.; Qi, T.; Qi, Y.; Fan, G. Physicochemical characterization and pharmacokinetics evaluation of β-caryophyllene/β-cyclodextrin inclusion complex. *Int. J. Pharm.* **2013**, *450*, 304–310. [CrossRef]
31. Lou, J.; Teng, Z.; Zhang, L.; Yang, J.; Ma, L.; Wang, F.; Tian, X.; An, R.; Yang, M.; Zhang, Q.; et al. β-Caryophyllene/Hydroxypropyl-β-Cyclodextrin Inclusion Complex Improves Cognitive Deficits in Rats with Vascular Dementia through the Cannabinoid Receptor Type 2—Mediated Pathway. *Front. Pharmacol.* **2017**, *8*, 2. [CrossRef]

32. Quintans-Júnior, L.J.; Araújo, A.A.; Brito, R.G.; Santos, P.L.; Quintans, J.S.; Menezes, P.P.; Serafini, M.R.; Silva, G.F.; Carvalho, F.M.; Brogden, N.K.; et al. β-caryophyllene; a dietary cannabinoid; complexed with β-cyclodextrin produced anti-hyperalgesic effect involving the inhibition of Fos expression in superficial dorsal horn. *Life Sci.* **2016**, *149*, 34–41. [CrossRef]
33. De Oliveira Neves, J.K.; Apolinário, A.C.; Alcantara Saraiva, K.L.; da Silva, D.T.C.; de Freitas Araújo Reis, M.Y.; de Lima Damasceno, B.P.G.; Pessoa, A.; Moraes Galvão, M.A.; Soares, L.A.L.; Veiga Júnior, V.F.; et al. Microemulsions containing Copaifera multijuga Hayne oil-resin: Challenges to achieve an efficient system for β-caryophyllene delivery. *Ind. Crops Prod.* **2018**, *111*, 185–192. [CrossRef]
34. Li, C.; Zhang, J.; Zu, Y.J.; Nie, S.F.; Cao, J.; Wang, Q.; Nie, S.P.; Deng, Z.Y.; Xie, M.Y.; Wang, S. Biocompatible and biodegradable nanoparticles for enhancement of anti-cancer activities of phytochemicals. *Chin. J. Nat. Med.* **2015**, *13*, 641–652. [CrossRef]
35. Akopian, D.; Kawashima, R.L.; Medh, J.D. Phosphatidylcholine-Mediated Aqueous Diffusion of Cellular Cholesterol Down-Regulatesthe ABCA1 Transporter in Human Skin Fibroblasts. *Int. J. Biochem. Res. Rev.* **2015**, *5*, 214–224. [CrossRef] [PubMed]
36. Nuñez-Garcia, M.; Gomez-Santos, B.; Buqué, X.; García-Rodriguez, J.L.; Romero, M.R.; Marin, J.J.G.; Arteta, B.; García-Monzón, C.; Castaño, L.; Syn, W.K.; et al. Osteopontin regulates the cross-talk between phosphatidylcholine and cholesterol metabolism in mouse liver. *J. Lipid Res.* **2017**, *58*, 1903–1915. [CrossRef]
37. Simons, K.; Ehehalt, R. Cholesterol lipid rafts and disease. *J. Clin. Investig.* **2002**, *110*, 597–603. [CrossRef]
38. Litz, J.P.; Thakkar, N.; Portet, T.; Keller, S.L. Depletion with Cyclodextrin Reveals Two Populations of Cholesterol in Model Lipid Membranes. *Biophys. J.* **2016**, *110*, 635–645. [CrossRef]
39. Sarpietro, M.G.; Di Sotto, A.; Accolla, M.L.; Castelli, F. Differential Scanning Calorimetry Study on the Interaction of β-Caryophyllene and β-Caryophyllene Oxide with Phospholipid Bilayers. *Thermochim. Acta* **2015**, *600*, 28–34. [CrossRef]

9

Preparation, Characterization and Preliminary In Vitro Testing of Nanoceria-Loaded Liposomes

Agostina Grillone [1,*], Tianshu Li [2], Matteo Battaglini [1,3], Alice Scarpellini [4], Mirko Prato [5], Shinji Takeoka [6] and Gianni Ciofani [1,7,*]

1. Smart Bio-Interfaces, Istituto Italiano di Tecnologia, Viale Rinaldo Piaggio 34, 56025 Pontedera, Italy; matteo.battaglini@iit.it
2. Research Organization for Nano & Life innovation, Waseda University, 2-2 Wakamatsu-cho, Shinjuku-ku, Tokyo 162-8480, Japan; tianshuli@aoni.waseda.jp
3. The Biorobotics Institute, Scuola Superiore Sant'Anna, Viale Rinaldo Piaggio 34, 56025 Pontedera, Italy
4. Electron Microscopy Facility, Istituto Italiano di Tecnologia, Via Morego 30, 16163 Genova, Italy; alice.scarpellini@iit.it
5. Materials Characterization Facility, Istituto Italiano di Tecnologia, Via Morego 30, 16163 Genova, Italy; mirko.prato@iit.it
6. Department of Life Science and Medical Bioscience, Graduate School of Advanced Science and Engineering (TWIns), Waseda University, 2-2 Wakamatsu-cho, Shinjuku-ku, Tokyo 162-8480, Japan; takeoka@waseda.jp
7. Department of Mechanical and Aerospace Engineering, Politecnico di Torino, Corso Duca degli Abruzzi 24, 10129 Torino, Italy

* Correspondence: agostina.grillone@iit.it (A.G.); gianni.ciofani@iit.it (G.C.);

Abstract: Cerium oxide nanoparticles (nanoceria), well known for their pro- and antioxidant features, have been recently proposed for the treatment of several pathologies, including cancer and neurodegenerative diseases. However, interaction between nanoceria and biological molecules such as proteins and lipids, short blood circulation time, and the need of a targeted delivery to desired sites are some aspects that require strong attention for further progresses in the clinical application of these nanoparticles. The aim of this work is the encapsulation of nanoceria into a liposomal formulation in order to improve their therapeutic potentialities. After the preparation through a reverse-phase evaporation method, size, Z-potential, morphology, and loading efficiency of nanoceria-loaded liposomes were investigated. Finally, preliminary in vitro studies were performed to test cell uptake efficiency and preserved antioxidant activity. Nanoceria-loaded liposomes showed a good colloidal stability, an excellent biocompatibility, and strong antioxidant properties due to the unaltered activity of the entrapped nanoceria. With these results, the possibility of exploiting liposomes as carriers for cerium oxide nanoparticles is demonstrated here for the first time, thus opening exciting new opportunities for in vivo applications.

Keywords: cerium oxide nanoparticles; liposomes; drug delivery

---

1. Introduction

In cerium oxide, Ce owns the peculiar ability to easily switch between two oxidation states, Ce^{3+} and Ce^{4+}, through the loss of electrons and/or oxygen, thus giving origin to crystalline defects or vacancies on the surface of the material [1]. At a nanoscale level, due to the higher surface/volume ratio, this phenomenon is more evident, thus making cerium oxide nanoparticles (nanoceria) more reactive with respect to the bulk material. The discovery of the excellent catalytic activities of nanoceria and their ability to act as free radicals scavengers have opened new perspectives in the biomedical fields and, more specifically, in all those scenarios where oxidative stress plays a crucial role in the pathogenesis of diseases [2]. Previous studies have shown that nanoceria are able to neutralize reactive oxygen species (ROS), including superoxide anions, peroxide radicals, and hydroxyl radicals, by mimicking the activity of enzymes involved in antioxidant defenses such as superoxide dismutase and catalase [3]. The biological activities of cerium oxide nanoparticles were assessed in vitro on several cell culture models such as cardiac [4], neuronal [5], and stem cells [6]; in vivo, nanoceria showed strong antioxidant properties by decreasing both nitric oxide and peroxynitrite formation in a murine model of ischemic cardiomyopathy [7], and they slowed down the progression of retinal degeneration in mouse and rat models [8,9], promoted the regression of retinal vascular lesions in mice [10], and inhibited weight gain in rats [11].

Another peculiar feature of cerium oxide nanoparticles is their ability to act as a pro-oxidant agent at acidic pH values [12]. Several research groups reported that, where tumor microenvironment is acidic, nanoceria triggers ROS accumulation [12], possess cytotoxic and anti-invasive properties [13,14], and sensitize cells to radiotherapy [15]. Anticancer activity of nanoceria was studied in vitro for the treatment of breast, pancreas, ovarian, lung, and colon cancer cells [15–17].

Despite the significant promises of nanoceria, several challenges still need to be addressed before a translational exploitation into clinical practice. First of all, nanoceria dispersions are often unstable in aqueous solutions and in high ionic media, quickly precipitating and forming aggregates that hinder their in vivo administration [18] or at least that heavily affect their transport and biodistribution [19]. The interaction of nanoparticles with proteins moreover triggers recognition by phagocytic cells, thus inducing retention in the reticuloendothelial system (mainly in the spleen and in the liver), with a consequent reduction of blood circulation half-life [20]. Additionally, proteins adsorbed on the surface of nanoceria may also modify their surface chemistry and thus their physicochemical properties, in addition to the hydrodynamic size and the surface charge that determine cellular uptake and subcellular localization [21–23].

The goal of this study is the investigation of the possibility of exploiting the advantages of a liposomal drug delivery system in order to increase the therapeutic index of nanoceria. Liposomes are promising vectors that allow for the incorporation of hydrophilic and hydrophobic drugs due to their amphiphilic nature and vescicular structure [24]. Liposomes composed of phospholipids are biocompatible and biodegradable, with a diameter in the range of 50–200 nm, and they generally do not undergo a rapid systemic clearance [24]. Surface modifications by means of polymeric chains as polyethylene glycol (PEG), in fact, provide a stealth layer that reduces their uptake by the immune system, thus prolonging the persistence of the liposomes in the blood circulation [24]. In addition, the use of liposomes can promote a selective delivery of the payload into targeted cells/tissues upon the functionalization of their surface with antibodies, antigens, or small molecules capable of binding specific receptors on the cell membrane [25,26]. Furthermore, such a targeting strategy can be also exploited for the crossing of biological barriers, thus allowing compartments otherwise inaccessible, such as the central nervous system, to be reached [27].

In this work, nanoceria-loaded liposomes were prepared through a reverse-phase evaporation method, extruded with membrane filters, and finally purified with gel permeation chromatography. Obtained hybrid nanovectors were extensively investigated in terms of lipid concentration, size distribution, Z-potential, morphology, and loading efficiency. Finally, preliminary in vitro studies have been carried out on normal human dermal fibroblasts to investigate biocompatibility and unaltered antioxidant activity of the entrapped nanoceria.

2. Results

2.1. Characterization of Liposomes

Empty liposomes and nanoceria-loaded liposomes were prepared by a reverse-phase evaporation method in order to obtain a high loading amount of nanoceria. Size and Z-potential were assessed before biological testing, and obtained results are summarized in Table 1. Free nanoceria present an average diameter of 12 ± 1 nm and a *Z*-potential of 32.0 ± 3.8 mV. Empty liposomes and nanoceria-loaded liposomes have a hydrodynamic size of about 165 ± 42 nm and 230 ± 10 nm, respectively. As expected, analyses revealed a negative *Z*-potential of −41.0 ± 11.2 mV for empty liposomes because of the presence of the anionic lipid (1,5-dihexadecyl-*N*-succinyl-L-glutamate, DHSG), while nanoceria-loaded liposomes present a positive surface charge of 30.8 ± 0.4 mV deriving from the adsorption of cerium oxide nanoparticles on the surface of negatively charged liposomes. Values obtained from inductively coupled plasma mass spectroscopy (ICP-MS) revealed 6 mg/mL of complexed nanoceria for a dispersion of 9 mg/mL of nanoceria-loaded liposomes, highlighting a loading efficiency of 12%. The samples were found stable for many weeks since the preparation, resulting into a variation of the hydrodynamic size <15% after one month of storage.

Morphology of the samples was confirmed by transmission electron microscopy (TEM) images. Figure 1a shows the monodispersed cerium oxide nanoparticles used in this work, while Figure 1b highlights the formation of well-defined spherical liposomes, and suggests the presence of cerium oxide nanoparticles complexed to the liposomes, both inside the lipid vesicles and on their surface, as also confirmed by the increment of the *Z*-potential.

The analysis of the total antioxidant capacity (TAC) of nanoceria-loaded liposomes and empty liposomes was assessed and expressed in terms of Trolox equivalents, a water-soluble vitamin E analog that serves as an antioxidant standard [28]. The TAC of 7 µg of nanoceria-loaded liposomes was found significantly higher (6.14 ± 0.34 nmol; * $p < 0.05$) with respect to the negligible effect of the same quantity of empty liposomes (0.09 ± 0.03 nmol), showing strong retained efficiency of the encapsulated nanoceria.

Table 1. Characterization of nanoceria, liposomes, and nanoceria-loaded liposomes dispersions.

Sample	Size (nm)	Polydispersity Index	*Z*-Potential (mV)
Nanoceria	12 ± 1	0.156 ± 0.010	32.0 ± 3.8
Empty liposomes	165 ± 42	0.147 ± 0.006	−41.0 ± 11.2
Nanoceria-loaded liposomes	230 ± 10	0.263 ± 0.023	30.8 ± 0.4

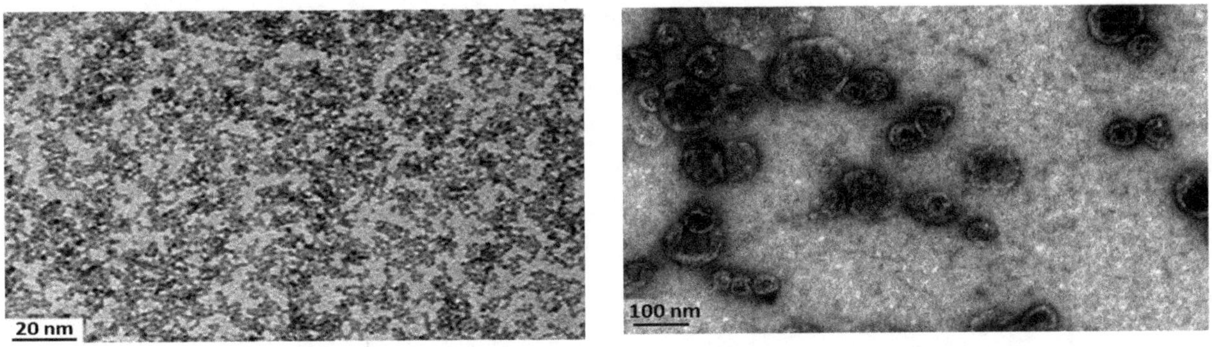

(**a**) (**b**)

Figure 1. TEM imaging of free nanoceria (**a**) and of nanoceria-loaded liposomes (**b**).

2.2. In Vitro Studies

Biocompatibility of empty liposomes and of nanoceria-loaded liposomes was investigated on normal human dermal fibroblast (NHDF) cell line by a PicoGreen assay. As shown in Figure 2a, results indicate good cytocompatibility for all the samples up to a concentration of 200 µg/mL and after 48 h of treatment. No significant variation of fluorescence intensity, and therefore of number of cells in the samples, was in fact detected in the different cultures, thus demonstrating no cytotoxic effects of all of the formulations.

Confocal microscopy was instead used to verify the cellular uptake of nanoceria-loaded liposomes, and Figure 2b clearly shows strong internalization by NHDF cells after 48 h of incubation, with a strong accumulation of nanoceria-loaded liposomes (in red) in the perinuclear area of the cells (cell membranes stained in green, nuclei in blue).

To demonstrate unaltered antioxidant activity of entrapped nanoceria, reactive oxygen species (ROS) formation was assessed. NHDF cells were stimulated with 1 mM H_2O_2 for the intracellular generation of ROS, after a pre-incubation with increasing concentrations of nanoceria-loaded liposomes and empty liposomes as a control. Figure 3 shows that the treatment for 45 min with 1 mM H_2O_2 induced an increase in the ROS production of about 56% with respect to non-treated cells, which was hindered by the pre-incubation with nanoceria-loaded liposomes in a dose-dependent manner. This demonstrates a maintained antioxidant activity of cerium oxide nanoparticles encapsulated in the liposomes.

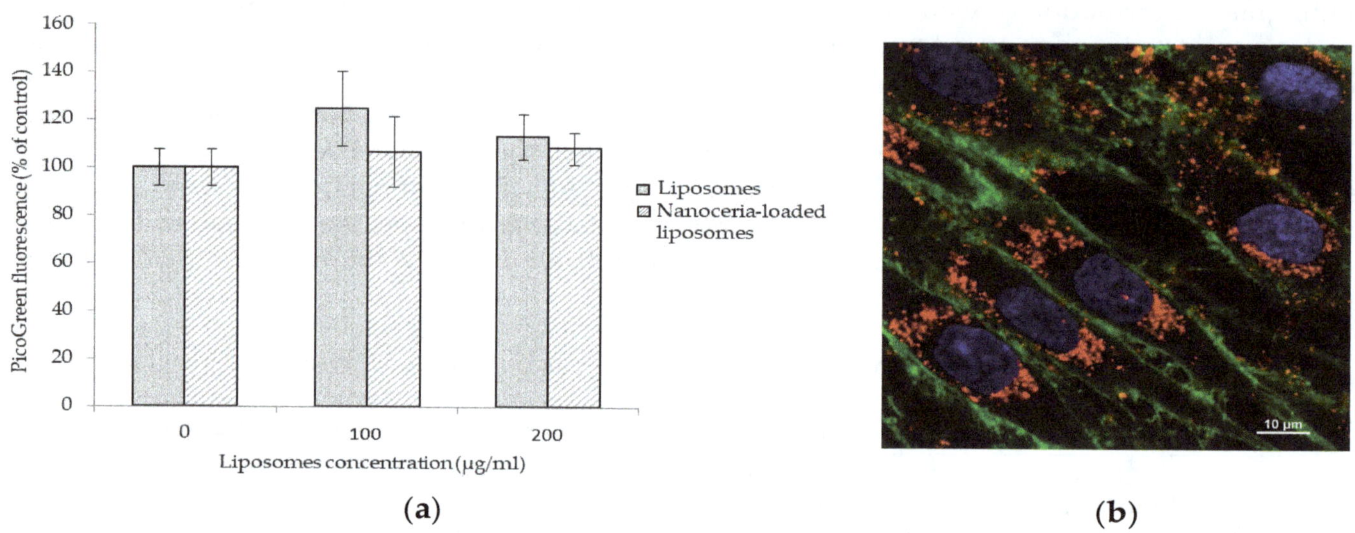

Figure 2. PicoGreen assay on NHDF cells after 48 h of incubation with increasing concentrations of empty liposomes and nanoceria-loaded liposomes (**a**); confocal image showing nanoceria-loaded liposomes (in red) up-taken by NHDF cells after 48 h of incubation; nanoceria-loaded liposomes are stained in red, cell membranes in green, and nuclei in blue (**b**).

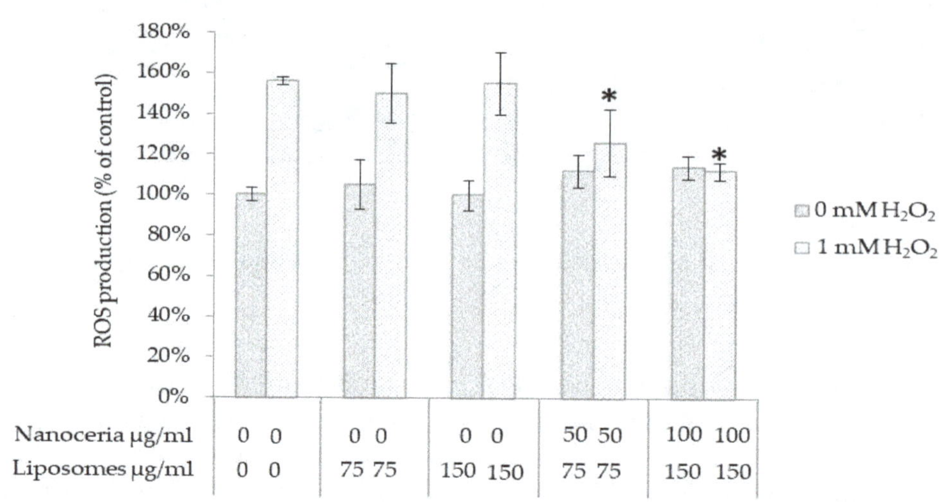

Figure 3. Quantitative evaluation of reactive oxygen species levels in NHDF cells treated with empty liposomes and nanoceria-loaded liposomes, with and without H_2O_2 pro-oxidant insult; * $p < 0.05$.

3. Discussion

The excessive and non-balanced production of free radicals, a process known as oxidative stress, can damage various cell components such as proteins, lipids, and DNA, causing many different diseases [29]. Neurodegenerative disorders, cancer, atherosclerosis, hypertensions, autoimmune diseases, diabetes, and obesity are just some of the pathological conditions associated with oxidative stress [30].

A way to restore the cell redox status could be the use of cerium oxide nanoparticles, the ability of which, as ROS scavengers, has been demonstrated by countless studies in the literature [31,32]. However, though efforts have been made to improve the stability and the biodistribution of nanoceria in vivo through polymeric coatings or surface modifications with ligand moieties, to date only one work reports the use of drug delivery systems as a multi-stage strategy for increasing the therapeutic potential of nanoceria [33]. In this research, the authors obtained cerium oxide nanoparticles encapsulation in poly(lactide-*co*-glycolide) microspheres, without however confirming the ROS scavenging activity of entrapped nanoceria in vitro [33].

As a similar approach, our objective was focused on the investigation of a strategy to load nanoceria into a drug delivery platform, namely, liposomes, that traditionally gained considerable interest in nanomedicine because of many advantageous features. Their high biocompatibility, the possibility of controlling their physicochemical properties, their ability to entrap molecules in both an aqueous core and a lipid bilayer, and, most importantly, the specific targeting to a desired site through an appropriate surface functionalization are only some of the properties that make liposomes an efficient drug carrier [34].

Most of the studies about the encapsulation of small inorganic nanoparticles in liposomes concern quantum dots [35], silica nanoparticles [35], and magnetic nanoparticles [36]. Extensively studied, megnetoliposomes are an interesting example of a multifunctional liposomes/nanoparticles hybrid platform, and they can be exploited as contrast agents in magnetic resonance imaging, for magnetically guided targeting delivery, or for generating heat when exposed to an alternating magnetic field [37].

A study of interaction between liposomes and nanoceria has been approached by Liu et al., who exploited phosphocoline-based liposomes as a model of the cell membrane, but focusing their investigations only on the interaction between nanoceria and biological membranes [38].

In the present work, we demonstrate for the first time that nanoceria can be encapsulated inside liposomes preserving their antioxidant activities. The final lipid composition has been the result of an extensive procedure of optimization, which took into account the stability of the preparation, the encapsulation yield, and the biocompatibility of the nanovectors. Particular attention has also been dedicated to the ease of purification of the final products. The presented formulation was an optimal compromise among all these considered factors.

Thus, nanoceria-loaded liposomes, well-tolerated by fibroblasts, can be extensively internalized by the cells and preserved strong antioxidant activities. The proposed strategy is therefore extremely promising for improving the biodistribution and the in vivo targeting: the encapsulation into liposomes could in fact protect nanoceria by the surface absorption of blood proteins that can affect the interaction with cells, while at the same time protecting the surface chemistry of the nanoparticles and therefore their catalytic activities. Moreover, the PEGylation of the liposome surface and their stability deriving from favorable electrostatic interactions could represent an advantage in overcoming the fast clearance from the blood circulation, by shielding liposomes from immunoglobulins and proteins of the complement system, which act as signals for recognition by the mononuclear phagocytic system. Liposomal lipids could also be used for several strategies of functionalization with targeting moieties, thus avoiding a direct link of ligands on the nanoparticle surface that could hinder their catalytic activities while, at the same time, enabling the targeting and crossing of biological barriers, such as the blood–brain barrier, which represents the major obstacle of nanoceria delivery to the central nervous system. Finally, the capacity of nanocarriers such as liposomes to act as multi-functional vectors for the delivery of multiple cargos offers an interesting stimulus for alternative therapeutic strategies. As an example, co-encapsulation of nanoceria and imaging contrast enhancers such as magnetic nanoparticles could make the liposomes an actual theranostic nanoplatform suitable in all those scenarios where nanoceria can play an important medical action.

4. Materials and Methods

4.1. Preparation of Lipid Mixture and Liposomes

For the liposome preparation, a lipid anionic mixture of 1,2-dipalmitoyl-sn-glycero-3-phosphocholine (DPPC), cholesterol, 1,5-dihexadecyl-*N*-succinyl-L-glutamate (DHSG), and 1,2-distearoylsn-glycero-3-phosphoethanolamine-*N*-[monomethoxy poly(ethylene glycol) (5000)] (PEG-DSPE) at a molar ratio of 5:5:1:0.03 was used. DPPC and cholesterol were purchased from Nippon Fine Chemicals (Osaka, Japan), PEG-DSPE from NOF Corporation (Tokyo, Japan), and DHSG was in-house synthesized in laboratory [39,40].

A mixture was prepared by dissolving those lipid components (total 100 mg) in *t*-butylalcohol (20 mL); the mixed solution was then freeze-dried overnight, and powder was then used for liposome preparation.

Nanoceria-loaded liposomes were prepared by a reverse-phase evaporation method. More specifically, 10 mg of mixed lipid powder was dissolved in ethanol, and 50 mg of nanoceria was then added (47,232 from Alfa Aesar, Ward Hill, MA, USA), presenting a Ce^{3+}/Ce^{4+} ratio of ~1.6, please see characterization reported in Figure S1, Supplementary Materials). After the solvent at 40 °C was removed by rotary evaporation under reduced pressure, the obtained dried lipid-nanoceria mixed film was hydrated and dispersed in 1 mL of water at room temperature for 3 h through stirring.

The liposome dispersion thereafter underwent two extrusion cycles through polycarbonate filters of a 200 nm pore size (Whatman® Nuclepore™ Track-Etched Membranes, Maidstone, UK). In order to separate un-loaded nanoceria from the liposome dispersion, suspension was purified through gel permeation chromatography using a Sephadex G-100 column and deionized water as eluent.

Each fraction containing liposomes was collected and analyzed in terms of size, *Z*-potential, nanoceria content, and lipid concentration. The same procedure was used for empty liposomes preparation, without nanoceria addition. Lipid concentration of the liposomes was calculated from the concentration of cholesterol using a cholesterol assessment kit (Abcam, Cambridge, UK) according to the manufacturer's instruction.

4.2. Liposomes Characterization

Particle size distribution and *Z*-potential of nanoceria, empty liposomes, and nanoceria-loaded liposomes were investigated with a Nano Z-Sizer (Malvern Instrument, Malvern, UK). For both analyses, each measurement was performed three times. Nanoceria content was calculated by means of elemental analysis performed through inductively coupled plasma mass spectroscopy (ICP-MS, Thermo Scientific, Waltham, MA) analysis, and the obtained value was used to determine the encapsulation efficiency through the following equation:

$$\%EE = [(\text{nanoparticles added} - \text{free nanoparticles})/\text{nanoparticles added}] \times 100, \quad (1)$$

Transmission electron microscopy (TEM) was performed in order to analyze sample morphology. For negative staining, 10 μL of the nanoceria-loaded liposomes dispersion or of free nanoceria solution was placed on carbon-coated 200 mesh copper grids for 5 min and then stained with a 1% uranyl acetate solution. Thereafter, grids were washed three times with water to remove the excess of staining and allowed to air-dry. Transmission electron microscopy of the samples was performed using a JEOL JEM-1011 microscope (JEOL Ltd., Tokyo, Japan) equipped with a tungsten thermionic gun operating at a 100 kV accelerating voltage. TEM images were acquired with a 11 Mp Orius 1000 CCD camera (Gatan, Pleasanton, CA, USA).

The antioxidant efficiency of nanoceria-loaded liposomes was evaluated through a specific assay (the Total Antioxidant Capacity Assay Kit, Sigma, Saint Louise, MO, USA) that allows for the determination of the antioxidant capacity of a substance in terms of Trolox equivalents. Trolox is a water-soluble vitamin E analog [28] and was used as a standard antioxidant in order to obtain a calibration curve following the manufacturer's instruction. A Cu^{2+} working solution was added to dispersions of empty liposomes, nanoceria-loaded liposomes (in both cases corresponding to an amount of 7 μg of nanovectors), and to all the Trolox standard samples. In the presence of antioxidants, Cu^{2+} ions are converted to Cu^{+} ions, which react with a colorimetric probe giving an absorbance peak at 570 nm. This peak, assessed after 90 min of incubation through a microplate reader (Victor3, PerkinElmer, Waltham, MA, USA), is proportional to the total antioxidant capacity.

4.3. Cell Cultures

The normal human dermal fibroblast (NHDF) cell line was purchased from Lonza (Basel, Switzerland) and cultured in Dulbecco's Modified Eagle's Medium (DMEM) supplemented with 10% fetal bovine serum (FBS) and 1% penicillin-streptomycin. Cells were grown at 37 °C in an atmosphere containing 5% CO_2 and passaged by trypsinization with 0.5% trypsin/ethylenediaminetetraacetic (EDTA).

4.4. Cytotoxicity of Nanoceria-Loaded Liposomes and Empty Liposomes

The biocompatibility of nanoceria-loaded liposomes and empty liposomes was tested in terms of cell proliferation by the Quant-IT™ PicoGreen® dsDNA assay (Molecular Probes, Eugene, OR, USA), enabling cell number quantification upon evaluation of nucleic acids concentration. Cells were seeded at a density of 6×10^3 cells/cm^2 in 24-well plates and incubated for 24 h at 37 °C and 5% CO_2. The medium was then replaced with fresh medium containing empty liposomes or nanoceria-loaded liposomes with different concentrations (0, 100, and 200 μg/mL). After 48 h since the beginning of the treatment, cells were lysed and incubated with the appropriate reagents according the manufacturer's instructions. Finally, fluorescence was measured in 96-well black plates through a microplate reader (Victor3, PerkinElmer, Waltham, MA; excitation 485 nm, emission 535 nm).

4.5. Cellular Uptake Investigation

Internalization of nanoceria-loaded liposomes into NHDF cells was investigated by confocal microscopy. Cells were seeded at a density of 3×10^3 cell/cm^2 in Ibidi μ-Dishes (35 mm, Ibidi) and after 24 h they were treated with nanoceria-loaded liposomes at a concentration of 100 μg/mL for 48 h. The liposomes were previously stained with a lipophilic red-fluorescent dye (1:200 dilution, Dil, Molecular Probes, Eugene, OR). Finally, cells were rinsed with PBS and treated for 10 min with CellMask, a green-fluorescent dye for labeling cell membranes (1:1000 dilution, Invitrogen, Carlsbad, CA, USA), and with Hoechst 33342 (5 μg/mL, Invitrogen) for nucleus counterstaining. A confocal microscope (C2s, Nikon, Tokyo, Japan) was therefore used for the acquisition of the images.

4.6. Intracellular Antioxidant Activity Evaluation

In order to investigate the antioxidant activity of nanoceria-loaded liposomes, 2′,7′-dichlorodihydrofluorescein diacetate (H_2DCF-DA) Cellular Reactive Oxygen Species Detection Assay Kit (Life Technologies) was used. H_2DCF-DA is a fluorogenic dye that is able to diffuse through cell membrane and to intracellularly interact with hydroxyl, peroxyl, and other ROS. More specifically, after its cell internalization, H_2DCF-DA is deacetylated by cellular esterases to a non-fluorescent compound, which is later oxidized by ROS into 2′,7′-dichlorofluorescein (DCF), a fluorescent compound that thus becomes a direct indicator of the intracellular ROS levels. NHDF cells were seeded in a 24-well plate at a density of 6×10^3 cell/cm^2, incubated for 24 h, and then treated for 48 h with dispersions of empty liposomes or nanoceria-loaded liposomes at different concentrations (0, 75, and 150 μg/mL), respectively containing 0, 50, and 100 μg/mL of nanoceria. In order to induce intracellular ROS accumulation, cells were treated with 1 mM H_2O_2 for 45 min at 37 °C in a complete medium, and finally incubated with 100 μM H_2DCF-DA in a serum-free medium at 37 °C in the dark for 30 min. After cell lysis through three freezing/thawing cycles, fluorescence was quantified with a microplate reader (Victor3, Perkin Elmer, Waltham, MA; excitation 485 nm, emission 535 nm).

4.7. Statistical Analyses

Data were analyzed with one-way ANOVA followed by Bonferroni's post hoc test or two-tailed unpaired t-test through KaleidaGraph (Synergy Software). In all experiments, performed in triplicate, data with a p-value < 0.05 were considered statistically significant.

5. Conclusions

Liposomes were demonstrated to be an excellent platform for nanoceria encapsulation without altering antioxidant properties of the nanoparticles. Nanoceria-loaded liposomes showed good biocompatibility, a regular spherical shape, nanometric size, and preserved antioxidant activity in vitro. Further investigations will be needed in order to modify the liposome surface with appropriate ligands for a targeted delivery. The encapsulation of nanoceria into a liposomal drug delivery system could improve the pharmacokinetic profile of nanoceria in vivo and represents a stimulus for new strategies of nanotechnology-based therapies.

Author Contributions: Agostina Grillone and Tianshu Li designed and performed experiments; Matteo Battaglini, Alice Scarpellini and Mirko Prato contributed to the analysis tools; Shinji Takeoka and Gianni Ciofani conceived experiments and wrote the paper.

References

1. Das, S.; Dowding, J.M.; Klump, K.E.; Mcginnis, J.F.; Self, W.; Seal, S. Cerium oxide nanoparticles: Applications and prospects in nanomedicine. *Nanomedicine* **2013**, *8*, 1483–1508. [CrossRef] [PubMed]
2. Karakoti, A.; Singh, S.; Dowding, J.M.; Seal, S.; Self, W.T. Redox-active radical scavenging nanomaterials. *Chem. Soc. Rev.* **2010**, *39*, 4422–4432. [CrossRef] [PubMed]
3. Celardo, I.; Pedersen, J.Z.; Traversa, E.; Ghibelli, L. Pharmacological potential of cerium oxide nanoparticles. *Nanoscale* **2011**, *3*, 1411–1420. [CrossRef] [PubMed]
4. Niu, J.; Wang, K.; Kolattukudy, P.E. Cerium oxide nanoparticles inhibits oxidative stress and nuclear factor-κB Activation in H9c2 cardiomyocytes exposed to cigarette smoke extract. *Pharmacology* **2011**, *338*, 53–61. [CrossRef]
5. Schubert, D.; Dargusch, R.; Raitano, J.; Chan, S.W. Cerium and yttrium oxide nanoparticles are neuroprotective. *Biochem. Biophys. Res. Commun.* **2006**, *342*, 86–91. [CrossRef] [PubMed]
6. Pagliari, F.; Mandoli, C.; Forte, G.; Magnani, E.; Pagliari, S.; Nardone, G.; Licoccia, S.; Minieri, M.; Di Nardo, P.; Traversa, E. Cerium oxide nanoparticles protect cardiac progenitor cells from oxidative stress. *ACS Nano* **2012**, *6*, 3767–3775. [CrossRef] [PubMed]
7. Niu, J.; Azfer, A.; Rogers, L.M.; Wang, X.; Kolattukudy, P.E. Cardioprotective effects of cerium oxide nanoparticles in a transgenic murine model of cardiomyopathy. *Cardiovasc. Res.* **2007**, *73*, 549–559. [CrossRef] [PubMed]
8. Kong, L.; Cai, X.; Zhou, X.; Wong, L.L.; Karakoti, A.S.; Seal, S.; McGinnis, J.F. Nanoceria extend photoreceptor cell lifespan in tubby mice by modulation of apoptosis/survival signaling pathways. *Neurobiol. Dis.* **2011**, *42*, 514–523. [CrossRef] [PubMed]
9. Chen, J.; Patil, S.; Seal, S.; McGinnis, J.F. Rare earth nanoparticles prevent retinal degeneration induced by intracellular peroxides. *Nat. Nanotechnol.* **2006**, *1*, 142–150. [CrossRef] [PubMed]

10. Zhou, X.; Wong, L.L.; Karakoti, A.S.; Seal, S.; McGinnis, J.F. Nanoceria inhibit the development and promote the regression of pathologic retinal neovascularization in the *Vldlr* knockout mouse. *PLoS ONE* **2011**, *6*. [CrossRef] [PubMed]
11. Rocca, A.; Moscato, S.; Ronca, F.; Nitti, S.; Mattoli, V.; Giorgi, M.; Ciofani, G. Pilot in vivo investigation of cerium oxide nanoparticles as a novel anti-obesity pharmaceutical formulation. *Nanomed. NBM* **2015**, *11*, 1725–1734. [CrossRef] [PubMed]
12. Wason, M.S.; Zhao, J. Cerium oxide nanoparticles: Potential applications for cancer and other diseases. *Am. J. Transl. Res.* **2013**, *5*, 126–131. [PubMed]
13. Alili, L.; Sack, M.; Karakoti, A.S.; Teuber, S.; Puschmann, K.; Hirst, S.M.; Reilly, C.M.; Zanger, K.; Stahl, W.; Das, S.; et al. Combined cytotoxic and anti-invasive properties of redox-active nanoparticles in tumor-stroma interactions. *Biomaterials* **2011**, *32*, 2918–2929. [CrossRef] [PubMed]
14. Alili, L.; Sack, M.; von Montfort, C.; Giri, S.; Das, S.; Carroll, K.S.; Zanger, K.; Seal, S.; Brenneisen, P. Downregulation of tumor growth and invasion by redox-active nanoparticles. *Antioxid. Redox Signal.* **2013**, *19*, 765–778. [CrossRef] [PubMed]
15. Wason, M.S.; Colon, J.; Das, S.; Seal, S.; Turkson, J.; Zhao, J.; Baker, C.H. Sensitization of pancreatic cancer cells to radiation by cerium oxide nanoparticle-induced ROS production. *Nanomed. NBM* **2013**, *9*, 558–569. [CrossRef] [PubMed]
16. Asati, A.; Santra, S.; Kaittanis, C.; Perez, J.M.; Florida, O. Surface-charge-dependent cell localization and cytotoxicity of cerium oxide nanoparticles. *Technology* **2010**, *32826*, 5321–5331. [CrossRef] [PubMed]
17. Lin, W.; Huang, Y.-W.; Zhou, X.-D.; Ma, Y. Toxicity of cerium oxide nanoparticles in human lung cancer cells. *Int. J. Toxicol.* **2006**, *25*, 451–457. [CrossRef] [PubMed]
18. Nanda, H.S. Surface modification of promising cerium oxide nanoparticles for nanomedicine applications. *RSC Adv.* **2016**, *6*, 111889–111894. [CrossRef]
19. Yokel, R.A.; Hussain, S.; Garantziotis, S.; Demokritou, P.; Castranova, V.; Cassee, F.R. The yin: An adverse health perspective of nanoceria: Uptake, distribution, accumulation, and mechanisms of its toxicity. *Environ. Sci. Nano* **2014**, *1*, 406–428. [CrossRef] [PubMed]
20. Wang, B.; He, X.; Zhang, Z.; Zhao, Y.; Feng, W. Metabolism of nanomaterials in vivo: Blood circulation and organ clearance. *Acc. Chem. Res.* **2013**, *46*, 761–769. [CrossRef] [PubMed]
21. Walkey, C.; Das, S.; Seal, S.; Erlichman, J.; Heckman, K.; Ghibelli, L.; Traversa, E.; McGinnis, J.F.; Self, W.T. Catalytic properties and biomedical applications of cerium oxide nanoparticles. *Environ. Sci. Nano* **2015**, *2*, 33–53. [CrossRef] [PubMed]
22. Patila, S.; Sandbergb, A.; Heckertc, E.; Selfc, W.; Seala, S. Protein adsorption and cellular uptake of cerium oxide nanoparticles as a function of zeta potential. *Biomaterials* **2007**, *28*, 4600–4607. [CrossRef] [PubMed]
23. Dowding, J.M.; Das, S.; Kumar, A.; Dosani, T.; McCormack, R.; Gupta, A.; Sayle, T.X.; Sayle, D.C.; von Kalm, L.; Seal, S.; et al. Cellular interaction and toxicity depend on physicochemical properties and surface modification of redox-active nanomaterials. *ACS Nano* **2013**, *7*, 4855–4868. [CrossRef] [PubMed]
24. Wang, X.; Wang, Y.; Chen, Z.G.; Shin, D.M. Advances of cancer therapy by nanotechnology. *Cancer Res. Treat.* **2009**, *41*, 1–11. [CrossRef] [PubMed]
25. Wicki, A.; Witzigmann, D.; Balasubramanian, V.; Huwyler, J. Nanomedicine in cancer therapy: Challenges, opportunities, and clinical applications. *J. Control. Release* **2015**, *200*, 138–157. [CrossRef] [PubMed]
26. Li, T.; Amari, T.; Semba, K.; Yamamoto, T.; Takeoka, S. Construction and evaluation of pH-sensitive immunoliposomes for enhanced delivery of anticancer drug to ErbB2 over-expressing breast cancer cells. *Nanomed. NBM* **2017**, *13*, 1219–1227. [CrossRef] [PubMed]
27. Jain, K.K. Nanobiotechnology-based strategies for crossing the blood—Brain barrier. *Nanomedicine* **2012**, *7*, 1225–1233. [CrossRef] [PubMed]
28. Poljsak, B.; Raspor, P. The antioxidant and pro-oxidant activity of vitamin C and trolox in vitro: A comparative study. *J. Appl. Toxicol.* **2008**, *28*, 183–191. [CrossRef] [PubMed]
29. Aruoma, O.I. Free radicals, oxidative stress, and antioxidants in human health and disease. *JAOCS* **1998**, *75*, 199–212. [CrossRef]
30. Emerit, J.; Edeas, M.; Bricaire, F. Neurodegenerative diseases and oxidative stress. *Biomed. Pharmacother.* **2004**, *58*, 39–46. [CrossRef] [PubMed]
31. Xu, C.; Qu, X. Cerium oxide nanoparticle: A remarkably versatile rare earth nanomaterial for biological applications. *NPG Asia Mater.* **2014**, *6*, e90. [CrossRef]

32. Nelson, C.B.; Johnson, M.E.; Walker, M.L.; Riley, K.R.; Sims, C.M. Antioxidant cerium oxide nanoparticles in biology and medicine. *Antioxidants* **2016**, *5*, 15. [CrossRef] [PubMed]
33. Singh, V.; Singh, S.; Das, S.; Kumar, A.; Self, W.T.; Seal, S. A facile synthesis of PLGA encapsulated cerium oxide nanoparticles: Release kinetics and biological activity. *Nanoscale* **2012**, *4*, 2597. [CrossRef] [PubMed]
34. Gregoriadis, G. Engineering liposomes for drug delivery: Progress and problems. *Trends Biotechnol.* **1995**, *13*, 527–537. [CrossRef]
35. Chen, C.S.; Yao, J.; Durst, R.A. Liposome encapsulation of fluorescent nanoparticles: Quantum dots and silica nanoparticles. *J. Nanopart. Res.* **2006**, *8*, 1033–1038. [CrossRef]
36. Pradhan, P.; Giri, J.; Rieken, F.; Koch, C.; Mykhaylyk, O.; Döblinger, M.; Banerjee, R.; Bahadur, D.; Plank, C. Targeted temperature sensitive magnetic liposomes for thermo-chemotherapy. *J. Control. Release* **2010**, *142*, 108–121. [CrossRef] [PubMed]
37. Kulshrestha, P.; Gogoi, M.; Bahadur, D.; Banerjee, R. In vitro application of paclitaxel loaded magnetoliposomes for combined chemotherapy and hyperthermia. *Colloids Surf. B Biointerfaces* **2012**, *96*, 1–7. [CrossRef] [PubMed]
38. Liu, Y.; Liu, J. Adsorption of nanoceria by phosphocholine liposomes. *Langmuir* **2016**, *32*, 13276–13283. [CrossRef] [PubMed]
39. Sou, K.; Naito, Y.; Endo, T.; Takeoka, S.; Tsuchida, E. effective encapsulation of proteins into size-controlled phospholipid vesicles using freeze-thawing and extrusion. *Biotechnol. Prog.* **2003**, *19*, 1547–1552. [CrossRef] [PubMed]
40. Takeoka, S.; Mori, K.; Ohkawa, H.; Sou, K.; Tsuchida, E. Synthesis and assembly of poly(ethylene glycol)—Lipids with mono-, di-, and tetraacyl chains and a poly(ethylene glycol) chain of various molecular weights. *J. Am. Chem. Soc.* **2000**, *122*, 7927–7935. [CrossRef]

10

Antimicrobial Effect of *Thymus capitatus* and *Citrus limon* var. *pompia* as Raw Extracts and Nanovesicles

Roberto Pinna [1,†], Enrica Filigheddu [1,†], Claudia Juliano [2], Alessandra Palmieri [3], Maria Manconi [4], Guy D'hallewin [5], Giacomo Petretto [2], Margherita Maioli [1,6], Carla Caddeo [4], Maria Letizia Manca [4], Giuliana Solinas [1], Antonella Bortone [7], Vincenzo Campanella [8] and Egle Milia [3,7,*]

1 Department of Biomedical Sciences, University of Sassari, 07100 Sassari, Italy; caesareus83@yahoo.it (R.P.); loran23@hotmail.it (E.F.); mmaioli@uniss.it (M.M.); gsolinas@uniss.it (G.S.)
2 Department of Chemistry and Pharmacy, University of Sassari, 07100 Sassari, Italy; julianoc@uniss.it (C.J.); gpetretto@uniss.it (G.P.)
3 Department of Medicine, Surgery and Experimental Science, University of Sassari, 07100 Sassari, Italy; luca@uniss.it
4 Department of Life and Environmental Sciences, University of Cagliari, 09124 Cagliari, Italy; manconi@unica.it (M.M.); caddeoc@unica.it (C.C.); mlmanca@unica.it (M.L.M.)
5 Institute of Science of Food Production UOS Sassari-CNR, 07040 Sassari, Italy; guy.dhallewin@gmail.com
6 Laboratory of Molecular Biology and Stem Cell Engineering, National Institute of Biostructures and Biosystems, 40129 Bologna, Italy
7 Dental Unite, Azienda Ospedaliero-Universitaria, 07100 Sassari, Italy; nennebortone@tiscali.it
8 Department of Clinical and Translational Medicine, Tor Vergata University of Rome, 00133 Rome, Italy; vincenzo.campanella@uniroma2.it
* Correspondence: emilia@uniss.it;
† These authors contributed equally to this work.

Abstract: In view of the increasing interest in natural antimicrobial molecules, this study screened the ability of *Thymus capitatus* (TC) essential oil and *Citrus limon* var. *pompia* (CLP) extract as raw extracts or incorporated in vesicular nanocarriers against *Streptococcus mutans* and *Candida albicans*. After fingerprint, TC or CLP were mixed with lecithin and water to produce liposomes, or different ratios of water/glycerol or water/propylene glycol (PG) to produce glycerosomes and penetration enhancer vesicles (PEVs), respectively. Neither the raw extracts nor the nanovesicles showed cytotoxicity against human gingival fibroblasts at all the concentrations tested (1, 10, 100 μg/mL). The disc diffusion method, MIC-MBC/MFC, time-kill assay, and transmission electron microscopy (TEM) demonstrated the highest antimicrobial potential of TC against *S. mutans* and *C. albicans*. The very high presence of the phenol, carvacrol, in TC (90.1%) could explain the lethal effect against the yeast, killing up to 70% of *Candida* and not just arresting its growth. CLP, rich in polyphenols, acted in a similar way to TC in reducing *S. mutans*, while the data showed a fungistatic rather than a fungicidal activity. The phospholipid vesicles behaved similarly, suggesting that the transported extract was not the only factor to be considered in the outcomes, but also their components had an important role. Even if other investigations are necessary, TC and CLP incorporated in nanocarriers could be a promising and safe antimicrobial in caries prevention.

Keywords: Oral antimicrobials; caries prevention; natural extracts; nanovesicles

1. Introduction

As proposed in the "ecological plaque hypothesis", a carious lesion develops under changed environmental conditions, producing a corresponding disturbance to the stability of the resident microflora [1]. Changes occur when the frequency of fermentable dietary carbohydrate intake is increased. In such a situation, the biofilm spends more time at low pH, allowing *Streptococcus mutans* to proliferate at the expense of the resident community. *S. mutans* contributes to the lowering of the pH and the growth of acidogenic species at the expense of the resident microflora [2,3]. This breakdown disrupts the de- and remineralization in teeth, pushing the equilibrium toward demineralization and tooth cavities. *Candida albicans* can appear in cariogenic biofilm when bonded to *S. mutans*, thus increasing the virulence of the biofilm and resulting in severe and recurrent caries in early childhood [4] and in salivary disorders [5].

In addition to fluorine, the capacity of which has been widely recognized as an anti-carious agent [5–7], a broad range of chemical agents have been used to reduce the cariogenicity of *S. mutans* in the biofilm [8]. Nevertheless, the increasing phenomenon of antibiotic resistance [9] necessitates the study of alternative therapeutic strategies to chemicals, and new substances, including natural extracts, have been widely investigated [10,11]. The antimicrobial capacity of biomolecules relies on the presence of chemical groups with distinct biosynthetic origins: Phenolic and polyphenols, terpenoids, alkaloids, lectins and polypeptides, and polyacetylenes [12,13]. In particular, terpenoids and flavonoids have demonstrated great potential against cariogenic bacteria and *C. albicans* [14–17]. Recently, encapsulation of natural molecules within lipid-based carriers has shown to increase their efficacy by protecting them from degradation [18], enhancing bioavailability [19], and delivering adequate concentration to the target tissues [20] or microorganisms [21].

Within lipid-based carriers, lamellar vesicles are composed of phospholipids, drugs, and, in some cases, additive components, such as surfactants and co-solvents. The identification of the appropriate combination of vesicle components is a matter of intensive study. Phospholipid nanovesicles having high concentrations of glycerol as co-solvent (glycerosomes), and penetration enhancer-containing vesicles (PEVs) have demonstrated a high efficacy in carrying polyphenols. Indeed, PEVs were able to promote the penetration of the active components of *S. insularis* essential oil in the skin, greater than that of control liposomes, and similarly, glycerosomes potentiated the aptitude of the pompia extract to counteract oxidative stress in both keratinocytes and fibroblasts, preventing their death [22,23]. Their versatility and absence of toxicity can make them suitable carriers for the delivery of antimicrobial molecules.

Among the enormous number of plant genera, various types of *Thymus* of the Lamiaceae family, and *Citrus* of the Rutaceae family have attracted attention for their bactericidal, fungicidal, and anti-inflammatory activities [14,16,24]. In this work, *Thymus capitatus* (TC) and *Citrus limon* var. *pompia* (CLP), typical species of Sardinia (Italy), were investigated. A great concentration of phenols has been identified in the essential oil of TC [25]. In addition, the high availability of flavonoids rich in polyphenolic rings [23] suggest great antimicrobial capacity for CLP.

Thus, in view of the increasing general interest in developing antimicrobials of natural origins, which could, more specifically, be useful in caries prevention, this study aimed to assess the antimicrobial efficacy of TC essential oil and CLP extract used as raw extracts or incorporated in vesicular nanocarriers in the neutralization of *S. mutans* and *C. albicans*.

2. Materials and Methods

2.1. Plant Collection

The aerial parts (flowers, leaves and stems) of TC were collected in North Sardinia (40°82′02″ N; 8°63′10″ E) from wild plants growing on marl soil over limestone. Harvesting took place in mid-June when the plants were fully flowering, in the so-called "balsamic time", which is the period of the plant growth cycle in which essential oil and/or specific metabolite production reaches its maximum.

CLP fruit was harvested in January from plants growing on alluvial soil located near Cedrino river in Orosei (40°37′75″ N; 9°71′23″ E). After harvest, the TC and CLP were immediately stored at 5 °C and processed within the following 24 h, as previously reported [23].

2.2. Extraction Procedures

The essential oil was extracted from the fresh aerial parts of TC. The collected parts were put into a heated (30 °C) ventilated armoire (Memmert 260, Spinea, Venice, Italy) until dry. Then, 150 g of the dried parts were powdered by milling the matrix with a ball-mill (Retsh Emax, Retsch GmbH, Haan, Germany) for 20 min, and steam-distilled for 2 h using a circulatory Clevenger-type apparatus (Merk KGaA, Dormstadt, Germany) according to the European Pharmacopoeia. The distillate was then dried over anhydrous sodium sulphate and the obtained essential oil was stored at low temperature until use. The chemical characterization of TC was conducted using a solution of the essential oil in hexane.

CLP fruit rind (flavedo and albedo) was removed within 24 h of harvest and subjected to extraction as previously reported [23]. Briefly, the rind was minced with a knife, dried, powdered, and dispersed in a water/ethanol (50:50 *v*/*v*) blend. After centrifugation, the supernatant was collected, ethanol was removed with a rotovapor (Buchi R 300, Buchi, Cornaredo, Italy), while water was removed by freeze-drying. A fine yellow powder was obtained, and vacuum stored until use. The chemical characterization of the extract was conducted using the powder dissolved in methanol (1:100 *w*/*v*).

2.3. Identification of TC and CLP Components

2.3.1. GC-MS Analysis of TC Essential Oil

The GC-MS analysis of a TC essential oil solution in hexane (dilution ratio 1:200 *v*/*v*, injection volume 1 μL) was carried out by using an Agilent 7890 GC (Palo Alto, CA, USA) equipped with a Gerstel MPS autosampler, coupled with an Agilent 7000C MSD detector (Palo Alto, CA, USA). The chromatographic separation was performed on a HP-5MS capillary column (30 m × 0.25 mm, film thickness of 0.17 μm), and the following temperature program was used: 60 °C hold for 3 min, increased to 210 °C at a rate of 4 °C/min, held at 210 °C for 15 min, increased to 300 °C at a rate of 10 °C/min, and finally held at 300 °C for 15 min. Helium was used as the carrier gas at a constant flow of 1 mL/min. The data was analyzed using a MassHunter Workstation B.06.00 SP1, with identification of the individual components performed by comparison with the co-injected pure compounds and by matching the MS fragmentation patterns and retention indices with literature data or commercial mass spectral libraries (NIST/EPA/NIH 2008; HP1607 purchased from Agilent Technologies, Palo Alto, CA, USA).

2.3.2. GC-FID Analysis of TC Essential Oil

The GC-FID analysis of a TC essential oil solution in hexane (dilution ratio 1:200 *v*/*v*, injection volume 1 μL) was carried out by using an Agilent 4890N (Palo Alto, CA, USA) equipped with a FID and an HP-5 capillary column (30 m × 0.25 mm, film thickness of 0.17 μm). The column temperature was held at 60 °C for 3 min, then increased to 210 °C at a rate of 4 °C/min and held at 210 °C for 15 min, then increased to 300 °C at a rate of 10 °C/min, and finally held at 300 °C for 15 min. Injector and detector temperatures were 250 °C. Helium was used as the carrier gas at a flow rate of 1 mL/min. The compound quantification in the essential oil was carried out by the internal normalization of FID chromatogram. Results were expressed as a relative percentage.

A hydrocarbon mixture of n-alkanes (C_9–C_{22}) was analyzed separately under the same chromatographic conditions to calculate the retention indexes with the generalized equation by Van del Dool and Kartz [26], $Ix = 100[(t_x - t_n)/(t_{n+1} - t_n) + n]$, where t_n and t_{n+1} are the retention times of the reference n-alkane hydrocarbons eluting immediately before and after chemical compound "X"; t_x is the retention time of compound "X".

2.3.3. Targeted LC-MS/MS Analysis of CLP Extract

Liquid chromatography was performed by using a Flexar UHPLC AS system (Perkin-Elmer, Shelton, CT, USA) equipped with a degasser, Flexar FX-10 pump, autosampler, and PE 200 column Oven interfaced to an AB Sciex (Foster City, CA, USA) API4000 Q-Trap instrument as in Manconi et al. [23]. Briefly, a CLP extract solution in methanol (dilution ratio 1:100 *w/v*) was filtered through 0.20 μm syringe PVDF filters (Whatmann International Ltd., Little Chalfont, Buckinghamshire, UK) and injected (5 μL) in the LC-MS/MS system. The chromatographic separation was carried out on a XSelect HSS C18 column (Waters, Milford, MA, USA) (100 × 2.1 mm i.d., 2.5 μm d). Mobile phase A was water containing 0.1% formic acid, while mobile phase B was acetonitrile containing 0.1% formic acid. Elution was carried out at 41 °C according to the following flow and solvent gradient: 0–4 min, isocratic 0% solvent B and the flow changes from 300 μL to 350 μL; 4–6 min, linear gradient 0–12% B and the flow achieves 400 μL/min; 6–12 min, linear gradient 12–20% B and flow constant at 400 μL/min; 16–17 min, linear gradient 20–100% B and flow retrieves to 300 μL/min.

All quantitative data were elaborated with the aid of the Analyst software. Results were expressed as μg/mg of the freeze-dried extract.

2.4. *Vesicle Preparation and Characterization*

Soybean lecithin was purchased from Galeno (Potenza, Italy). Glycerol, propylene glycol, and all other products were purchased from Sigma-Aldrich (Milan, Italy).

2.4.1. Vesicle Preparation

The TC essential oil or CLP extract were incorporated into liposomes, glycerosomes, and propylen glycol-penetration enhancer containing vesicles (PG-PEVs) using an environmentally-friendly technique avoiding the use of organic solvents (Table 1).

Table 1. Composition of TC essential oil and CLP extract loaded liposomes, glycerosomes, and PG-PEVs.

Sample	Soy Lecithin (mg)	Essential Oil/Extract (mg)	Water (mL)	Glycerol (mL)	PG (mL)
TC liposomes	60	10	1.0	–	–
TC glycerosomes	60	10	0.5	0.5	–
TC PG-PEVs	60	10	0.5	–	0.5
CLP liposomes	60	10	1.0	–	–
CLP glycerosomes	60	10	0.5	0.5	–
CLP PG-PEVs	60	10	0.5	–	0.5

Liposomes were formulated by dispersing lecithin (60 mg/mL) and TC essential oil or CLP extract (10 mg/mL) in bidistilled water. The dispersions were sonicated (30 cycles, 5 s ON and 2 s OFF; 13 microns of probe amplitude) by using a Soniprep 150 (MSE Crowley, London, UK).

Glycerosomes were formulated by dispersing lecithin (60 mg/mL) and TC essential oil or CLP extract (10 mg/mL) in a water:glycerol blend (50:50 *v/v*). The dispersions were sonicated (30 cycles, 5 s ON and 2 s OFF; 13 microns of probe amplitude) by using a Soniprep 150 (MSE Crowley, London, UK).

PG-PEVs were formulated by dispersing lecithin (60 mg/mL) and TC essential oil or CLP extract (10 mg/mL) in a water:propylene glycol blend (50:50 *v/v*). The dispersions were sonicated (30 cycles, 5 s ON and 2 s OFF; 13 microns of probe amplitude) by using a Soniprep 150 (MSE Crowley, London, UK).

2.4.2. Vesicle Characterization

The average diameter and polydispersity index (PI; a measure of width of the size distribution) of the vesicles were determined by Photon Correlation Spectroscopy using a Zetasizer nano (Malvern Instruments, Worcestershire, UK). Samples ($n = 6$) were backscattered by a helium-neon laser (633 nm) at an angle of 173° and a constant temperature of 25 °C. The zeta potential of the vesicles, an indicator of the stability of vesicular dispersions, was estimated by using the Zetasizer nano by means of the M3-PALS (phase analysis light scattering) technique, which measures the particle electrophoretic mobility. Prior to the analysis, the samples (10 µL) were diluted with the appropriate mixture (i.e., water or water/glycerol or water/propylene glycol, 10 mL). A long-term stability study was performed by monitoring the vesicle size, polydispersity index, and zeta potential over 60 days at 4 °C.

2.5. *Cytotoxicity Assay*

Human gingival fibroblasts (HGFs) were isolated from biopsies of gingiva from human adult patients, all informed and consenting (ethical approval by ethics committee review boards for human studies in Sassari, ref. number 2034/2014). The samples were disinfected in poly(vinylpyrrolidone)–iodine solution (PVP-I, Sigma Aldrich Chemie GmbH, Munich, Germany) for 3 min and washed twice in Hank's balanced salt solution (HBSS; Sigma Aldrich Chemie GmbH, Munich, Germany). Dissociation was then performed by mechanical fragmentation and enzymatic digestion in 0.1% type I collagenase (Gibco Life Technologies, Grand Island, NY, USA) for 120 min at 37 °C in Hanks balanced salt solution (HBSS; Sigma Aldrich Chemie GmbH, Munich, Germany). The cell suspension was filtered through a 70 µm cell strainer (Euroclone, Milano, Italy) and centrifuged at 1800 rpm for 10 min. Then, the cells were transferred in culturing medium containing DMEM medium (Invitrogen, Carlsbad, CA, USA) supplemented with 10% heat-inactivated fetal bovine serum (FBS, Invitrogen, Carlsbad, CA, USA), 200 U/mL penicillin, and 0.1 mg/mL streptomycin. The cells seeded in culture flasks were placed at 37 °C in a humidified atmosphere containing 5% CO_2. The MTT assay was used to analyze the cytotoxic effect of the two extracts on fibroblasts, according to recently published papers [27,28]. In total, 1×10^4 cells were suspended in 96-well plates diluted in 200 µL of medium. After attachment, the cells were incubated for 48 h with 200 µL of medium containing the different compounds to be tested at different concentrations (1, 10, 100 µg/mL). After 48 h, the medium was removed and 100 µL of 0.65 mg/mL MTT were added in each well and incubated for 3 h. The MTT (yellow tetrazolium salt) was enzymatically converted into purple formazan precipitate by viable cells. The concentration of formazan represents an indicator of viable cells. After removing the medium, 100 µL of DMSO was added to dissolve the formazan participates. Finally, absorbance was detected at the 570 nm wavelength by an ELISA plate reader (Gemini EM Microplate Reader; Molecular devices, San Jose, CA, USA). Control untreated cells were incubated for 48 h with the medium alone (100% viability).

The relative viability of the cells, as compared to the control, was calculated using the following formula:

$$\%\ \text{cell viability} = (\text{OD570 of treated cells}) \times 100\%/(\text{OD570 of control cells}).$$

The data were entered using SPSS Version 2.0 (IBM SPSS, 2013). An ANOVA test was used to analyze the data obtained, and the level of significance was set at $p < 0.001$.

2.6. *Antimicrobial Assays*

Antimicrobial analysis was conducted using the following planktonic microorganisms: *S. mutans* (ATCC 35668); *C. albicans* (ATCC 10231).

2.6.1. Preparation of the Microbial Inocula

Stock culture of each tested microorganisms maintained at −20 °C was recovered by subculturing on nutrient agar plates using Mueller Hinton Agar (MHA) (Sigma-Aldrich) with the addition of sheep blood for *S. mutans*, while for *C. albicans*, Sabouraud Destrose (IFU) was used in accordance with the European Committee on Antimicrobial Susceptibility Testing. One or two colonies of the same morphological type were selected from the plates and aseptically transferred into test tubes containing

2 mL of sterile saline by means of a sterile loop. McFarland standard was used as a reference to adjust the turbidity of the bacterial suspensions to the required range for bioassays (1–2 × 10^8 UFC/mL).

2.6.2. Disc Diffusion Method

The assessment of the antimicrobial activity of the raw extracts and that of the corresponding extracts incorporated in the nanovesicles was carried out using the disc diffusion method [12]. Sterile Whatman filter paper discs of a 6 mm diameter were impregnated with 15 μL of each sample in a sterile biological safety cabinet. The discs were then aseptically placed in the center of inoculated petri plates (9 cm in diameter) uniformly spread with 0.1 mL of the overnight culture of each microorganism. The plates were refrigerated at 4 °C for 2 h to allow the samples to diffuse into the agar medium and then incubated upside down at 37 °C for 48 h. The tests were conducted in triplicate and the measurement of the inhibition zones was read at 24 and 48 h. A paper disc without antimicrobials was used as a positive control for the growth of the microorganisms. Gentamycin (10 mg/disc; Gibco) and Ketoconazole (10 mg/disc; Janssen Pharmaceutics) were used as negative controls for bacterial and fungal strains, respectively. The scale applied for the measurement of the antimicrobial activity as the zone of inhibition was as follows (disc diameter included): Not sensitive (−) for total zone diameters ≤ 12 mm; sensitive (+) for diameters ranging between 12 and 19 mm; extremely sensitive (+++) for zone diameters ≥ 20 mm. The bioassays were conducted in a biological safety cabinet in accordance with the protocols of Clinical and Laboratory Standards Institute (CLSI), formerly National Committee for Clinical Laboratory Standards [29].

2.6.3. Minimum Inhibitory Concentration (MIC), Minimum Bactericidal Concentration (MBC), and Minimum Fungicidal Concentration (MFC)

The MIC, MBC, and MFC of the raw extracts and that of the nanovesicles against *S. mutans* and *C. albicans* were determined using a broth microdilution method according to standard guidelines [30,31]. In 96-well microtiter trays, each sample was subjected to two-fold serial dilutions (2.5–0.078 mg/mL) in MHA or Sabouraud Destrose Liquid Medium for bacteria and yeasts, respectively, and the wells were inoculated with 10^3 to 10^4 bacteria or yeast cells from 24 h broth cultures; the plates were then incubated at 37 °C for 24 h. The MIC was defined as the lowest concentration of each sample that completely inhibited microorganisms' growth. MBCs and MFCs were determined by sub-culturing small aliquots (10 μL) of the suspensions from wells not showing microbial onto solid media (MHA and Sabouraud Dextrose Agar for the bacteria and the yeast, respectively). The MBC and MFC values were defined as the lowest concentrations that produced no colonies on the agar plates.

2.6.4. Microbial Killing Rates by Time-Kill Assay

Time-dependent killing of the raw extracts and the nanovesicles were identified against standardized microbial inocula of *S. mutans* and *C. albicans* in a liquid medium not supporting cell growth [32]. Microorganisms in a logarithmic phase of growth were centrifuged at 2000 rpm for 10 min, washed in phosphate-buffered saline (PBS, Dulbecco A; pH 7.3), and resuspended at the density of 5 × 10^5 to 1 × 10^6 colony-forming units (cfu)/mL in appropriate volumes of PBS containing suitable concentrations of each bioactive agent. An inoculum of microorganisms in PBS without any antimicrobial was used as a control and was included in each assay. After the inoculation, the suspensions were incubated at 37 °C. At time zero and at predetermined intervals (1, 2, and 3 h), 0.5 mL of the mixtures were aseptically removed and subjected to serial 10-fold dilution in PBS; aliquots of 1 mL of the appropriate dilutions were then placed in petri dishes (90 mm diameter) and 19 mL of molten MHA or Sabouraud Dextrose were added for *S. mutans* and *C. albicans*, respectively, swirling thoroughly. The plates were then incubated for 48 h at 37 °C; the number of viable microorganisms at each time was evaluated by counting plates with 30 to 300 colonies. These evaluations were done in duplicate.

2.7. Transmission Electron Microscopy

The ultramorphology of *S. mutans* and *C. albicans* after contact with the raw extracts and the extract loaded vesicles, using MIC values, was studied using transmission electron microscopy (TEM). Cell suspensions of *S. mutans* and *C. albicans* were aseptically removed from the cultures. Each culture was divided into two groups, one of which was left untreated (control), while the other group (treated) was further subdivided into four subgroups for microorganism species, each of which was treated at the MIC of each bioactive agent as for the time-kill assay. Thereafter, both the subgroups and the controls were incubated for 24 h at 37 °C. Subsequently, all the cell material was harvested by centrifugation and prefixed with a 2.5% glutaraldehyde solution overnight at 4 °C. As in previous studies under TEM [33–35], the pellets were washed in cacodylate buffer, pH 7.4, post-fixed in 1% osmium tetroxide for 30 min, and washed twice in cacodylate buffer, dehydrated using ethanol in increasing concentrations (25–100%), embedded in epoxy resin to make the blocks of the cell pellets, cut into ultra-thin sections (80 µm in thickness) using a Diatome diamond knife, and stained with lead citrate and uranyl acetate. Samples were placed on 50 mesh copper grids and observed under TEM (Zeiss 109 EM Turbo, Königsallee, Göttingen, Germany).

3. Results

3.1. Chemical Composition

After GC-MS analysis, a total of 14 compounds were identified, representing 99% of the whole TC essential oil. The chemical composition was dominated by carvacrol, which represents 90% of the total active ingredients contained in the essential oil (Table 2).

Table 2. Main components of TC essential oil as analyzed by GC/GC-MS techniques. Results are expressed as relative percentages obtained by internal normalization of FID chromatogram. RI: experimental retention indexes on HP5 column.

Main Components of TC Essential Oil	A%	RI
p-cymene	1.1	1022.9
limonene	0.2	1026.5
1,8-cineole	0.6	1028.8
γ-terpinene	0.4	1066.5
linalool	1.6	1100.9
camphor	0.1	1142.5
borneol	0.7	1165.1
terpinen-4-ol	1.1	1176.9
α-terpineol	0.2	1192.7
Thymol	0.5	1294.6
carvacrol	90.1	1306.5
carvacrol acetate	0.1	1375.3
cariophyllene	1.0	1419.3
cariophyllene oxide	1.3	1586.2

The chemical characterization of CLP extract was carried out by targeted LC-MS/MS analysis. Thirteen compounds belonging to flavanones and phenolic acids were identified and quantified, as previously reported [23]. The main compound detected in the extract was quinic acid with a concentration that matched 220 µg/mg of freeze-dried extract.

3.2. Vesicles Characterization

TC essential oil and CLP extract were incorporated in different types of phospholipid vesicles, namely liposomes, glycerosomes, and PG-PEVs (Table 1), aiming at protecting the bioactive components from possible degradation and controlling their release.

The physical characteristics of the different vesicle systems are reported in Table 3. TC essential oil and CLP extract loaded liposomes were around 86 and 137 nm, respectively. The addition of glycerol (glycerosomes) or propylene glycol (PG-PEVs) led to an increase in size, which was more significant when using TC essential oil. Regardless of the composition of the vesicles, the polydispersity index, which is a dimensionless measure of the broadness of the size distribution, was always ≤0.3, thus indicating a homogeneous distribution of the vesicle size in the dispersions. The zeta potential of the vesicles was generally highly negative, predicting a good stability of the vesicle dispersions during storage. Indeed, the long-term stability studies (60 days at 4 °C) showed that the variation in the vesicle size, polydispersity index, and zeta potential were never greater than 10%.

Table 3. The main physico-chemical properties of TC and CLP loaded liposomes, glycerosomes, and PG-PEVs are reported: Mean diameter (MD), polydispersity index (PI), and zeta potential (ZP) estimated by dynamic and electrophoretic light scattering. Mean values ± standard deviations were obtained from 8 replicates.

Sample	MD (nm)	PI	ZP (mV)
TC liposomes	86 ± 12	0.25	−72 ± 12
TC glycerosomes	479 ± 40	0.23	−49 ± 3
TC PG-PEVs	337 ± 45	0.24	−50 ± 1
CLP liposomes	137 ± 16	0.26	−43 ± 4
CLP glycerosomes	180 ± 16	0.30	−51 ± 9
CLP PG-PEVs	218 ± 28	0.30	−65 ± 5

3.3. Cytotoxicity Assay

HGFs were treated or not (control) with different concentrations of TC and CLP for 48 h. The cell viability in the presence of the investigated compounds was assayed. Using one-way ANOVA, no significant differences ($p < 0.001$) were found between the treated cells and control cells. In addition, both TC liposome (100 μg/mL) and TC PG-PEVs (100 μg/mL), as well as CLP liposome (100 μg/mL) treated cells exhibited a significant increase in cell viability, as compared to untreated cells (Figures 1 and 2), indicative of a proliferative effect.

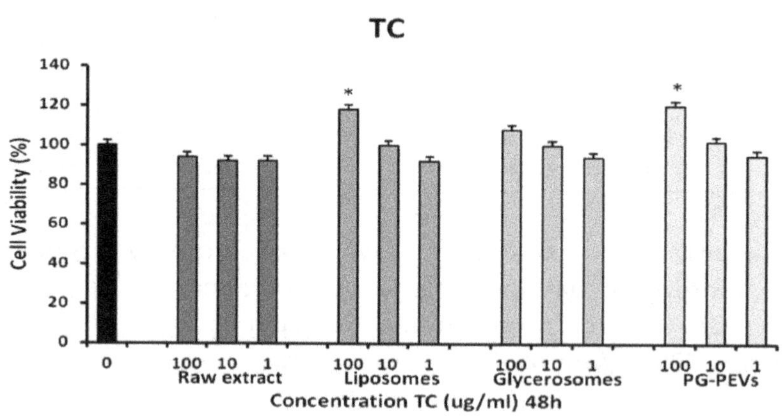

Figure 1. MTT assay after 48 h exposure to different concentrations (100, 10, 1 μg/mL) of TC essential oil, TC liposomes, TC glycerosomes, and TC PG-PEVs. ANOVA analysis showed high significance values (* $p < 0.001$) for liposomes and PG-PEVs at 100 μg/mL vs. the untreated control (0; 100% viability).

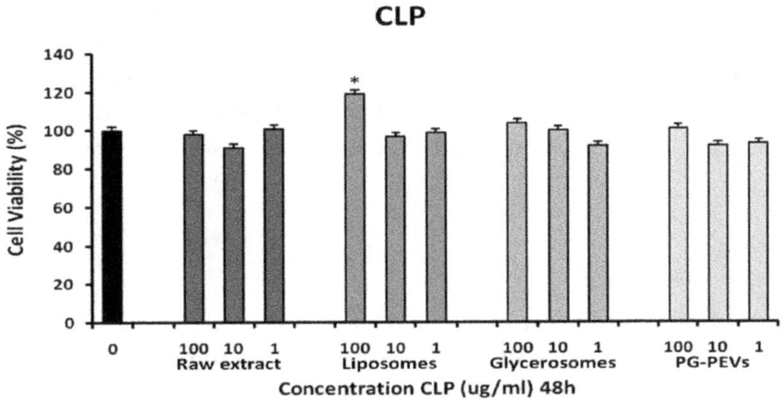

Figure 2. MTT assay after 48 h exposure to different concentrations (100, 10, 1 μg/mL) of CLP essential oil, TC liposomes, TC glycerosomes, and TC PG-PEVs. ANOVA analysis showed high significance values (* $p < 0.001$) for liposomes at 100 μg/mL vs. the untreated control (0; 100% viability).

3.4. Disc Diffusion Method

Antimicrobial susceptibility tests on discs impregnated with 15 μL of each sample showed that TC had an inhibition capacity towards the tested microorganisms. Also, this preliminary screening demonstrated that TC in the nanovesicles had similar antibacterial effects to the raw essential oil. The raw CLP extract did not display any antimicrobial activity, neither against *S. mutans* nor *C. albicans*. Conversely, when CLP extract was delivered by the nanovesicles, the antimicrobial activity against *S. mutans* increased, while it remained ineffective against *C. albicans*. In Tables 4 and 5, the antimicrobial activity and 95% CI of the halo inhibition diameters (mm) against *S. mutans* and *C. albicans* are reported.

Table 4. Descriptive statistics for the antimicrobial activity of TC essential oil against the microorganisms using the disc diffusion assay.

TC Essential Oil	*S. mutans*		*C. albicans*	
	Mean ± SD	95%CI	Mean ± SD	95%CI
Raw oil	12 ± 0	12–12	12 ± 0.5	10.76–13.24
Liposomes	13 ± 0	13–13	0 ± 0	0–0
Glycerosomes	11 ± 0	11–11	11.83 ± 0.29	11.12–12.6
PG-PEVs	0 ± 0	0–0	9 ± 1.73	4.69–13.30
Gentamicin	14 ± 0	14–14	-	-
Ketoconazole	-	-	11.33 ± 0.58	9.89–12.77

Table 5. Descriptive statistics for the antimicrobial activity of CLP extract against the microorganisms using the Disc Diffusion assay.

CLP Extract	*S. mutans*		*C. albicans*	
	Mean ± SD	95%CI	Mean ± SD	95%CI
Raw extract	0 ± 0	0–0	0 ± 0	0–0
Liposomes	8.97 ± 0.58	8.82–9.11	0 ± 0	0–0
Glycerosomes	14 ± 0	14.0–14.0	0 ± 0	0–0
PG-PEVs	10 ± 0	10–10	0 ± 0	0–0

3.5. MIC-MBC/MFC

Raw TC essential oil showed high activity against *S. mutans* with an MIC and MBC of 0.5 mg/mL (Table 6). Raw CLP extract inhibited *S. mutans* with an MIC and MBC of 0.625 mg/mL. However, TC essential oil and CLP extract loaded in liposomes were not effective against the bacteria with an MIC range >2.5 mg/mL, whereas MICs for TC essential oil and CLP extract loaded in glycerosomes and PG-PEVs were <0.078 mg/mL, meaning that no bacterial growth was achieved even at the lower concentrations. Regarding *C. albicans*, MIC and MFC values for the raw TC essential oil were the most effective among the samples tested (Table 7). TC essential oil loaded vesicles were not effective against the yeast (MIC and MBC >2.5 mg/mL), regardless of how they were formulated. MIC and MFC values for raw CLP against *C. albicans* were 0.625 mg/mL, while all vesicles loading CLP extract were not able to inhibit the yeast.

Table 6. Minimum inhibitory concentrations (MICs), minimum bactericidal concentrations (MBCs), and minimum fungicidal concentrations (MFCs) (expressed as mg/mL) of TC essential oil and TC loaded in nanovesicles against *S. mutans* and *C. albicans* determined by the broth microdilution method.

Strain	Raw Essential Oil		Liposomes		Glycerosomes		PG-PEVs	
	MIC	MBC/MFC	MIC	MBC/MFC	MIC	MBC/MFC	MIC	MBC/MFC
S. mutans	0.5	0.5	>2.5	>2.5	<0.078	<0.078	<0.078	<0.078
C. albicans	0.25	0.5	>2.5	>2.5	>2.5	>2.5	>2.5	>2.5

Table 7. Minimum inhibitory concentrations (MICs), minimum bactericidal concentrations (MBCs), and minimum fungicidal concentrations (MFCs) (expressed as mg/mL) of CLP extract and CLP loaded in nanovesicles against *S. mutans* and *C. albicans* determined by the broth microdilution method.

Strain	Raw Essential Oil		Liposomes		Glycerosomes		PG-PEVs	
	MIC	MBC/MFC	MIC	MBC/MFC	MIC	MBC/MFC	MIC	MBC/MFC
S. mutans	0.625	0.625	>2.5	>2.5	<0.078	<0.078	<0.078	<0.078
C. albicans	0.625	0.625	>2.5	>2.5	>2.5	>2.5	>2.5	>2.5

3.6. Time-Kill Assay

A time-kill assay was used to further evaluate the antimicrobial activities of the samples. Despite its subjective character, the MIC assay is used to judge the performance of the other methods of susceptibility testing [36]. In our case, MICs for raw TC essential oil and loaded in nanovesicles against *S. mutans* ranged from <0.078 mg/mL to >2.5 mg/mL, while MICs against *C. albicans* ranged from 0.25 mg/mL to >2.5 g/mL. Thus, because of the wide range of MICs, we identified the MICs of raw TC against *S. mutans* (0.5 mg/mL) and *C. albicans* (0.25 mg/mL) as suitable concentrations to conduct a time-course of microbial viability for TC essential oil loaded in vesicles (Figure 3). Similarly, microbial viability for non-incorporated CLP extract and that loaded in vesicles against the target microorganisms was conducted as MICs for the bacteria and the yeast (0.625 mg/mL). The results demonstrated that the inoculum of *S. mutans* was reduced to 11% within 3 h after the addition of raw TC essential oil; and *C. albicans'* viability was inhibited to 30% after 3 h of exposure to the raw oil. Raw CLP extract reduced the viability of *S. mutans* to 18%, whereas it was not able to inhibit the yeast significantly within the 3 h of this experimentation. The nanovesicles, regardless of the loaded TC essential oil or CLP extract, at the tested concentrations of MICs could arrest neither the growth of *S. mutans* nor that of *C. albicans*, except for CLP in PG-PEVs, which showed an inhibition ability towards the yeast (Figure 3).

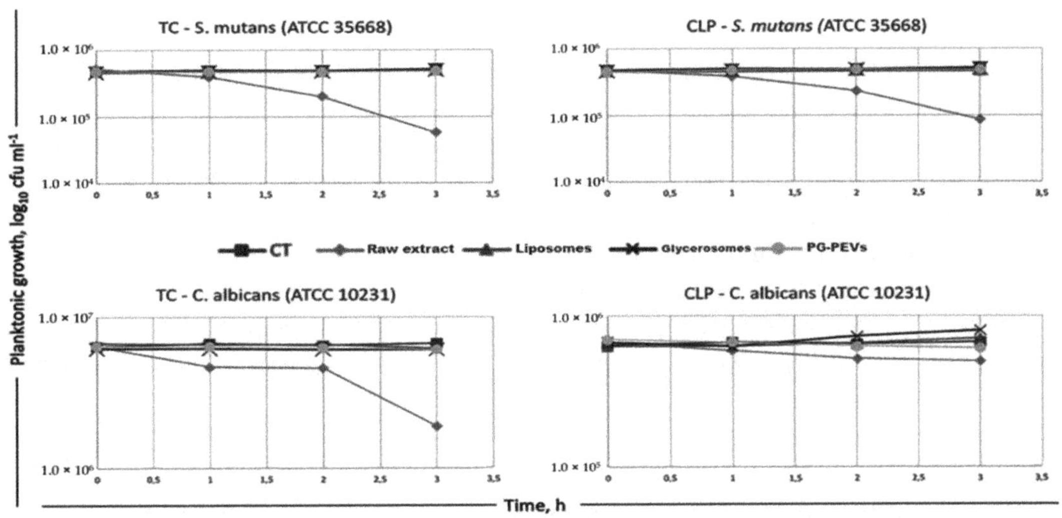

Figure 3. Time-kill curves of *S. mutans* and *C. albicans* treated with TC essential oil, CLP extract, and their nanovesicles.

3.7. Transmission Electron Microscopy (TEM)

3.7.1. Untreated *S. mutans*

Under TEM, untreated *S. mutans* appeared in clusters and showed an intact and well-defined cell wall (CW), plasma membrane (PM), and cytoplasmic space. The nucleoid could be seen in some cells located in an eccentric position in the cytoplasm (Figure 4A).

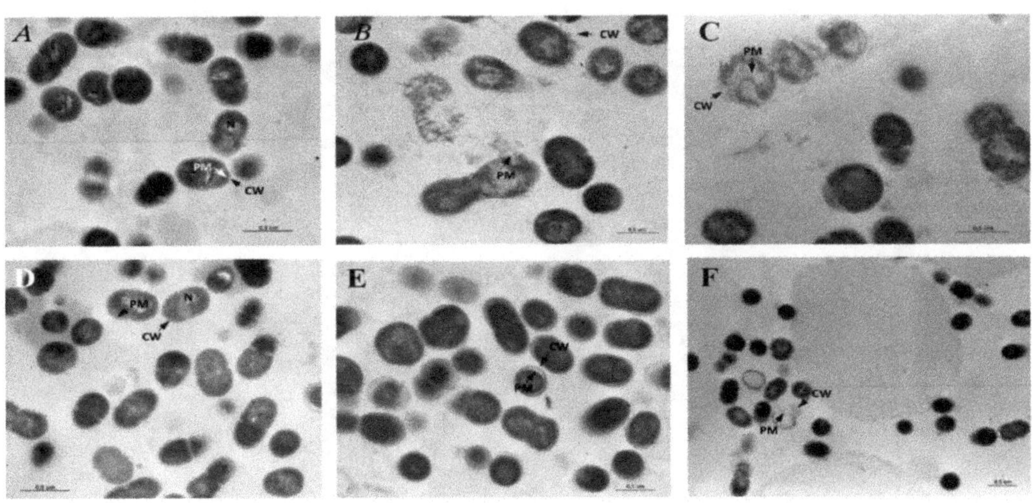

Figure 4. (**A**) Untreated S. mutans shows an intact and well-defined cell wall (CW), plasma membrane (PM), and cytoplasmic space with a nucleoid (N). (**B**) When treated with TC essential oil, S. mutans appears swollen and degenerated with clear evidence of rupture of the CW and PM up to cell disintegration. (**C**) After contact with CLP extract, S. mutans displays features of degeneration comparable to those described in the cells treated with TC essential oil.(**D**) Regardless of the extract loaded, after contact with liposomes, S. mutans showed a well-conserved morphology in comparison to the control, whereas (**E**) after contact with glycerosomes, the cells appear swollen and show the enlargement of the wideness between CW and PM, and (**F**) after contact with PG-PEVs, the cells are surrounded by dense globules infiltrating the CW with perforation of the CW and PM. Other cells appear clearly disintegrated in the cluster.

3.7.2. Treated *S. mutans*

When treated with TC essential oil, the cluster of *S. mutans* showed a high range of degenerated cells. The cells appeared swollen and deformed with a clearly observed rupture of CW and PM in addition to cytoplasm degeneration up to cell disintegration (Figure 4B). After contact with CLP extract, *S. mutans* showed morphological aspects of degeneration comparable to those described in the cells treated with TC essential oil (Figure 4C). After contact with liposomes (Figure 4D), *S. mutans* showed a well-conserved morphology in comparison to the control, whereas after contact with glicerosomes (Figure 4E), the cells showed characteristic enlargement of the wideness between the CW and PM, and after PG-PEV contact (Figure 4F), the cells appeared surrounded by dense globules infiltrating the CW and displayed perforation of the CW and membrane. Occasional aspects of cell degeneration were also reported using PG-PEVs.

3.7.3. Untreated *C. albicans*

The ultrastructure of the yeast shows a prominent and amorphous CW surrounding the inner PM and the dark intracytoplasmatic space (Figure 5A). Microfibrils of β glucans could be seen in the outer layer of the membrane. Microfibrils formed a wide-meshed network of fibrils extending into the cell wall (Figure 5B).

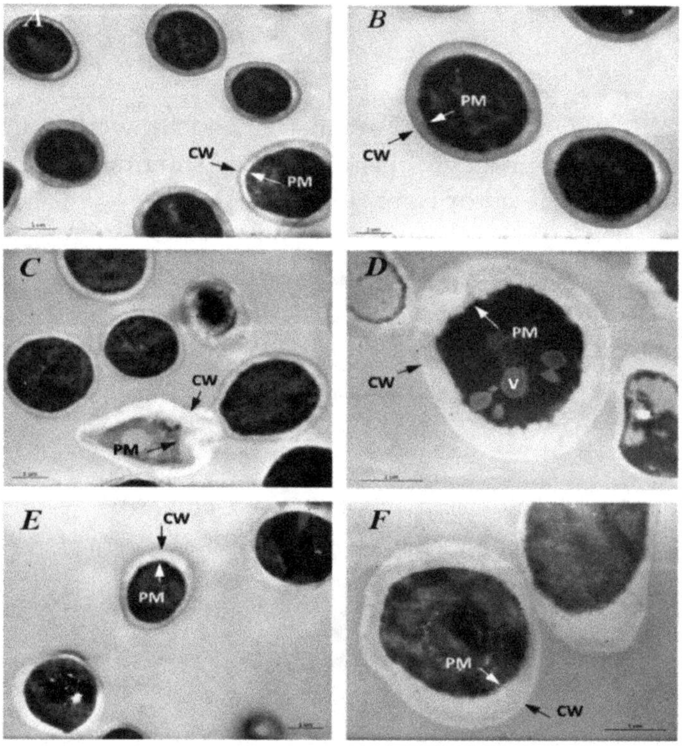

Figure 5. (**A**) Untreated *C. albicans* shows a prominent and amorphous CW surrounding the PM and the dark intracytoplasmatic space. (**B**) Characteristic microfibrils of β glucans can be observed in the outer layer of the membrane. Microfibrils are intermeshed into thicker bundles, forming a wide-meshed network of fibrils extending into the cell wall. (**C**) After 24 h of contact with TC essential oil, the yeast show features compatible with a fungicidal activity. The photograph shows alteration in the shape and wideness of the CW with rupture of the PM and cytoplasm fragmentation of the yeast. (**D**) In other cells, the PM appears ruffled and vacuoles of medium density and shape could be detected within the cytoplasm. (**E**) Protoplasms treated with CLP extract show an enlargement of the wideness between the CW and PM. (**F**) No morphological alterations could be observed neither in the PM nor in the cytoplasm, suggesting a fungistatic rather than a fungicidal effect of CPL extract.

3.7.4. Treated *C. albicans*

After 24 h contact with TC essential oil, *C. albicans* showed an alteration in the shape and wideness of the CW with rupture of the PM together with cytoplasm fragmentation and features compatible with cell death (Figure 5C). Other cells showed an irregularly ruffled PM with vacuoles (V) of medium density and shape in the cytoplasm (Figure 5D). Protoplasms treated with CLP extract showed an enlargement of the wideness between the CW and PM (Figure 5E). However, no morphological alterations could be observed, neither in the PM nor in the cytoplasm, suggesting a fungistatic rather than a fungicidal effect of CPL towards *C. albicans* (Figure 5F). After contact with liposomes (Figure 6A), the cells showed a quite conserved morphology in comparison to the control, while after contact with glycerosomes (Figure 6B) and PG-PEVs (Figure 6C), halos of different thicknesses delimiting and infiltrating the CW were commonly observed in addition to occasional aspects of cell degeneration using PG-PEVs.

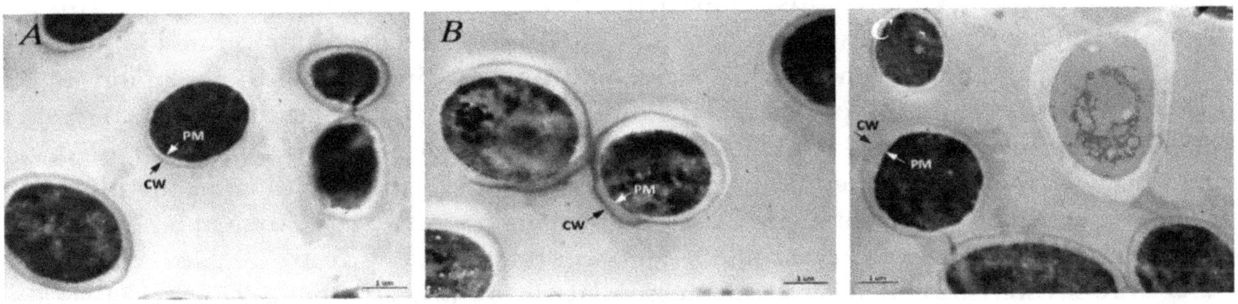

Figure 6. (**A**) After contact with liposomes, the cells show quite conserved morphology in comparison to the control, while (**B**) after contact with glycerosomes and (**C**) PG-PEVs, halos of different thicknesses delimiting and infiltrating the CW are common features in the cells, with some occasional aspects of cell degeneration using PG-PEVs.

4. Discussion

Despite developments in the understanding of biological and physico-chemical mechanisms, dental caries remains one of the most common diseases of our era, affecting 60% to 90% of children and 100% of adults worldwide [37]. The main methods of prevention have been based on the daily use of fluoride toothpaste, a reduction in both the amount and regularity of sugar intake, and drinking fluoridated water [6,38,39]. However, the effect of fluorine is mainly to increase resistance to demineralization and promote remineralization in teeth, while its antimicrobial activity has not generally been considered significant [40,41]. Hence, antimicrobial agents, directly interfering with the metabolism of dental plaque, are required in addition to mechanical cleaning [8,42]. In particular, the poor specificity of chemical agents [43] and global antimicrobial resistance [44–46] require new and safe molecules able to target microorganisms selectively [47].

Given this context, we chose to study the antimicrobial capacity of TC essential oil and CLP extract with the intention of identifying new natural agents taken from Sardinia's biodiversity, which could be useful against *S. mutans* and *C. albicans*. The extracts were incorporated in different phospholipid nanovesicles with the intent to protect the bioactive molecules from degradation and volatility, while modulating their delivery over time and improving its bioavailability and potency at the target site [48]. Because in previous studies we had found that glycerosomes and PG-PEVs were effective in transporting bioactive polyphenols [22,23], this study had the intention to test the possibility that the same carriers would be useful in delivering antimicrobial TC essential oil and CPL extract. The vesicle systems used in this experiment demonstrated a homogeneous distribution of particle size (PI ≤ 0.3) and a highly negative zeta potential, which, as a result of the index of the magnitude of repulsive interaction between the colloidal particles, ensured the high stability of the nanodispersions [23,49]. Regardless of their antimicrobial aggressiveness, none of the samples examined, at the concentrations used, showed cytotoxicity in gingival fibroblasts. This outcome confirms the use of Thyme biomolecules as safe compounds (GRAS) [50] and contributes to the understanding of Citrus flavonoids in the field of modern medicine. In addition, the data confirm the possible use of phospholipid nanovesicles as oral systems [51].

The data also suggest that at selected doses, there will be a selective cytotoxicity of the natural extracts towards microbes due to the fundamental differences in composition and structure of the host cells, compared to those of bacteria and yeasts [52]. TC essential oil was the most effective antimicrobial. The very high presence of the phenol carvacrol in TC essential oil (90.1%) could explain the major activity of this fraction against *S. mutans* and *C. albicans* [15,17,53,54]. However, a synergistic interaction of the oxigenate, terpene (1.1%); the bicyclic sesquiterpene, caryophyllene oxide (1.3%); the terpenes, p-cymene and terpinen-4-ol (1.1%); and thymol (1.1%) could also be involved in the antimicrobial ability [55,56]. In addition, a direct effect of caryophyllene oxide has been reported against *Streptococcus* [57]. With regards to carvacrol, its high toxicity against microorganisms derives from its hydrophobicity and allows it to partition the lipids of the cell membrane [58], making the membrane destabilized and permeable [53,59,60], and thus leading to the leakage of ions and other cell constituents, the impairment of several enzyme systems [17,61], and also endoplasmic reticulum stress [15]. Toxicity requires a $pH < pKa$, in which case the peptide is fully positively charged, capable of interacting with the anionic membrane of the cells [58], and thus able to enter the phospholipid bilayer of the membrane. Accordingly, we used culture media with a pH range of $5.7–7 \pm 0.1$, which allowed the pH dependence of carvacrol [53,59], pKa phenolic OH group ~10.9 [62]. *S. mutans* and *C. albicans* were severely inhibited by the raw essential oil as shown by the MBC-MFC/MIC ratio and the time-kill kinetics (Tables 6 and 7, Figure 3). In particular, the MIC and MFC, in addition to the killing kinetics, demonstrated that the TC essential oil was the most effective fungicidal, killing up to 70% of the yeasts and not just arresting their growth. These data were supported by the morphological analysis of *S. mutans* and *C. albicans* showing cell features compatible to lethal and not inhibitory effects.

Regarding CLP extract, the chromatographic technique coupled with mass spectrometry revealed it was rich in flavanones, flavones, and phenolic acid mainly represented by quinic acid (219.7 μg/mg), followed by neoeriocitrin (46.5 μg/mg), neohesperidin (44.6 μg/mg), naringin (23.8 μg/mg), and sinapic acid (30.1 μg/mg) [23]. Although the compounds in CLP extract belong to a different class with respect to the components found in TC essential oil, they exerted the antimicrobial activity in a similar way by reducing the growth and viability of *S. mutans*, as demonstrated by the MIC and time-kill assays. This result is not in agreement with the disc diffusion assay, which seemed to demonstrate that CLP extract was unable to inhibit *S. mutans*. We could explain the data as a misinterpretation of the therapeutic efficacy of the extract using the agar disc. In fact, it is well known that the inhibition halo is an effect of the capacity of the antimicrobial agent to diffuse into the agar, inhibiting germination and growth of the test microorganism. However, it is also possible that antimicrobial cationic agents could combine with the anionic agar polysaccharide gel [63], making this method imprecise in effectively predicting the capacity of a compound. Despite its bactericidal ability, CLP extract was not effective as fungicidal compound, as was evidenced by the MIC and time-kill assay (Table 7 and Figure 3). These data, in addition to the TEM images, could suggest a fungistatic rather than a fungicidal effect of CLP extract towards *C. albicans*. To explain the different susceptibility of the yeast to the extracts, a specific toxicity of some of the TC essential oil's active fractions, in particular, carvacrol [15,17,53,54], could be supposed. A proteic partner in the phospholipid bilayer of the fungal membrane has been proposed for carvacrol. This interplay is similar to most antifungal therapies, e.g., azoles among others, which lead to a fungistatic effect [64]. In addition, antifungal therapies have side effects in humans and cause an increase in *Candida* resistance [64–68]. Thus, although further studies are necessary, among them an assessment of whether emerging resistance could be developed using multiple exposures to TC essential oil, the fungicidal ability of this natural drug should be considered as a safe alternative to chemicals.

Regarding phospholipid vesicles, TC essential oil and CLP extract loaded in liposomes did not display any antibacterial activity against *S. mutans* (MIC > 2.5 mg/mL). Conversely, TC essential oil and CLP extract loaded in glycerosomes and PG-PEVs resulted in MICs that were unquantifiable, meaning that no bacteria growth was detectable under these experimental conditions, even at the lowest concentrations. Thus, it could be possible that glycerosomes and PG-PEVs exerted their antibacterial activities after the 3 h time limit of the kill assay, at which point the raw extracts were effective against the bacteria. It is likely that in some way, the vesicles might slow the release of the loaded bioactive molecules within that time. In addition, we could suppose that the extract transported by the vesicles was not the only factor in determining the toxicity against *S. mutans*. Under TEM, the prime target of glycerosomes and PG-PEVs seemed to be the bacterial CW, which was surrounded by dense halos with a tendency to reach the bacterial membrane. Although the vesicles may be too large to penetrate the bacterial envelope, it is likely that the co-surfactant molecules partition the lipid compartments of the bacterial cells. This may occur either directly (from the vesicles to the bacteria) or indirectly (through the aqueous phase). As larger, lipophilic co-solvent molecules, such as glycerol and propylenglycol, have a higher affinity for lipidic compartments than smaller, more hydrophilic compounds, they might have contributed to the activity of the system [69]. This consideration may explain the different abilities and morphological features of phospholipid vesicles against *S. mutans*.

Regarding the antimicrobial activity against *C. albicans*, glycerosomes and PG-PEVs displayed a fungistatic activity, highlighting a greater resistance of the yeast membrane in comparison to that of the bacteria.

5. Conclusions

On the bases of the data obtained in this study, TC essential oil possesses the highest antimicrobial capacity against *S. mutans* and *C. albicans*. CLP extract showed bactericidal properties against *S. mutans*, but it was not effective as a fungicidal compound. Regardless of the extract loaded, glycerosomes and PG-PEVs behaved similarly against both the bacterium and the yeast.

Author Contributions: Conceptualization and investigation: E.M., M.M. (Maria Manconi), G.D.; formal analysis: R.P., G.D. and G.P.; formal analysis, writing—review and editing: M.M. (Maria Manconi), C.C. and M.L.M.; investigation: M.M. (Margherita Maioli); formal analysis: C.J. and A.P.; formal analysis: G.S.; writing—review and editing: E.F., A.B. and V.C.; writing—review and editing, supervision: E.M.

Acknowledgments: Egle Milia thanks Salvatore Marceddu, Inst. of Biomolecular Chemistry, CNR, Sassari, Italy, for his technical support in the TEM analysis.

References

1. Marsh, P.D. Sugar, fluoride, pH and microbial homeostasis in dental plaque. *Proc. Finn. Dent. Soc.* **1991**, *87*, 515–525.
2. Marsh, P.D. Plaque as a biofilm: Pharmacological principles of drug delivery and action in the sub- and supragingival environment. *Oral Dis.* **2003**, *9* (Suppl. 1), 16–22. [CrossRef] [PubMed]
3. Flemming, H.-C.; Wingender, J.; Szewzyk, U.; Steinberg, P.; Rice, S.A.; Kjelleberg, S. Biofilms: An emergent form of bacterial life. *Nat. Rev. Microbiol.* **2016**, *14*, 563–575. [CrossRef] [PubMed]
4. Falsetta, M.L.; Klein, M.I.; Colonne, P.M.; Scott-Anne, K.; Gregoire, S.; Pai, C.-H.; Gonzalez-Begne, M.; Watson, G.; Krysan, D.J.; Bowen, W.H.; et al. Symbiotic relationship between Streptococcus mutans and Candida albicans synergizes virulence of plaque biofilms in vivo. *Infect. Immun.* **2014**, *82*, 1968–1981. [CrossRef] [PubMed]
5. Pinna, R.; Campus, G.; Cumbo, E.; Mura, I.; Milia, E. Xerostomia induced by radiotherapy: An overview of the physiopathology, clinical evidence, and management of the oral damage. *Ther. Clin. Risk Manag.* **2015**, *11*, 171–188. [CrossRef] [PubMed]

6. Cagetti, M.G.; Campus, G.; Milia, E.; Lingström, P. A systematic review on fluoridated food in caries prevention. *Acta Odontol. Scand.* **2013**, *71*, 381–387. [CrossRef] [PubMed]
7. Milia, E.; Castelli, G.; Bortone, A.; Sotgiu, G.; Manunta, A.; Pinna, R.; Gallina, G. Short-term response of three resin-based materials as desensitizing agents under oral environmental exposure. *Acta Odontol. Scand.* **2013**, *71*, 599–609. [CrossRef] [PubMed]
8. Marsh, P.D. Controlling the oral biofilm with antimicrobials. *J. Dent.* **2010**, *38*, S11–S15. [CrossRef]
9. World Health Organization. *Antimicrobial Resistance: Global Report on Surveillance*; World Health Organization: Geneva, Switzerland, 2014; ISBN 9789241564748.
10. Waikedre, J.; Dugay, A.; Barrachina, I.; Herrenknecht, C.; Cabalion, P.; Fournet, A. Chemical Composition and Antimicrobial Activity of the Essential Oils from New Caledonian Citrus macroptera and Citrus hystrix. *Chem. Biodivers.* **2010**, *7*, 871–877. [CrossRef] [PubMed]
11. Verkaik, M.J.; Busscher, H.J.; Jager, D.; Slomp, A.M.; Abbas, F.; van der Mei, H.C. Efficacy of natural antimicrobials in toothpaste formulations against oral biofilms in vitro. *J. Dent.* **2011**, *39*, 218–224. [CrossRef] [PubMed]
12. Cowan, M.M. Plant products as antimicrobial agents. *Clin. Microbiol. Rev.* **1999**, *12*, 564–582. [CrossRef]
13. Cushnie, T.P.T.; Lamb, A.J. Antimicrobial activity of flavonoids. *Int. J. Antimicrob. Agents* **2005**, *26*, 343–356. [CrossRef]
14. Hooper, S.J.; Lewis, M.A.O.; Wilson, M.J.; Williams, D.W. Antimicrobial activity of Citrox® bioflavonoid preparations against oral microorganisms. *Br. Dent. J.* **2011**, *210*, E22. [CrossRef] [PubMed]
15. Chaillot, J.; Tebbji, F.; Remmal, A.; Boone, C.; Brown, G.W.; Bellaoui, M.; Sellam, A. The Monoterpene Carvacrol Generates Endoplasmic Reticulum Stress in the Pathogenic Fungus Candida albicans. *Antimicrob. Agents Chemother.* **2015**, *59*, 4584–4592. [CrossRef] [PubMed]
16. Marchese, A.; Orhan, I.E.; Daglia, M.; Barbieri, R.; Di Lorenzo, A.; Nabavi, S.F.; Gortzi, O.; Izadi, M.; Nabavi, S.M. Antibacterial and antifungal activities of thymol: A brief review of the literature. *Food Chem.* **2016**, *210*, 402–414. [CrossRef] [PubMed]
17. Khan, S.T.; Khan, M.; Ahmad, J.; Wahab, R.; Abd-Elkader, O.H.; Musarrat, J.; Alkhathlan, H.Z.; Al-Kedhairy, A.A. Thymol and carvacrol induce autolysis, stress, growth inhibition and reduce the biofilm formation by Streptococcus mutans. *AMB Express* **2017**, *7*, 49. [CrossRef]
18. Silva, P.; Bonifácio, B.; Ramos, M.; Negri, K.; Maria Bauab, T.; Chorilli, M. Nanotechnology-based drug delivery systems and herbal medicines: A review. *Int. J. Nanomed.* **2013**, *9*, 1. [CrossRef] [PubMed]
19. Saraf, S.; Jain, A.; Hurkat, P.; Jain, S.K. Topotecan Liposomes: A Visit from a Molecular to a Therapeutic Platform. *Crit. Rev. Ther. Drug Carr. Syst.* **2016**, *33*, 401–432. [CrossRef]
20. Matougui, N.; Boge, L.; Groo, A.-C.; Umerska, A.; Ringstad, L.; Bysell, H.; Saulnier, P. Lipid-based nanoformulations for peptide delivery. *Int. J. Pharm.* **2016**, *502*, 80–97. [CrossRef]
21. Wang, L.; Wang, Y.; Wang, X.; Sun, L.; Zhou, Z.; Lu, J.; Zheng, Y. Encapsulation of low lipophilic and slightly water-soluble dihydroartemisinin in PLGA nanoparticles with phospholipid to enhance encapsulation efficiency and in vitro bioactivity. *J. Microencapsul.* **2016**, *33*, 43–52. [CrossRef] [PubMed]
22. Castangia, I.; Manca, M.L.; Caddeo, C.; Maxia, A.; Murgia, S.; Pons, R.; Demurtas, D.; Pando, D.; Falconieri, D.; Peris, J.E.; et al. Faceted phospholipid vesicles tailored for the delivery of Santolina insularis essential oil to the skin. *Coll. Surf. B Biointerfaces* **2015**, *132*, 185–193. [CrossRef]
23. Manconi, M.; Manca, M.L.; Marongiu, F.; Caddeo, C.; Castangia, I.; Petretto, G.L.; Pintore, G.; Sarais, G.; D'Hallewin, G.; Zaru, M.; et al. Chemical characterization of Citrus limon var. pompia and incorporation in phospholipid vesicles for skin delivery. *Int. J. Pharm.* **2016**, *506*, 449–457. [CrossRef] [PubMed]
24. Karimi, M.; Ghasemi, A.; Sahandi Zangabad, P.; Rahighi, R.; Moosavi Basri, S.M.; Mirshekari, H.; Amiri, M.; Shafaei Pishabad, Z.; Aslani, A.; Bozorgomid, M.; et al. Smart micro/nanoparticles in stimulus-responsive drug/gene delivery systems. *Chem. Soc. Rev.* **2016**, *45*, 1457–1501. [CrossRef]
25. Cosentino, S.; Tuberoso, C.I.G.; Pisano, B.; Satta, M.; Mascia, V.; Arzedi, E.; Palmas, F. In-vitro antimicrobial activity and chemical composition of Sardinian Thymus essential oils. *Lett. Appl. Microbiol.* **1999**, *29*, 130–135. [CrossRef] [PubMed]
26. Van Den Dool, H.; Kratz, P.D. A generalization of the retention index system including linear temperature programmed gas—Liquid partition chromatography. *J. Chromatogr. A* **1963**, *11*, 463–471. [CrossRef]

27. Cruciani, S.; Santaniello, S.; Garroni, G.; Fadda, A.; Balzano, F.; Bellu, E.; Sarais, G.; Fais, G.; Mulas, M.; Maioli, M.; et al. Myrtus Polyphenols, from Antioxidants to Anti-Inflammatory Molecules: Exploring a Network Involving Cytochromes P450 and Vitamin D. *Molecules* **2019**, *24*, 1515. [CrossRef]
28. Ferhi, S.; Santaniello, S.; Zerizer, S.; Cruciani, S.; Fadda, A.; Sanna, D.; Dore, A.; Maioli, M.; D'hallewin, G.; Ferhi, S.; et al. Total Phenols from Grape Leaves Counteract Cell Proliferation and Modulate Apoptosis-Related Gene Expression in MCF-7 and HepG2 Human Cancer Cell Lines. *Molecules* **2019**, *24*, 612. [CrossRef] [PubMed]
29. Tenover, F.C.; Mohammed, M.J.; Stelling, J.; O'Brien, T.; Williams, R. Ability of laboratories to detect emerging antimicrobial resistance: Proficiency Testing and Quality Control results from the World Health Organization's External Quality Assurance System for Antimicrobial Susceptibility Testing. *J. Clin. Microbiol.* **2001**, *39*, 241–250. [CrossRef] [PubMed]
30. Ghannoum, M.A.; Rice, L.B. Antifungal agents: Mode of action, mechanisms of resistance, and correlation of these mechanisms with bacterial resistance. *Clin. Microbiol. Rev.* **1999**, *12*, 501–517. [CrossRef] [PubMed]
31. Hacek, D.M.; Dressel, D.C.; Peterson, L.R. Highly reproducible bactericidal activity test results by using a modified National Committee for Clinical Laboratory Standards broth macrodilution technique. *J. Clin. Microbiol.* **1999**, *37*, 1881–1884.
32. Juliano, C.; Demurtas, C.; Piu, L. In vitro study on the anticandidal activity of Melaleuca alternifolia (tea tree) essential oil combined with chitosan. *Flavour Fragr. J.* **2008**, *23*, 227–231. [CrossRef]
33. Milia, E.; Lallai, M.R.; García-Godoy, F. In vivo effect of a self-etching primer on dentin. *Am. J. Dent.* **1999**, *12*, 167–171. [PubMed]
34. Milia, E.; Cumbo, E.; Cardoso, R.J.A.; Gallina, G. Current dental adhesives systems. A narrative review. *Curr. Pharm. Des.* **2012**, *18*, 5542–5552. [CrossRef]
35. Milia, E.; Pinna, R.; Castelli, G.; Bortone, A.; Marceddu, S.; Garcia-Godoy, F.; Gallina, G. TEM morphological characterization of a one-step self-etching system applied clinically to human caries-affected dentin and deep sound dentin. *Am. J. Dent.* **2012**, *25*, 321–326.
36. Andrews, J.M. Determination of minimum inhibitory concentrations. *J. Antimicrob. Chemother.* **2001**, *48* (Suppl. 1), 5–16. [CrossRef]
37. National Institute of Health Consensus Development Panel. National Institutes of Health Consensus Development Conference statement. Diagnosis and management of dental caries throughout life. *J. Am. Dent. Assoc.* **2001**, *132*, 1153–1161. [CrossRef]
38. Marinho, V.C.; Chong, L.Y.; Worthington, H.V.; Walsh, T. Fluoride mouthrinses for preventing dental caries in children and adolescents. *Cochrane Database Syst. Rev.* **2016**, *7*, CD002284. [CrossRef]
39. Pitts, N.B.; Zero, D.T.; Marsh, P.D.; Ekstrand, K.; Weintraub, J.A.; Ramos-Gomez, F.; Tagami, J.; Twetman, S.; Tsakos, G.; Ismail, A. Dental caries. *Nat. Rev. Dis. Prim.* **2017**, *3*, 17030. [CrossRef] [PubMed]
40. Marsh, P.D. Microbial Ecology of Dental Plaque and its Significance in Health and Disease. *Adv. Dent. Res.* **1994**, *8*, 263–271. [CrossRef]
41. Rmaile, A. Mechanical Properties and Disruption of Dental Biofilms. Ph.D. Thesis, University of Southampton, Southampton, UK, 2013.
42. Marsh, P.D. Dental plaque as a biofilm and a microbial community—Implications for health and disease. *BMC Oral Health* **2006**, *6*, S14. [CrossRef]
43. Jeon, J.-G.; Rosalen, P.L.; Falsetta, M.L.; Koo, H. Natural Products in Caries Research: Current (Limited) Knowledge, Challenges and Future Perspective. *Caries Res.* **2011**, *45*, 243–263. [CrossRef] [PubMed]
44. Norrby, S.R.; Nord, C.E.; Finch, R.; European Society of Clinical Microbiology and Infectious Diseases. Lack of development of new antimicrobial drugs: A potential serious threat to public health. *Lancet Infect. Dis.* **2005**, *5*, 115–119. [CrossRef]
45. Valeriani, F.; Protano, C.; Gianfranceschi, G.; Cozza, P.; Campanella, V.; Liguori, G.; Vitali, M.; Divizia, M.; Romano Spica, V. Infection control in healthcare settings: Perspectives for mfDNA analysis in monitoring sanitation procedures. *BMC Infect. Dis.* **2016**, *16*, 394. [CrossRef]
46. Ríos, J.L.; Recio, M.C. Medicinal plants and antimicrobial activity. *J. Ethnopharmacol.* **2005**, *100*, 80–84. [CrossRef]
47. Campanella, V.; Syed, J.; Santacroce, L.; Saini, R.; Ballini, A.; Inchingolo, F. Oral probiotics influence oral and respiratory tract infections in pediatric population: A randomized double-blinded placebo-controlled pilot study. *Eur. Rev. Med. Pharmacol. Sci.* **2018**, *22*, 8034–8041. [CrossRef] [PubMed]

48. Sherry, M.; Charcosset, C.; Fessi, H.; Greige-Gerges, H. Essential oils encapsulated in liposomes: A review. *J. Liposome Res.* **2013**, *23*, 268–275. [CrossRef] [PubMed]
49. Caddeo, C.; Sales, O.D.; Valenti, D.; Saurí, A.R.; Fadda, A.M.; Manconi, M. Inhibition of skin inflammation in mice by diclofenac in vesicular carriers: Liposomes, ethosomes and PEVs. *Int. J. Pharm.* **2013**, *443*, 128–136. [CrossRef]
50. Smith, R.L.; Cohen, S.M.; Doull, J.; Feron, V.J.; Goodman, J.I.; Marnett, L.J.; Portoghese, P.S.; Waddell, W.J.; Wagner, B.M.; Hall, R.L.; et al. A procedure for the safety evaluation of natural flavor complexes used as ingredients in food: Essential oils. *Food Chem. Toxicol.* **2005**, *43*, 345–363. [CrossRef]
51. Bergsson, G.; Arnfinnsson, J.; Steingrimsson, O.; Thormar, H. In Vitro Killing of Candida albicans by Fatty Acids and Monoglycerides. *Antimicrob. Agents Chemother.* **2001**, *45*, 3209–3212. [CrossRef]
52. Mai, S.; Mauger, M.T.; Niu, L.; Barnes, J.B.; Kao, S.; Bergeron, B.E.; Ling, J.; Tay, F.R. Potential applications of antimicrobial peptides and their mimics in combating caries and pulpal infections. *Acta Biomater.* **2017**, *49*, 16–35. [CrossRef] [PubMed]
53. Ultee, A.; Slump, R.A.; Steging, G.; Smid, E.J. Antimicrobial activity of carvacrol toward Bacillus cereus on rice. *J. Food Prot.* **2000**, *63*, 620–624. [CrossRef] [PubMed]
54. Coimbra, M.; Isacchi, B.; van Bloois, L.; Torano, J.S.; Ket, A.; Wu, X.; Broere, F.; Metselaar, J.M.; Rijcken, C.J.F.; Storm, G.; et al. Improving solubility and chemical stability of natural compounds for medicinal use by incorporation into liposomes. *Int. J. Pharm.* **2011**, *416*, 433–442. [CrossRef] [PubMed]
55. Barra, A.; Coroneo, V.; Dessi, S.; Cabras, P.; Angioni, A. Characterization of the volatile constituents in the essential oil of Pistacia lentiscus l. from different origins and its antifungal and antioxidant activity. *J. Agric. Food Chem.* **2007**, *55*, 7093–7098. [CrossRef]
56. Zengin, H.; Baysal, A.H. Antibacterial and antioxidant activity of essential oil terpenes against pathogenic and spoilage-forming bacteria and cell structure-activity relationships evaluated by SEM microscopy. *Molecules* **2014**, *19*, 17773–17798. [CrossRef]
57. Pieri, F.A.; de Castro Souza, M.C.; Vermelho, L.L.R.; Vermelho, M.L.R.; Perciano, P.G.; Vargas, F.S.; Borges, A.P.B.; da Veiga-Junior, V.F.; Moreira, M.A.S. Use of β-caryophyllene to combat bacterial dental plaque formation in dogs. *BMC Vet. Res.* **2016**, *12*, 216. [CrossRef]
58. Malmsten, M. Interactions of Antimicrobial Peptides with Bacterial Membranes and Membrane Components. *Curr. Top. Med. Chem.* **2016**, *16*, 16–24. [CrossRef]
59. Ultee, A.; Gorris, L.G.; Smid, E.J. Bactericidal activity of carvacrol towards the food-borne pathogen Bacillus cereus. *J. Appl. Microbiol.* **1998**, *85*, 211–218. [CrossRef] [PubMed]
60. Gallucci, M.N.; Carezzano, M.E.; Oliva, M.M.; Demo, M.S.; Pizzolitto, R.P.; Zunino, M.P.; Zygadlo, J.A.; Dambolena, J.S. In vitro activity of natural phenolic compounds against fluconazole-resistant Candida species: A quantitative structure-activity relationship analysis. *J. Appl. Microbiol.* **2014**, *116*, 795–804. [CrossRef] [PubMed]
61. De Galvão, L.C.C.; Furletti, V.F.; Bersan, S.M.F.; Da Cunha, M.G.; Ruiz, A.L.T.G.; Carvalho, J.E.D.; Sartoratto, A.; Rehder, V.L.G.; Figueira, G.M.; Teixeira Duarte, M.C.; et al. Antimicrobial activity of essential oils against Streptococcus mutans and their antiproliferative effects. *Evid. Based Complement. Altern. Med.* **2012**, *2012*, 751435. [CrossRef]
62. Friedman, M. Chemistry and multibeneficial bioactivities of carvacrol (4-isopropyl-2-methylphenol), a component of essential oils produced by aromatic plants and spices. *J. Agric. Food Chem.* **2014**, *62*, 7652–7670. [CrossRef] [PubMed]
63. Sutherland, I.W. The biofilm matrix—An immobilized but dynamic microbial environment. *Trends Microbiol.* **2001**, *9*, 222–227. [CrossRef]
64. Pappas, P.G.; Kauffman, C.A.; Andes, D.; Benjamin, D.K.; Calandra, T.F.; Edwards, J.E., Jr.; Filler, S.G.; Fisher, J.F.; Kullberg, B.; Ostrosky-Zeichner, L.; et al. Clinical Practice Guidelines for the Management of Candidiasis: 2009 Update by the Infectious Diseases Society of America. *Clin. Infect. Dis.* **2009**, *48*, 503–535. [CrossRef] [PubMed]
65. Stana, A.; Vodnar, D.C.; Tamaian, R.; Pîrnău, A.; Vlase, L.; Ionuț, I.; Oniga, O.; Tiperciuc, B. Design, synthesis and antifungal activity evaluation of new thiazolin-4-ones as potential lanosterol 14α-demethylase inhibitors. *Int. J. Mol. Sci.* **2017**, *18*, 177. [CrossRef] [PubMed]
66. Akins, R.A. An update on antifungal targets and mechanisms of resistance in Candida albicans. *Med. Mycol.* **2005**, *43*, 285–318. [CrossRef]

67. Perlin, D.S. Resistance to echinocandin-class antifungal drugs. *Drug Resist. Updat.* **2007**, *10*, 121–130. [CrossRef] [PubMed]
68. Shapiro, R.S.; Robbins, N.; Cowen, L.E. Regulatory Circuitry Governing Fungal Development, Drug Resistance, and Disease. *Microbiol. Mol. Biol. Rev.* **2011**, *75*, 213–267. [CrossRef]
69. Umerska, A.; Cassisa, V.; Matougui, N.; Joly-Guillou, M.-L.; Eveillard, M.; Saulnier, P. Antibacterial action of lipid nanocapsules containing fatty acids or monoglycerides as co-surfactants. *Eur. J. Pharm. Biopharm.* **2016**, *108*, 100–110. [CrossRef] [PubMed]

11

Increased Loading, Efficacy and Sustained Release of Silibinin, a Poorly Soluble Drug Using Hydrophobically-Modified Chitosan Nanoparticles for Enhanced Delivery of Anticancer Drug Delivery Systems

Cha Yee Kuen [1,2], Sharida Fakurazi [3], Siti Sarah Othman [1] and Mas Jaffri Masarudin [1,2,*]

1 Department of Cell and Molecular Biology, Faculty of Biotechnology and Biomolecular Sciences, Universiti Putra Malaysia, 43400 Serdang, Selangor, Malaysia; yeekuen_91@hotmail.com (C.Y.K.); sarahothman@upm.edu.my (S.S.O.)
2 Cancer Research Laboratory, Institute of Biosciences, Universiti Putra Malaysia, 43400 Serdang, Selangor, Malaysia
3 Department of Human Anatomy, Faculty of Medicine and Health Sciences, Universiti Putra Malaysia, 43400 Serdang, Selangor, Malaysia
* Correspondence: masjaffri@upm.edu.my;

Abstract: Conventional delivery of anticancer drugs is less effective due to pharmacological drawbacks such as lack of aqueous solubility and poor cellular accumulation. This study reports the increased drug loading, therapeutic delivery, and cellular accumulation of silibinin (SLB), a poorly water-soluble phenolic compound using a hydrophobically-modified chitosan nanoparticle (pCNP) system. In this study, chitosan nanoparticles were hydrophobically-modified to confer a palmitoyl group as confirmed by 2,4,6-Trinitrobenzenesulfonic acid (TNBS) assay. Physicochemical features of the nanoparticles were studied using the TNBS assay, and Attenuated total reflectance Fourier transform infrared spectroscopy (ATR-FTIR) analyses. The FTIR profile and electron microscopy correlated the successful formation of pCNP and pCNP-SLB as nano-sized particles, while Dynamic Light Scattering (DLS) and Field Emission-Scanning Electron Microscopy (FESEM) results exhibited an expansion in size between pCNP and pCNP-SLB to accommodate the drug within its particle core. To evaluate the cytotoxicity of the nanoparticles, a Methylthiazolyldiphenyl-tetrazolium bromide (MTT) cytotoxicity assay was subsequently performed using the A549 lung cancer cell line. Cytotoxicity assays exhibited an enhanced efficacy of SLB when delivered by CNP and pCNP. Interestingly, controlled release delivery of SLB was achieved using the pCNP-SLB system, conferring higher cytotoxic effects and lower IC_{50} values in 72-h treatments compared to CNP-SLB, which was attributed to the hydrophobic modification of the CNP system.

Keywords: chitosan nanoparticles; hydrophobically-modified CNP; slibinin; nanobiotechnology

---

1. Introduction

Over the last decade, radiation, chemotherapy and surgery have become important methods to treat cancer patients. Among these methods, chemotherapy remains the most significant treatment, with synthetic drugs being the most potent chemotherapeutic drugs used [1]. The main obstacle faced by current treatments is the inefficient delivery of drugs to target cells. Thus, conventional treatment often leads to side effects in patients due to non-specific interaction of the drugs with non-cancerous cells in the body. Silibinin, also known as silybin, is a major active constituent obtained from the seeds of the milk thistle plant, *Silybum marianum*. It exists as a polyphenolic flavonolignan with hepatoprotective and antioxidant activity. Substantial evidence from current research has demonstrated its clinical use in medical therapies especially in Asia, Europe, and the USA [2–4]. It has been suggested that silibinin is an extremely utilizable natural compound for cancer studies [5,6]. Additionally, there have been increasing research endeavors conducted to elucidate the potential anticancer properties of silibinin against numerous cancer models, including lung [7,8], skin [9,10], prostate [11,12], colon [13], and bladder [14]. Silibinin is preferentially advantageous for development as a candidate therapeutic agent as it is considered remarkably safe in cytotoxicity studies, as it confers low toxicity even in acute administration dosages in both humans and animals, and there are no LD_{50} values for the flavonolignan reported in laboratory studies. However, its widespread application in medical therapy has been marred by its low bioavailability due to low solubility in water (0.4 mg/mL) [15–18]. This restriction was due to its multiple ring structure, which is too large to be absorbed by simple diffusion, which leads to poor water solubility, poor bioavailability and thus poor intestinal absorption [19].

In order to circumvent such a disadvantage, numerous methods for its synthesis have been proposed in order to increase the solubility and bioavailability of silibinin. This has included the implementation of solid lipid nanoparticles via encapsulation [20], incorporation in solid dispersion systems [21], and complexation with phospholipids [22]. A previous study by Zhang et al. utilized stearic acid as a colloidal carrier for the encapsulation of silibinin. This modification successfully incorporated silibinin into solid lipid nanoparticles with anticipated shape, size and entrapment efficiency. However, the systemic adoption of solid lipid nanoparticles for the encapsulation of silibinin is currently limited to the inherent rapid in vivo clearance by the reticuloendothelial system (RES) which decreases the persistence of the silibinin-nanoparticle complex from blood circulation. Considering the nano-scale dimensions of nanoparticles, they can be adapted to utilize the enhanced permeability and retention effects (EPR) of tumor vasculatures to increase the accumulation of chemotherapeutic drugs. Nanoparticles have been demonstrated to exhibit 200 times higher drug accumulation in tumor cells compared to normal tissues, such as kidney, muscle and heart [23].

Chitosan (CS) is a linear polysaccharide linked by a β-(1-4)-linked-D-glucosamine backbone with randomly acetylated amine groups. It is a product of the partial deacetylation of chitin and can be acquired from numerous sources including the exoskeleton of crustaceans [24]. CS is known for its superior features such as biocompatibility, biodegradable and non-toxicity, which makes it an excellent candidate to be utilized in agriculture, biomedicine, food industries and many other fields. A previous study by Kang et al. [25] has successfully synthesized chitosan nanoparticles (CNP) loaded with albendazole, a poorly water-soluble but extremely permeable anthelmintic drug, where a stable nanoparticle system was established. Besides this, Chai et al. [26] also demonstrated that CNP can function as a drug delivery system for Doxorubicin, an anticancer drug. The study showed that Doxorubicin was successfully coated by chitosan and alginate with a good combination and showed controlled release properties. Thus, CNP can be hydrophobically-modified to incur hydrophobic–hydrophobic interactions with drugs to encapsulate them into the nanoparticles, which can potentially increase the solubility of low bioavailability drugs, and protect and stabilize the drugs from the surrounding environment.

This study demonstrates the enhanced encapsulation efficiency of silibinin in hydrophobically-modified chitosan nanoparticles as compared with traditional chitosan nanoparticles, in order to enhance the therapeutic efficacy in the A549 human lung cancer cell line. Based on the background and objectives, perhaps novel, effective and safe hydrophobically-modified chitosan nanoparticles for the enhanced therapeutic delivery of silibinin is proposed. Findings from this study can perhaps be used to further increase the efficacy of silibinin in anti-cancer applications.

2. Results and Discussion

2.1. Particle Size and Polydispersity of Nanoparticle Samples

The formation of CNP occurred through ionic crosslinking between protonated amine groups of CS and anionic phosphate groups of the cross linker, Sodium Tripolyphosphate (TPP) [27,28]. When cross linking occurs, the protonated amine groups will associate with the anionic phosphate groups of TPP to form nanoparticles where the CS polymer will start to form spherical, nano-scaled particles. Figures 1 and 2 depict the particle size distribution (PSD) and polydispersity index (PDI) of nanoparticles formed by the crosslinking of 600 μL CS with different volumes of TPP. The graph suggested that the formation of nanoparticles occurred at the minimal addition of 100 μL TPP for pCNP and 150 μL for CNP. Figures 1 and 2 show where the size of the pCNP experienced a noticeable drop from 4583.00 ± 244.62 nm to 228.11 ± 119.06 nm, while the PDI dropped from 0.577 nm to 0.113 nm with the addition of 50 μL and 100 μL of TPP; the size of the CNP decreased from 761.40 ± 399.73 nm to 49.14 ± 3.98 nm, while the PDI decreased from 0.71 ± 0.18 nm to 0.36 ± 0.07 nm with the addition of 100 μL and 150 μL of TPP. This observation was similar to the earlier study of Masarudin et al. (2015), where a 50 μL addition of TPP was suggested as the minimal volume required to form CNP.

The smallest size of nanoparticles was obtained using 150 μL of TPP for CNP (49.14 ± 3.98 nm) and 200 μL for pCNP (77.08 ± 6.50 nm), respectively. The lowest PDI of nanoparticles was obtained using 250 μL of TPP for CNP (0.15 ± 0.07) and 200 μL for pCNP (0.14 ± 0.08), respectively. The PDI was used as an indication of nanoparticle homogeneity, which depicts the stability of the samples in the colloidal suspension [29]. The PDI showed a similar trend as PSD, where the value dropped at the TPP ranges of 50–150 μL. Both the PSD and PDI data suggested that a decrease in nanoparticle size occurred with an increase of the cross linker, while in turn increasing the monodispersity of the nanoparticles up to 200 μL of TPP addition. This trend was most probably contributed to by the increased volumes of TPP that provided more anionic phosphate groups to form electrostatic interactions with the protonated CS chain [30]. As more TPP was added, the cross-linking degree of the nanoparticles was augmented to where a compact particle structure is thought to occur, leading to the production of smaller-sized nanoparticles [31].

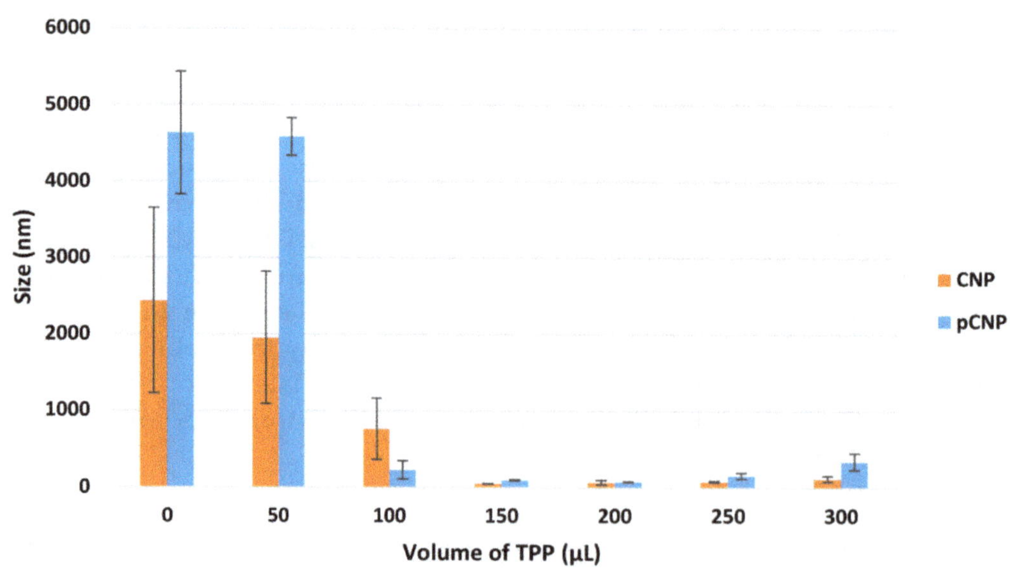

Figure 1. The PSD of nanoparticles at different TPP volumes. The smallest size of nanoparticles was obtained with the addition of 150 μL TPP for CNP and 200 μL for pCNP. Error bars represent the SEM averaged from three independent replicates of the experiment. The one-way analysis of variance (ANOVA) was performed with a p value of the particle size at 0.0002 and <0.0001 for CNP and pCNP, indicating that there was a significant effect of TPP volume on the particle size formed.

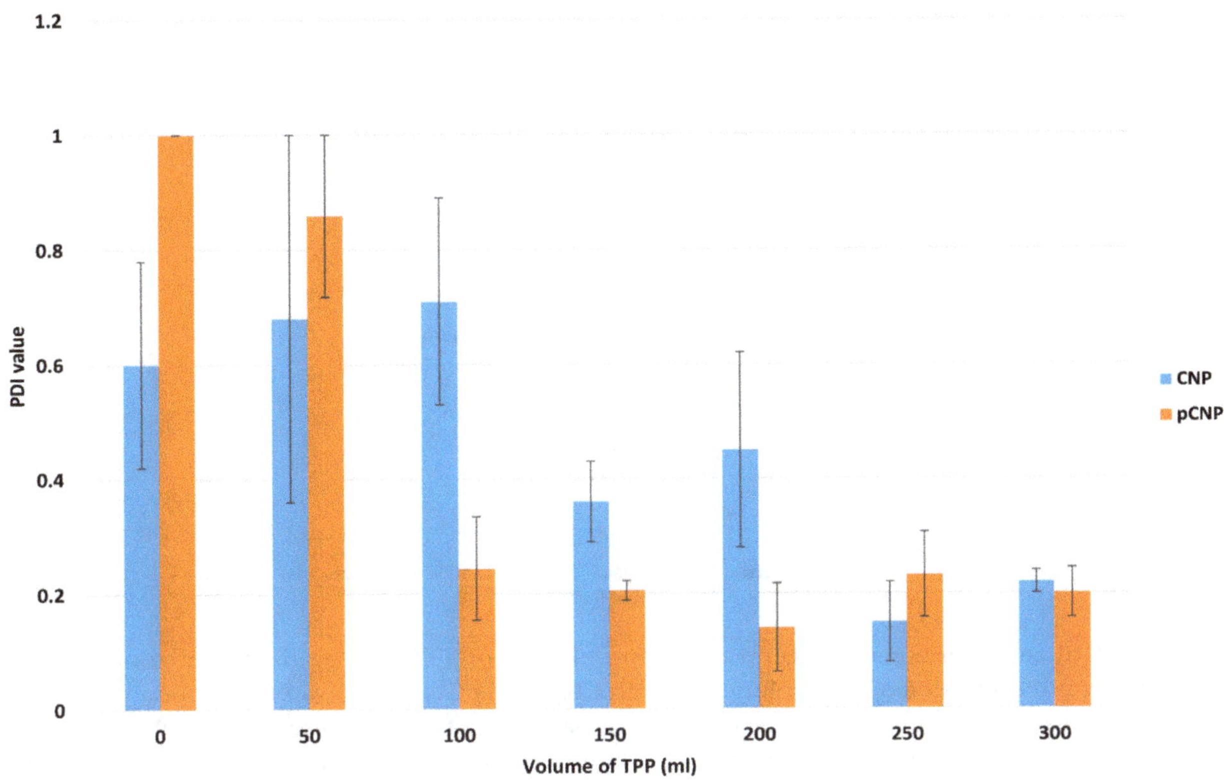

Figure 2. PDI of nanoparticles at different TPP volumes. The lowest PDI of nanoparticles was obtained with the addition of 250 µL TPP for CNP and 200 µL for pCNP. Error bars represent the SEM averaged from three independent replicates of the experiment. The one-way analysis of variance (ANOVA) was performed with *p* value of particle size <0.0001 for both CNP and pCNP indicating that there was a significant effect of TPP volume on the PDI of the nanoparticles formed.

Interestingly, when the TPP volume exceeded 200 µL, both the particle size and PDI increased to above 100 nm and 0.2, respectively. It possibly indicates that agglomeration between the nanoparticles occurred. The addition of anionic TPP beyond the optimum volume will attract more CS chains due to the increase in the degree of cross-linking, and will possibly attract the neighboring nanoparticles causing agglomeration [32], which suggests that 200 µL of TPP and 600 µL of pCS can form nanoparticles of optimum size and PDI.

2.2. Utilization of the Free Amine Group by Nanoparticles Formation

The formation of CNP and pCNP was suggested to be due to the ionic crosslinking interactions between protonated free amine group of CS/pCS and the anionic phosphate group of TPP. When the amount of cross-linker added was increased, the amount of amine groups being utilized will also increase, which in turn decreases the amount of free amine group available in a constant volume of CS/pCS. Figure 3 shows that the percentage of utilized amine groups of chitosan increased in direct proportion to the increased volume of TPP added to the CS/pCS, from 0 up to 22.20 $\pm$ 1.02 and 37.17 $\pm$ 1.397 for CNP and pCNP, respectively, and upon addition of 300 µL of TPP. The data suggested that cross-linking occurred between CS/PCS and TPP on the formation of CNP and pCNP. This increases postulates that CNP and pCNP were successfully constructed, which is similar to the observation reported by a previous study [29]. A higher percentage of utilized amine groups was detected in the pCNP compared to CNP, probably due to the interaction of palmitic acid with the CS prior to the TPP. The palmitic acid will conjugate to the amine group of the CS to form pCS, where utilization of the amine group occurs, and is then only further cross-linked with TPP to form pCNP, which explains the higher percentage of utilization compared to CNP.

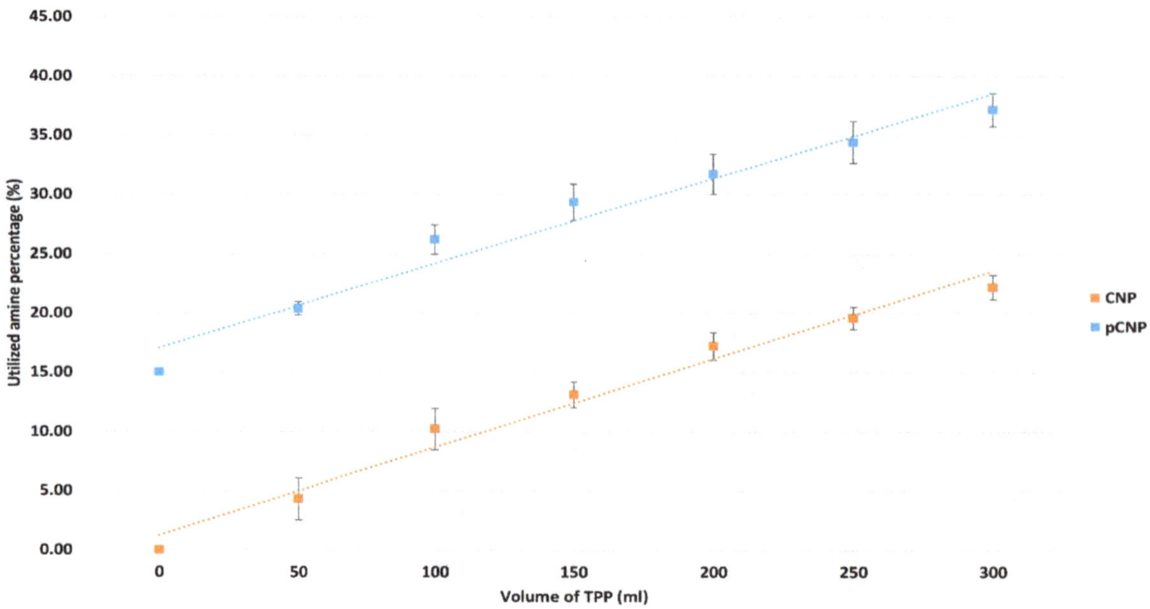

Figure 3. Utilized amine percentage at different volumes of TPP. The utilized amine percentage increased with the addition of TPP volume for both CNP and pCNP. The graph data are presented as mean ± SEM from three independent experiments. A paired *t*-test was performed with a *p* value below 0.0001, which indicates that CNP and pCNP have extremely significant differences on the percentage of free NH_2 group.

2.3. Formation of pCNP and pCNP-SLB

The encapsulation efficiency (% E.E) of pCNP were approximately 49.33 ± 1.45%, which suggests that when approximately 50% of the SLB had been loaded into the pCNP, there was about a 2.5-fold increase of the particle size increment. Anyway, the % E.E of CNP were approximately only 24.58 ± 2.06%, which suggests that only half of the SLB will be loaded into the CNP compared to the pCNP. A higher % E.E was achieved by the pCNP compared with the CNP, probably due to the hydrophobic anchor possessed by the palmitic acid that conjugated with the CS, forming a hydrophobic core, where the SLB will associate with the core instead of the hydrophilic surface. It suggested that the pCNP system is a great carrier candidate that can increase the loading of hydrophobic load. The study of Marchiori et al. [33], performed nanoencapsulation by using interfacial deposition of the preformed polymer method with pomegranate oil as an oil core for the encapsulation of SLB. In their study, a high % E.E was achieved, credited to the higher affinity of SLB with the oil core than the aqueous phase. These results was similar to the findings of our study, where higher % E.E was obtained in pCNP compared to CNP, as the SLB is suggested to have associated with the pCNP by hydrophobic–hydrophobic interaction.

On the other hand, the study of Shankar and Argawal successfully encapsulated SLB by using polymeric micelles. Polymeric micelles are self-assembled, amphiphilic copolymers where the hydrophilic part usually forms the shell and hydrophobic part forms the core, which is similar to the structure of pCNP. The study also achieved a high % E.E, suggesting that amphiphilic nanoparticles are a great candidate for hydrophobic SLB [34]. The size and PDI of the pNCP-SLB are shown in Figure 4. It is important to optimally obtain small-size nanoparticles as well as encapsulated nanoparticles, because the nano-scaled particles are able to extravasate through the endothelium in the epithelium, inflammatory sites, and tumors, or penetrate the microcapillaries. This possesses an advantageous effect in which the nanoparticles permit efficient uptake by many different cell types in addition to selective drug accumulation at target sites [35].

Particle size date showed an expansion of about 270%, from 77.08 ± 6.50 nm to 208.43 ± 12.02 nm, upon SLB loading (300 μM). Similarly, the PDI of the pCNP increased from 0.14 ± 0.08 to 0.30 ± 0.02

after encapsulation, suggesting the successful encapsulation of SLB in pCNP. The expansion in size indicated the successful incorporation of SLB within the core of the nanoparticles. The slight changes in PDI occurred due to the decrease of the uniformity in the size of the nanoparticles following encapsulation, which consist of a population of free pCNPs of smaller size (<100 nm) and pCNP-SLBs of larger size (>100 nm). The expansion in size was correlated with the encapsulation efficiency (% E.E) of the nanoparticles shown in Table 1.

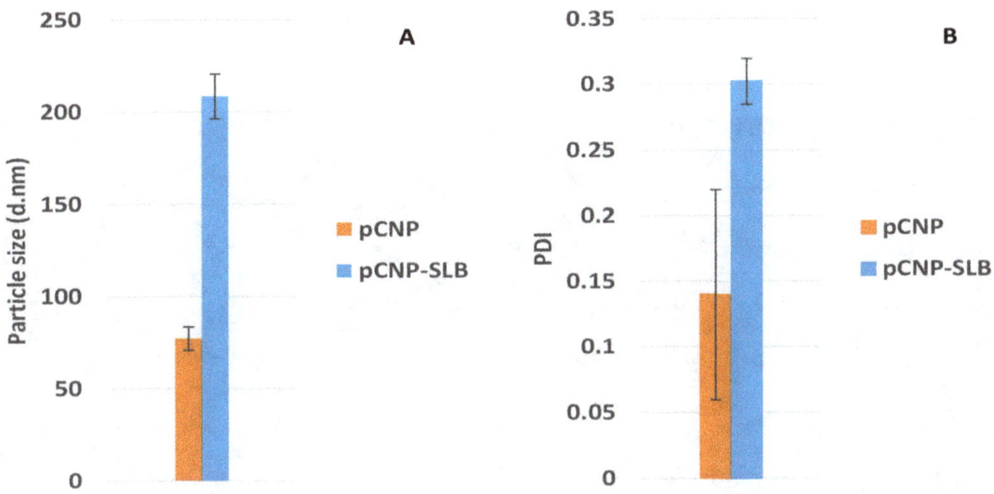

Figure 4. (**A**) PSD and (**B**) PDI of pCNP after SLB encapsulation. The particle size and PDI of pCNP increased after the encapsulation of SLB. The graph data is presented as mean ± SEM from three independent experiments. A p value below 0.05 was obtained, indicating significant differences in particle size between pCNP and pCNP-SLB as measured by paired t-test.

Table 1. % E.E of CNP-SLB and pCNP-SLB at 300 μM SLB. The results show that the % E.E of pCNP-SLB is about two-fold higher that CNP-SLB. The graph data are presented as mean ± SEM from three independent experiments.

Sample	% E.E CNP-SLB	% E.E pCNP-SLB
1	22.46	50.12
2	28.70	51.35
3	22.58	46.51
Average	24.58 ± 2.06	49.33 ± 1.45

2.4. Morphological Analysis of Nanoparticles by FESEM

A morphological analysis was performed using FESEM to ascertain the structure, size and polydispersity of CNP, pCNP and pCNP-SLB. As shown in Figure 5, the nanoparticles are generally spherical in shape, with a size ranging from below 100 nm before encapsulation and up to 200–300 nm post-encapsulation. As described in the study of Ariff et al., the CS or pCS in this study appeared to have an irregular shape when they stood alone, and to form spherically-shaped nanoparticles with the addition of TPP, indicating the success of the CNP/pCNP formation [36]. Blank CNP particles conferred sizes in the range of 64.1 nm to 84.7 nm, whilst pCNP was slightly larger at 87.9 nm to 110.0 nm diameter.

When SLB was encapsulated into the nanoparticles, the expansion in size detected from the DLS was made morphologically evident using FESEM. The pCNP-SLB samples existed as larger particles with sizes approximately 215.8 nm to 243.3 nm. It was postulated that the increase in size of pCNP was attributed to the incorporation of palmitic acid within its core, which led to a significant expansion after the encapsulation of SLB in pCNP. This result was similar to the results observed previous by

Ariff et al., where the size of nanoparticles expanded post-encapsulation [34]. A previous study by Leena et al. [18], utilized chitosan nanoparticles loaded with different concentrations of SLB and incorporated alginate/gelatin scaffolds for bone formation in vitro. The particle size of CNP-SLB obtained from the study was about 264 $\pm$ 51 nm post-encapsulation with 100 µM of SLB. Regarding the pCNP-SLB in this study, where an initial SLB concentration of 300 µM was used for encapsulation, a smaller size of nanoparticles with a higher % E.E was obtained in our study. This further suggests that pCNP is a better nano-carrier for SLB. Anyway, some agglomeration was observed in Figure 5, which can possibly be attributed to the drying process used while preparing the samples for FESEM imaging [37].

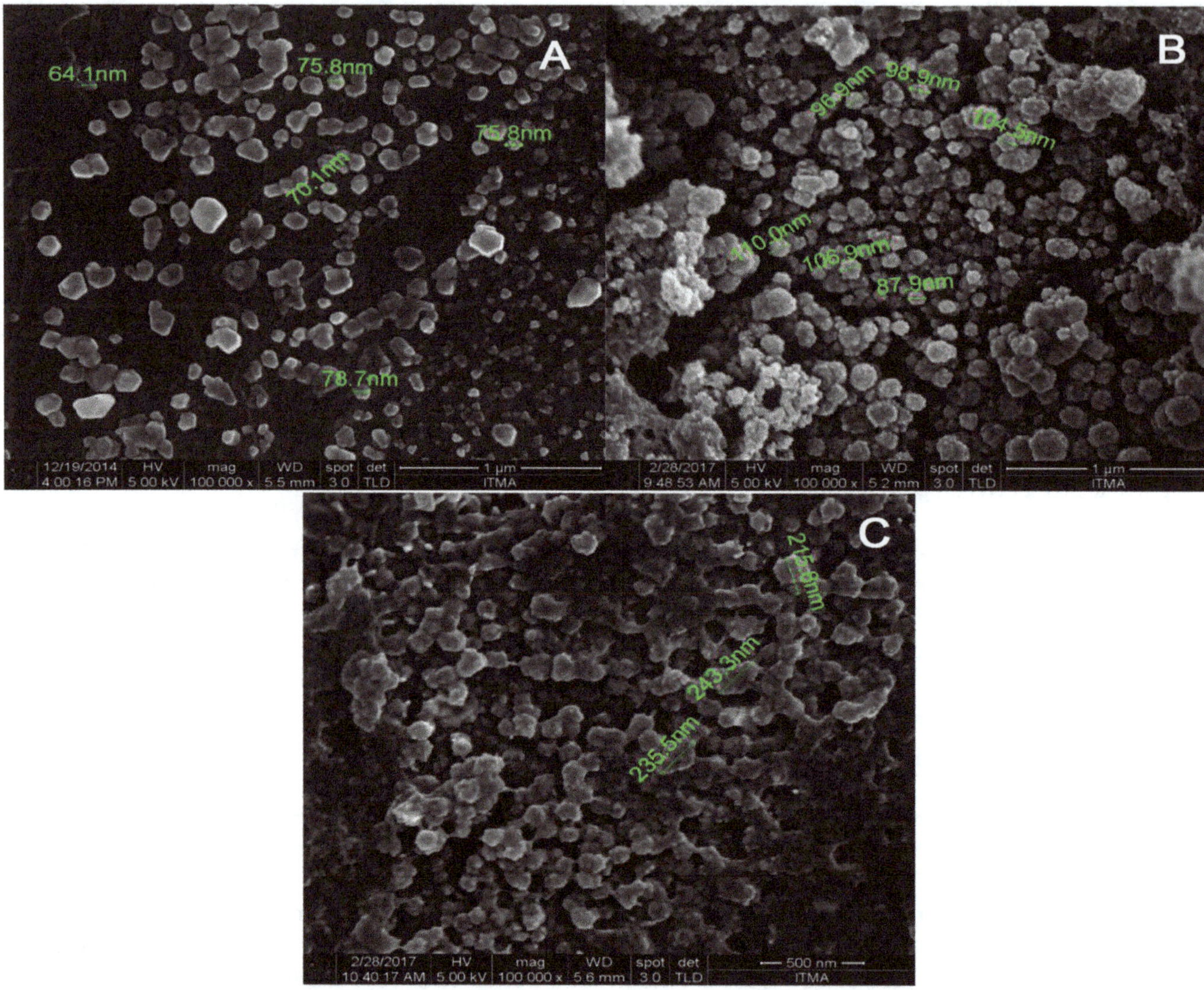

Figure 5. The figure shows the morphological structure of (**A**) CNP, (**B**) pCNP and (**C**) pCNP-SLB. The CNP shows a particle size of 64.1 nm to 84.7 nm, the pCNP shows a particle size of 87.9 nm to 110.0 nm, and the pCNP-SLB shows a particle size ranging from 215.8 nm to 243.3 nm.

2.5. Identification of Characteristic Functional Groups in Nanoparticle Samples

In order to study the formation of drug-encapsulated pCNP-SLB, an FTIR analysis was performed to study the presence of important functional groups belonging to SLB and pCNP that occurred in pCNP-SLB. According to Coates [38] every single molecule has a unique vibrational spectrum which can be utilized as a fingerprint to be compared between an "unknown" and a "known" spectra.

Thus, by comparing the peaks of the "known" spectra of SLB and pCNP with the "unknown" spectra of pCNP-SLB, we can deduce the formation of pCNP-SLB. The infrared spectra for SLB, pCNP, and pCNP-SLB is as shown in Figure 6, while a summary of the important characteristic functional groups detected is depicted in Table 2.

There are several characteristic peaks shown by pCNP: a broad peak at 3353 cm^{-1}, corresponding to the hydrogen-bonded O–H stretching vibration and N–H stretching from the primary amine overlapped in the same region; a peak at 1632 cm^{-1}, corresponding to the amide II carbonyl stretch; and a peak at 1067 cm^{-1}, corresponding to the inorganic phosphate group of TPP [39]. Besides this, several characteristic peaks are also possessed by SLB: at 3446 cm^{-1}, due to –OH stretching; at 2936 cm^{-1}, due to –CH stretching; at 1626 cm^{-1}, due to –C=O stretching; at 1507 and 1461 cm^{-1}, due to –C=C skeleton vibrations of aromatic ring stretching; and at 1268 cm^{-1}, due to –C–O–C stretching. From the table, the percentage of transmittance at the peak of 3353 cm^{-1} of pCNP and SLB was 49.62% and 49.98%, respectively, but this increased to 85.97% after encapsulation, indicating a decrease in the primary amine group. It shows that upon encapsulation, the free primary amine group was utilized and led to the shift in the peak from 3353 cm^{-1} in pCNP to 3416 cm^{-1} in pCNP-SLB. A similar observation was shown by the study of Kafshgari et al. [40] where the amine group of CS was shifted from the wavenumber of 3413 cm^{-1} to 3395 cm^{-1} upon encapsulation of bovine serum albumin due to the utilization of amine groups.

However, the inorganic phosphate group of pCNP detected at wavenumber of 1067 cm^{-1} and 1081 cm^{-1} for pCNP-SLB, with increased transmittance after encapsulation, indicated the utilization of the functional group. The characteristic peak for alkyl groups at 2888 cm^{-1} and 2936 cm^{-1} was detected in pCNP and SLB, respectively. After encapsulation, this peak appeared at 2851 cm^{-1}, with a decrease of transmittance, indicating that more active alkyl groups are present upon encapsulation, possibly due to the introduction of SLB in the pCNP [41]. Meanwhile, the peaks attributed to carbonyl groups of pCNP and SLB were detected at the 1632 cm^{-1} and 1626 cm^{-1} wavenumber, respectively, and shifted to 1635 cm^{-1} after encapsulation, also with an increase of transmittance, which shows the interaction between pCNP and SLB that utilized the C=O bond; these results were similar to the previous study of Tan et al. [42]. The C–O–C stretching that happened only in SLB was also observed in pCNP-SLB, with an increase in transmittance from 10 to 67.95%, indicating the utilization of the functional group after encapsulation.

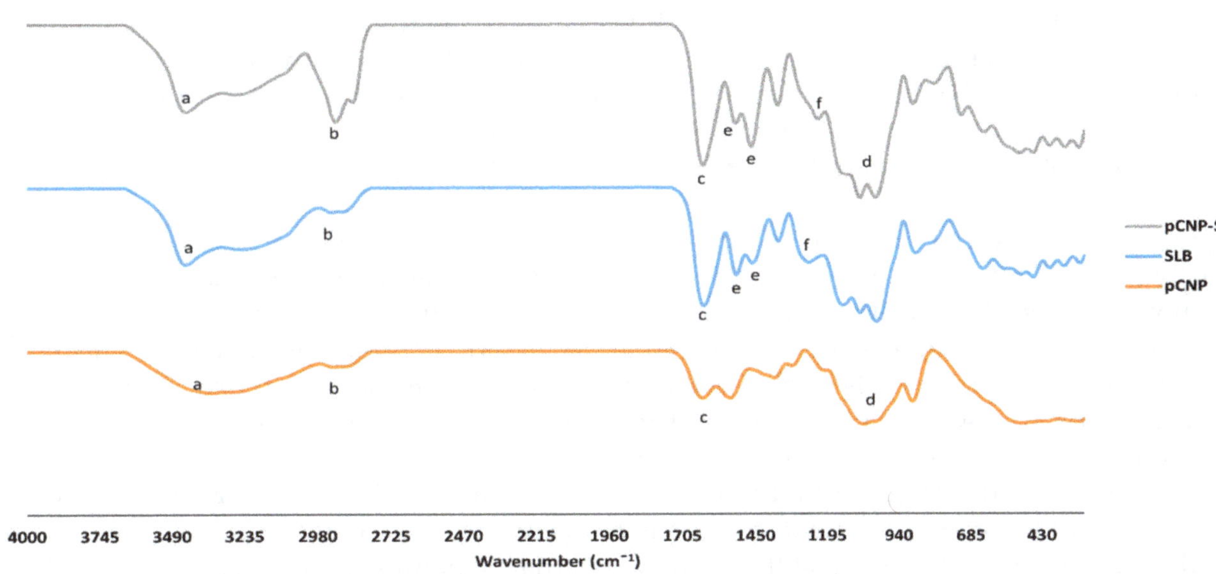

Figure 6. FTIR spectra of pCNP, SLB and pCNP-SLB. The characteristic functional groups are labeled for (**a**) amine group, (**b**) alkyl group, (**c**) carbonyl group, (**d**) inorganic phosphate group, (**e**) aromatic ring and (**f**) ether group.

Table 2. The functional groups present in pCNP, SLB and pCNP-SLB. All the characteristic functional groups of pCNP, SLB and pCNP-SLB are listed in the table at their respective wavenumber and percentage of transmittance.

Functional Group	Wavelength	Percentage Transmittance	Sample
Amine (a) (N–H)	3353	49.62	pCNP
	3446	49.98	SLB
	3416	85.97	pCNP-SLB
Alkyl group (b) (–CH, CH_2)	2888	80.94	pCNP
	2936	88.91	SLB
	2851	24.92	pCNP-SLB
Carbonyl group (c) (C=O)	1632	42.10	pCNP
	1626	12.62	SLB
	1635	71.46	pCNP-SLB
Inorganic Phosphate (d) (P=O)	1067	10	pCNP
	1081	40.15	pCNP-SLB
Aromatic ring (e) (C=C)	1507 & 1461	38.53 & 30.42	SLB
	1536 & 1465	81.63 & 41.83	pCNP-SLB
Ether (f) (C–O–C)	1268	10	SLB
	1223	67.95	pCNP-SLB

The characteristic functional groups are labeled for (**a**) amine group, (**b**) alkyl group, (**c**) carbonyl group, (**d**) inorganic phosphate group, (**e**) aromatic ring and (**f**) ether group.

2.6. CNP and pCNP Cytotoxicity in A549 Cell Lines

CNP is generally considered as non-cytotoxic to cells, due to its proven biodegradable and biocompatible properties [43]. In order to assess the effectiveness of its hydrophobically-modified counterpart, pCNP as a safe carrier for SLB delivery, an MTT cytotoxicity assay was performed in the A549 cell line against the nanoparticle system. MTT is used to assess initial cytotoxicity because we need to ensure that that vectors itself do not exert cytotoxicity effects. After incubation, those metabolically-active viable cells will produce purple formazon salts and can be read at 570 nm by using a spectrophotometer as an indicator for viable cells [44].

Figure 7 shows the viability of A549 cells after being treated by CNP and pCNP to compare the cytotoxicity of pCNP after hydrophobic modification, and the results demonstrate a similar cytotoxicity effect by both carriers where no IC_{50} was found. As mentioned in the previous study of Masarudin [45] there is no significant deviation between CNP and pCNP in term of size, morphology and also content. Thus, we also assumed that there is no substantial difference in terms of the cytotoxicity effect, and this was postulated by the results. It is important to verify the non-toxic effects of pCNP so that the delivery efficacy of SLB will not be affected by the vector in the later assay. The previous study of Zhang et al. [46] utilized hydrophobically-modified oleoyl-chitosan (OCH) as carriers for doxorubicin, and the vector did not confer cytotoxicity effects to A549 cell lines, which is similar to our results. Besides this, the study of Chiu et al. [47], also revealed that N-palmitoyl chitosan nanoparticles with different degrees of substitution had no significant cytotoxicity effect in HT1080 cells, which further indicated that pCNP is a good candidate for a delivery vector.

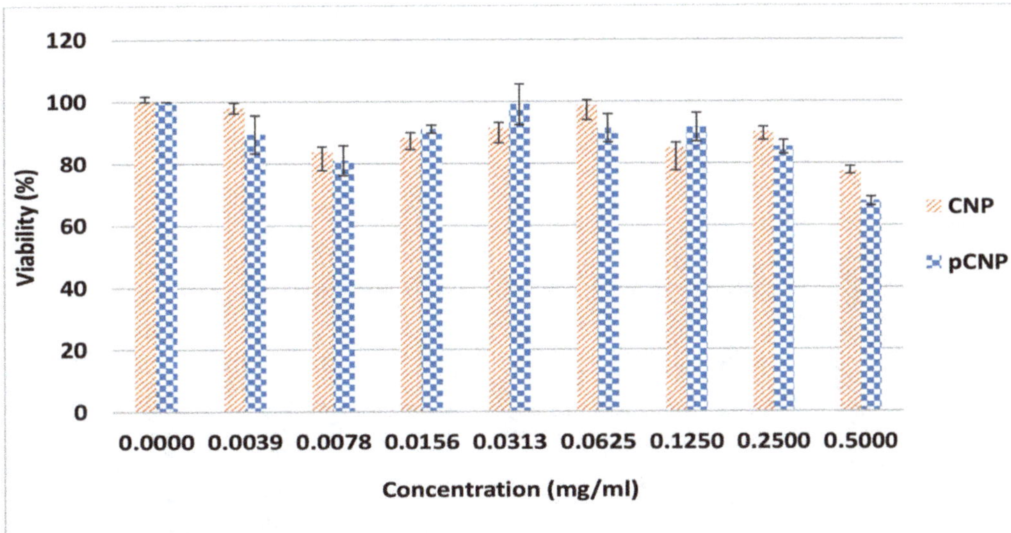

Figure 7. The percentage of viability assessed by CNP and pCNP using an MTT assay. CNP and pCNP have similar cytotoxicity effects where no IC_{50} was found. Data are presented as mean ± SEM from three independent experiments. One-way ANOVA was performed with $p = 0.1097$, which indicated that both CNP and pCNP had no significant difference in cytotoxicity effect in A549 cell lines. The experiment was not conducted with a further time point study because it showed no cytotoxicity effects in the 24 h study.

2.7. Nanoparticle-Mediated Cell Cytotoxicity of SLB CNP-SLB and pCNP-SLB in A549 Cell Lines

The MTT assay was repeated to assess the efficacy of SLB in A549 cells using CNP-SLB and pCNP-SLB systems to discern whether a nanoparticle-mediated delivery system can augment its in vitro efficiency. Approximately 300 μM of SLB was used for the encapsulation of CNP and pCNP to form CNP-SLB and pCNP-SLB, as suggested by the study of Mateen et al. [48], where 10–75 μM of SLB was able to inhibit the cell growth of non-small cell lung cancer (NSCLC) [49]. Based on the E.E data obtained from Table 1, both CNP-SLB and pCNP-SLB contained approximately 75 μM (24.57% E.E) and 150 μM (49.34% E.E) of SLB respectively, and the final concentration for cell treatment was 37.5 μM. Figure 8 shows the percentage of cell viability for cells treated with SLB, CNP-SLB, and pCNP-SLB, which generally revealed a substantial improvement in efficacy for SLB delivered using CNP and pCNP 48 h post treatment. Since the concentration of SLB encapsulated in pCNP was two-fold greater compared to CNP, it was initially thought that a lower IC50 would be obtained 48 h post-treatment. The IC_{50} calculated was 18.36 μM and 18.69 μM for CNP-SLB and pCNP-SLB, respectively. At this time point, the difference is thought to be less significant between CNP and its hydrophobically-modified version.

Interestingly, after 72 h of treatment, the IC_{50} for pCNP-SLB decreased to 6.058 μM, and that of CNP-SLB decreased to 12.77 μM, which is about 211% difference, as shown in Figure 9. This change was postulated to demonstrate the effectiveness of using pCNP as a controlled-release carrier, where the SLB was shown to be released slowly from the nanoparticle core upon treatment. Consequently, the efficacy of SLB for the first 48 h post-treatment was similar for both CNP and pCNP systems, but significantly differed for treatment of 72 h. This was most probably due to the fact that most of the SLB encapsulated in CNP was fully released at 48 h post-treatment, compared to pCNP, due to a greater association of SLB to the hydrophobic core in pCNP. This suggests that pCNP is great candidate for controlled-release properties, coupled with a higher % E.E for SLB. A previous study by Mateen et al. [48] demonstrated that an SLB treatment of 10–75 μM will cause growth inhibition in large cell carcinoma cells (H1299 and H460) and a bronchioalveolar carcinoma cell line (H322), which is similar to the findings of our study. However, the results of SLB delivery was improved by using pCNP, which shown by the low IC_{50}.

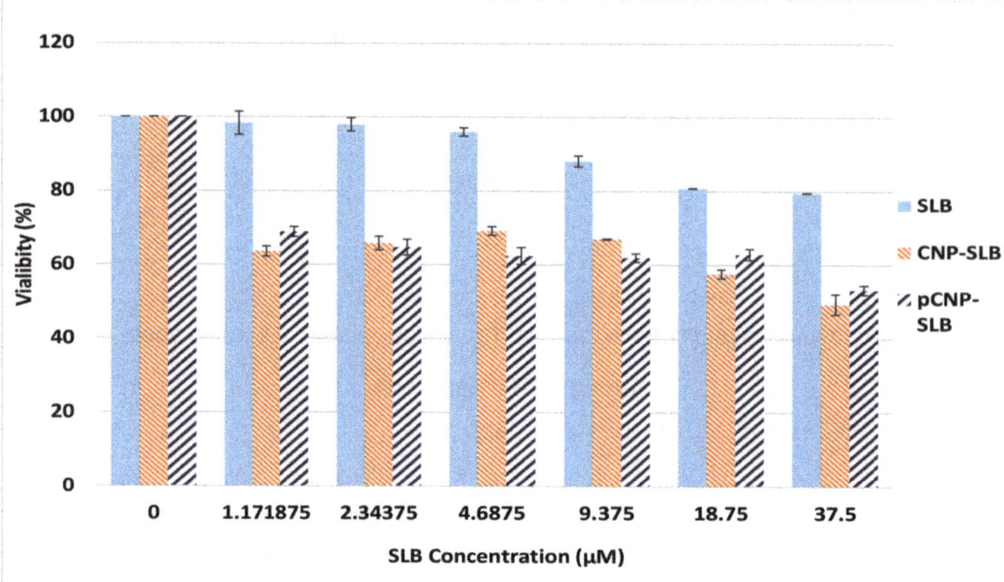

Figure 8. Cytotoxic effect of SLB, CNP-SLB and pCNP-SLB after 48 h of treatment. A similar SLB efficacy for CNP-SLB and pCNP-SLB was observed where both are significantly higher than SLB alone. Data are presented as mean ± SEM from three independent experiments. One-way ANOVA was performed with a p value below 0.05 for both between SLB and CNP-SLB and between SLB and pCNP-SLB, which indicated a significant difference of efficacy between SLB alone and SLB delivered by vector, and $p = 0.9995$ between CNP-SLB and pCNP-SLB, which indicated no significant difference of efficacy between them.

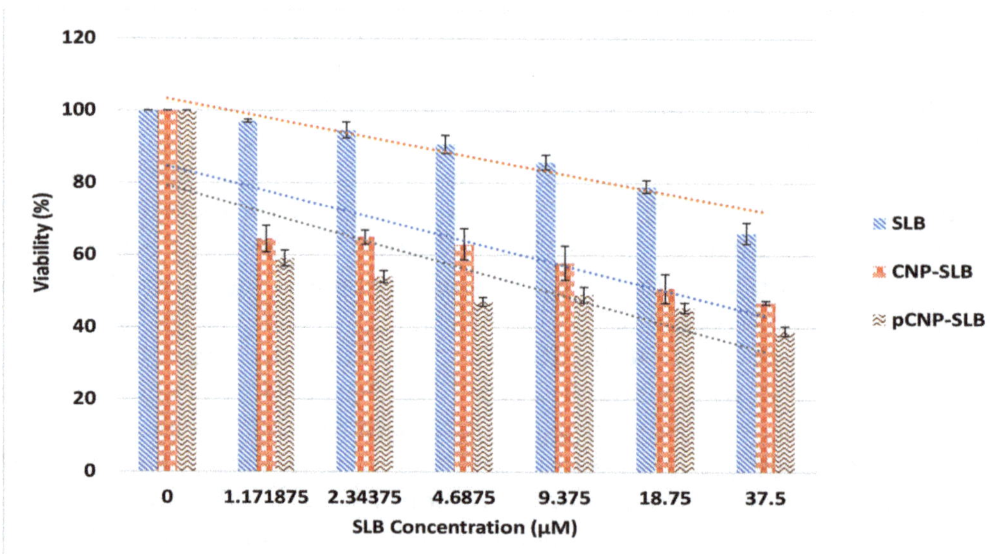

Figure 9. Cytotoxic effect of SLB, CNP-SLB and pCNP-SLB after 72 h of treatment. The highest efficacy was shown by pCNP-SLB, followed by CNP-SLB and SLB alone. Data are presented as mean ± SEM from three independent experiments. A one-way ANOVA was performed and a p value below 0.05 indicated a significant difference of efficacy between them.

The incorporation of palmitic acid into CNP formed pCNP, which provides a hydrophobic anchor to associate with SLB through a hydrophobic-hydrophobic interaction. As proposed by Masarudin [45], a higher drug efficacy was obtained when [^{14}C]-doxorubicin was delivered using pCNP compared to CNP as a carrier, which is comparable with the results in this study. The pCNP was able to achieve a higher % E.E when more SLB was encapsulated into the hydrophobic core, attributed to the hydrophobic-hydrophobic interaction and then delivered and released in a slower manner for longer duration compared to CNP. This explained why the efficacy of SLB for the first 48 h post treatment was similar, but differed considerably for the treatment of 72 h.

3. Materials and Methods

Chitosan (CS, low molecular weight), sodium tripolyphosphate (TPP), palmitic acid N-hydroxy-succinimide ester (NHS-palmitate), silibinin and dimethyl sulfoxide (DMSO) were acquired in powder form from Sigma-Aldrich (St. Louis, MO, USA). Roswell Park Memorial Institute-1640 medium (RPMI-1640), fetal bovine serum (FBS), 0.25% trypsin-EDTA (1×) and Antibiotic-Antimycotic (100×) were purchased from Gibco Life Technologies (Grand island, NY, USA). Glacial acetic acid, sodium hydroxide and hydrochloric acid (analytical grade) were obtained from Friendemann Schmidt Chemicals (Parkwood, Western Australia). Absolute ethanol was purchased from Nacalai Tesque, Inc. (Kyoto, Japan). All reagents, unless otherwise stated, were used without further purification.

3.1. *Synthesis of Chitosan Nanoparticles (CNP) and Palmitoyl Chitosan Nanoparticles (pCNP)*

3.1.1. Chitosan Nanoparticles (CNP)

CNPs were synthesized by ionic gelation methods as described by Masarudin et al. (2015) [29]. CS and TPP were prepared to a concentration of 1.0 mg/mL in 50 mL centrifuge tubes before subsequently diluted to 0.5 mg/mL and 0.7 mg/mL respectively, and adjusted to pH 5 and pH 2 using 1 M NaOH and 1 M HCl. The CNPs were formed by adding increasing volumes of TPP solution (0 μL to 300 μL) to 600 μL of CS solution. The CNPs were then purified by centrifugation at 13,000 rpm for 20 min. After centrifugation, 40% of the total CNP supernatant volume were mixed with 60% of deionized water (dH_2O) corresponding to the 40% supernatant volume and utilized for further analyses.

3.1.2. Hydrophobically-Modified Chitosan Nanoparticles (pCNP)

The 1.0 mg/mL CS was prepared as mentioned above and adjusted to pH 6. Separately, NHS-palmitate was prepared in absolute ethanol to a concentration of 0.9 mg/mL. NHS-palmitate was then added to the CS solution through dropwise addition at a 2:1 volume ratio, before being left to react for 20 h at 50 °C. Following incubation, the hydrophobically-modified chitosan (pCS) was precipitated from the solution by adjusting the pH to pH 9. The precipitate was subsequently separated from the solution by centrifugation at 4000 rpm for 45 min. The precipitate was washed once with a solution of acetone: ethanol (50:50) and then thrice with dH_2O, and left to dry in the oven. The pCS was then used to prepare pCNP using similar methods as previously described for CNP.

3.1.3. Synthesis of Silibinin-Encapsulated pCNP (pCNP-SLB)

5 mg of Silibinin was dissolved in 50% DMSO and 50% dH_2O to prepare a 10 mM master stock. It was then further diluted by mixing 100 μL of master stock with 100 μL of dH_2O until it became 5 mM and was added dropwise to 600 μL of pCS with continuous mixing until a final concentration of 300 μM was then added with 200 μL of TPP.

3.2. Physicochemical Characterization of Nanoparticle Samples

3.2.1. Analysis of Particle Size Distribution and Polydispersity

The size and distribution of synthesized CNPs, pCNPs, CNP-SLB and pCNP-SLB were ascertained using dynamic light scattering on a Malvern Zetasizer Nano S Instrument (Malvern Instruments, Worcestershire, UK). About 1000 µL of samples was loaded into a disposable cuvette, and the particle size was measured in triplicate readings for each sample to ensure the stability of the sample. All data were recorded as mean ± standard error of mean (SEM). The significant alteration of particle sizes between the CNP and pCNP samples was subsequently evaluated by one way analysis of variance (ANOVA), with a p value < 0.05 considered as significant.

3.2.2. Morphological and Surface Topological Analyses

The surface morphologies and size of pCNP and pCNP-SLB were further examined using field-emission scanning electron microscopy (FESEM) analysis. Nanoparticles were diluted prior to analysis by mixing 100 µL of samples with 500 µL of dH_2O. A drop of each diluted samples was then placed onto an aluminum stub and left to dry in an oven for three days. The sample-loaded stubs were then gold-coated in a vacuum before being observed under an electron microscope (FEI NOVA nanoSEM 230, Thermo Fisher, Hillsboro, OR, USA).

3.2.3. Fourier Transform Infrared (FTIR) Analysis with Attenuated Total Reflectance (ATR-FTIR)

FTIR analysis was performed for SLB, pCNP and pCNP-SLB samples. Prior to analysis, the samples were freeze dried using a Coolsafe 95-15 PRO freeze drier (ScanVac, Lynge, Denmark) for 48 h. Next, the samples in powder form was analyzed using a Spectrum 100 (Perkin Elmer, Waltham, MA, USA) using the attenuated total reflectance (ATR) method at an infrared frequency range of 200 to 4000 cm^{-1}.

3.3. Determination of Free Amine Groups in Nanoparticle Samples Using the 2,4,6-Trinitrobenzene Sulfonic Assay

Prior to the assay, 0.05% (v/v) TNBS reagent, 0.1 M $NaHCO_3$, 10% (w/v) SDS and 1.0 M HCl were prepared in a 15 mL centrifuge tube. CS standards were prepared by serially diluting 50 µL of 0.5 mg/mL CS solution using 0.1 M $NaHCO_3$. Approximately 50 µL of 0.05% (v/v) TNBS solution was then added to each sample in Eppendorf tubes. pCS standards were subsequently prepared using similar methods as for CS. Next, 100 µL of nanoparticle samples at different TPP volume additions were aliquoted into Eppendorf tubes and mixed with 100 µL 0.05% (v/v) TNBS solution. All the standard and sample tubes were then incubated for 3 h at 37 °C. Following incubation, 100 µL of the standard/samples were transferred into a 96-well plate. Approximately 100 µL of 10% SDS and 75 µL of 1 M HCl were added into each well and mixed, and the absorbance was read at a wavelength of 405 nm. The utilized amine percentage was then calculated using the following equation:

$$\text{Free amine percentage (\%)} = \frac{A_{405} \text{ of CNP /pCNP}}{\begin{array}{c} A_{405} \text{ of CS/pCS} \\ \text{(at same concentration used)} \end{array}} \times 100\% \quad (1)$$

The significant alteration of utilized amine percentage of CNP and pCNP samples was subsequently evaluated by paired t-test, with a p value < 0.05 considered as significant.

3.4. Encapsulation Efficiency of Silibinin in Nanoparticle Samples

The encapsulation efficiency (% EE) was calculated by comparing the difference in absorbance at 288 nm between free SLB and the supernatant of encapsulated SLB. The CNP-SLB and pCNP-SLB samples were centrifuged at 13,000 rpm for 20 min. The supernatant was then collected and the absorbance at

288 nm was read using a UV/VIS spectrophotometer (NP80, Implen, München, Germany). The % EE was then calculated using the following equation:

$$\% \text{ EE} = \frac{A_{288}\text{of free SLB} - A_{288} \text{ of SLB in supernatant}}{A_{288} \text{ of free SLB}} \times 100\% \quad (2)$$

The absorbance of free SLB at 288 nm was used to deduct the absorbance of SLB that remained in the supernatant post-encapsulation and divided by the absorbance of free SLB, then multiplied by 100 percent to get the percentage of encapsulation (% E.E).

3.5. Determination of In Vitro Cellular Efficacy Using Nanoparticle-Mediated Delivery of Silibinin

The A549 cell line was established by culturing in a T-25 flask with growth media consisting of 90% of 1× RPMI medium 1640 and 10% FBS. Approximately 100 µL of cells were seeded into a 96-wells plate. Cells were seeded at a density of 7×10^3 cells per well for 48-h treatments and 4×10^3 for 72-h treatment, whilst cells were treated with 100 µL of CNP, pCNP, SLB, CNP-SLB and pCNP-SLB. At the end of each time point, the wells were decanted and replaced with 170 µL fresh growth media. Separately, 5 mg/mL MTT solution was prepared in 1× PBS and sterilely filtered with 0.22 µm nylon filter. Approximately 30 µL of the MTT solution was then added into each well, mixed and incubated for a further 4 h. Following incubation, 150 µL of solution was removed and 100 µL of DMSO was added to each well. The absorbance was then read at 570 nm using a Bio-Rad iMark™ Microplate Absorbance Reader (Bio-Rad, Hercules, CA, USA). Cell viability was determined using the following equation:

$$\% \text{ viability} = \frac{A_{570} \text{ of treated cells}}{A_{570} \text{ of untreated cells}} \times 100\% \quad (3)$$

The significant efficacy of nanoparticles, SLB and SLB-encapsulated nanoparticles was subsequently evaluated by one way analysis of variance (ANOVA), with a p value < 0.05 considered as significant.

4. Conclusions

The present study showed the successful hydrophobic-modification of CNP and encapsulation of SLB. In addition, pCNP was found to be a better delivery vector compared to CNP due to the incorporation of NHS-palmitic acid, which is non-toxic and possesses a hydrophobic-hydrophobic interaction with SLB, achieving a higher encapsulation efficiency and higher efficacy effect in the A549 cell line compared to CNP. Hence, the pCNP system established in this study shows great potential for imminent customization and studies as a delivery vector, especially for low bioavailability drugs for cancer therapeutics.

Acknowledgments: The author Cha Yee Kuen would like to acknowledge Universiti Putra Malaysia (UPM) for provisions of a Graduate Research Fellowship. The author Mas Jaffri Masarudin would like to acknowledge Universiti Putra Malaysia for research funding under the UPM-IPB funds Vot No. 9425801 to conduct this research.

Author Contributions: Cha Yee Kuen and Mas Jaffri Masarudin conceived and designed the experiments; Cha Yee Kuen performed the experiments; Sharida Fakurazi, Siti Sarah Othman and Mas Jaffri Masarudin analyzed the data and contributed reagents/materials/analysis tools; Cha Yee Kuen wrote the paper. All authors read and edited the paper before submission.

References

1. Chalasani, S.; Prakash, K.V.; Pulla, R.P.; Tekula, R.; Manasa, E.; Umasankar, B. Development and validation of doxorubicin hcl in bulk and its pharmaceutical dosage form by visible spectrophotometry. *Int. J. Pharm. Sci.* **2013**, *3*, 216–218.
2. Wellington, K.; Jarvis, B. Silymarin: A review of its clinical properties in the management of hepatic disorders. *BioDrugs* **2001**, *15*, 465–489. [CrossRef] [PubMed]

3. Kim, N.C.; Graf, T.N.; Sparacino, C.M.; Wani, M.C.; Wall, M.E. Complete isolation and characterization of silybins and isosilybins from milk thistle (*Silybum marianum*). *Org. Biomol. Chem.* **2003**, *1*, 1684–1689. [CrossRef] [PubMed]
4. Tyagi, N.; De, R.; Begun, J.; Popat, A. Cancer therapeutics with epigallocatechin-3-gallate encapsulated in biopolymeric nanoparticles. *Int. J. Pharm.* **2017**, *518*, 220–227. [CrossRef] [PubMed]
5. Ramasamy, K.; Agarwal, R. Multitargeted therapy of cancer by silymarin. *Cancer Lett.* **2008**, *269*, 352–362. [CrossRef] [PubMed]
6. Mateen, S.; Raina, K.; Agarwal, R. Chemopreventive and Anti-cancer Efficacy of Silibinin against Growth and Progression of Lung Cancer. *Nutr. Cancer* **2013**, *65*, 3–11. [CrossRef] [PubMed]
7. Sharma, G.; Singh, R.P.; Chan, D.C.; Agarwal, R. Silibinin induces growth inhibition and apoptotic cell death in human lung carcinoma cells. *Anticancer Res.* **2003**, *23*, 2649–2655. [PubMed]
8. Chu, S.C.; Chiou, H.L.; Chen, P.N.; Yang, S.F.; Hsieh, Y.S. Silibinin inhibits the invasion of human lung cancer cells via decreased productions of urokinase-plasminogen activator and matrix metalloproteinase-2. *Mol. Carcinog.* **2004**, *40*, 143–149. [CrossRef] [PubMed]
9. Mohan, S.; Dhanalakshmi, S.; Mallikarjuna, G.U.; Singh, R.P.; Agarwal, R. Silibinin modulates UVB-induced apoptosis via mitochondrial proteins, caspases activation, and mitogen-activated protein kinase signaling in human epidermoid carcinoma A431 cells. *Biochem. Biophys. Res. Commun.* **2004**, *320*, 183–189. [CrossRef] [PubMed]
10. Dhanalakshmi, S.; Mallikarjuna, G.U.; Singh, R.P.; Agarwal, R. Dual efficacy of silibinin in protecting or enhancing ultraviolet B radiation-caused apoptosis in HaCaT human immortalized keratinocytes. *Carcinogenesis* **2004**, *25*, 99–106. [CrossRef] [PubMed]
11. Deep, G.; Agarwal, R. Anti-metastatic Efficacy of Silibinin: Molecular Mechanisms and Therapeutic Potential against Cancer. *Cancer Metastasis Rev.* **2010**, *29*, 447–463. [CrossRef] [PubMed]
12. Ting, H.; Deep, G.; Agarwal, R. Molecular Mechanisms of Silibinin-Mediated Cancer Chemoprevention with Major Emphasis on Prostate Cancer. *AAPS J.* **2013**, *15*, 707–716. [CrossRef] [PubMed]
13. Kumar, S.; Raina, K.; Agarwal, C.; Agarwal, R. Silibinin strongly inhibits the growth kinetics of colon cancer stem cell-enriched spheroids by modulating interleukin 4/6-mediated survival signals. *Oncotarget* **2014**, *5*, 4972–4989. [CrossRef] [PubMed]
14. Wu, K.; Ning, Z.; Zeng, J.; Fan, J.; Zhou, J.; Zhang, T.; Zhang, L.; Chen, Y.; Gao, Y.; Wang, B.; et al. Silibinin inhibits β-catenin/ZEB1 signaling and suppresses bladder cancer metastasis via dual-blocking epithelial-mesenchymal transition and stemness. *Cell Signal.* **2013**, *25*, 2625–2633. [CrossRef] [PubMed]
15. Morazzoni, P.; Bombardelli, E. Silybum marianum (*Carduus marianus*). *Fitoterapia* **1995**, *66*, 3–42.
16. Basaga, H.; Poll, G.; Tekkaya, C.; Aras, I. Free radical scavenging and antioxidative properties of "silibin" complexs on microsomal lipid peroxidation. *Cell Biochem. Funct.* **1997**, *15*, 27–33. [CrossRef]
17. Skottov, N.; Kreeman, V.; Vaoa, R.; Chmela, Z.; Ulrichov, J.; Simanek, V. Effect of silymarin and silibinin-phosphatidylcholine complex on plasma and lipoprotein cholesterol, and oxidation of LDL in rats fed on high cholesterol diet supplemented with current oil. *Acta Univ. Palacki. Olomuc. Fac. Med.* **2000**, *144*, 55–58. [CrossRef]
18. Leena, R.S.; Vairamani, M.; Selvamurugan, N. Alginate/Gelatin scaffolds incorporated with Silibinin-loaded Chitosan nanoparticles for bone formation in vitro. *Colloids Surf. B Biointerfaces* **2017**, *158*, 308–318. [CrossRef] [PubMed]
19. Kidd, P.; Head, K. A review of the bioavailability and clinical efficacy of milk thistle phytosome: A silybin-phosphatidylcholine complex (Siliphos). *Altern. Med. Rev.* **2005**, *10*, 193–203. [PubMed]
20. Zhang, J.Q.; Liu, X.; Li, X.L.; Jasti, B.R. Preparation and Characterization of Solid Lipid Nanoparticles Containing Silibinin. *Drug Deliv.* **2007**, *14*, 381–387. [CrossRef] [PubMed]
21. Yang, G.; Zhao, Y.; Feng, N.; Zhang, Y.; Liu, Y.; Dang, B. Improved dissolution and bioavailability of silymarin delivered by a solid dispersion prepared using supercritical fluids. *Asian J. Pharm. Sci.* **2015**, *10*, 194–202. [CrossRef]
22. Yanyu, X.; Yunmei, S.; Zhipeng, C.; Qineng, P. The preparation of silybin—Phospholipid complex and the study on its pharmacokinetics in rats. *Int. J. Pharm.* **2006**, *307*, 77–82. [CrossRef] [PubMed]
23. Greish, K. Enhanced permeability and retention (EPR) effect for anticancer nanomedicine drug targeting. *Cancer Nanotechnol.* **2010**, *624*, 25–37.
24. Hirano, S. Chitin and chitosan as novel biotechnological materials. *Polym. Int.* **1999**, *48*, 732–734. [CrossRef]

25. Kang, B.S.; Lee, S.E.; Ng, C.L.; Kim, J.K.; Park, J.S. Exploring the Preparation of Albendazole-Loaded Chitosan-Tripolyphosphate Nanoparticles. *Materials* **2015**, *8*, 486–498. [CrossRef] [PubMed]
26. Chai, F.; Sun, L.; He, X.; Li, J.; Liu, Y.; Xiong, F.; Ge, L.; Webster, T.J.; Zheng, C. Doxorubicin-loaded poly (lactic-co-glycolic acid) nanoparticles coated with chitosan/alginate by layer by layer technology for antitumor applications. *Int. J. Nanomed.* **2017**, *12*, 1791–1802. [CrossRef] [PubMed]
27. Shu, X.Z.; Zhu, K.J. The influence of multivalent phosphate structure on the properties of ionically cross-linked chitosan films for controlled drug release. *Eur. J. Pharm. Biopharm.* **2012**, *54*, 235–243. [CrossRef]
28. Hassan, U.A.; Hussein, M.Z.; Masarudin, M.J. Synthesis of a nanoparticle system for the enhanced accumulation of fluorescently-labelled amino acids encapsulated in monodispersed chitosan nanoparticle system. *Malays. Appl. Biol.* **2017**, *46*, 171–175.
29. Masarudin, M.J.; Cutts, S.M.; Evison, B.J.; Phillips, D.R.; Pigram, P.J. Factors determining the stability, size distribution, and cellular accumulation of small, monodisperse chitosan nanoparticles as candidate vectors for anticancer drug delivery: Application to the passive encapsulation of [^{14}C]-doxorubicin. *Nanotechnol. Sci. Appl.* **2015**, *8*, 67–80. [CrossRef] [PubMed]
30. Ravikumara, N.R.; Madhusudhan, B. Chitosan nanoparticles for tamoxifen delivery and cytotoxicity to MCF-7 and Vero cells. *Pure Appl. Chem.* **2011**, *83*, 2027–2040. [CrossRef]
31. Liu, H.; Gao, C. Preparation and properties of ionically crosslinked chitosan nanoparticles. *Polym. Adv. Technol.* **2009**, *20*, 613–619. [CrossRef]
32. Fan, W.; Yan, W.; Xu, Z.; Ni, H. Formation mechanism of monodisperse, low molecular weight chitosan nanoparticles by ionic gelation technique. *Colloids Surf. B Biointerfaces* **2012**, *90*, 21–27. [CrossRef] [PubMed]
33. Marchiori, M.C.L.; Rigon, C.; Copetti, P.M.; Sagrillo, M.R.; Cruz, L. Nanoencapsulation Improves Scavenging Capacity and Decreases Cytotoxicity of Silibinin and Pomegranate Oil Association. *AAPS PharmSciTech* **2017**, *18*, 3236–3246. [CrossRef] [PubMed]
34. Shankar, G.; Agrawal, Y.K. Formulation and evaluation of polymeric micelles for a poorly absorbed drug. *Res. J. Pharm. Biol. Chem. Sci.* **2015**, *6*, 1314–1321.
35. Singh, R.; Lillard, J.W. Nanoparticle-based targeted drug delivery. *Exp. Mol. Pathol.* **2009**, *86*, 215–223. [CrossRef] [PubMed]
36. Ariff, S.A.Y.; Yusoff, K.; Masarudin, M.J. Encapsulation of mirna in chitosan nanoparticles as a candidate for an anti-metastatic agent in cancer therapy. *Malays. Appl. Biol.* **2017**, *46*, 165–170.
37. Gomathi, T.; Prasad, P.S.; Sudha, P.N.; Anil, S. Size optimization and in vitro biocompatibility studies of chitosan nanoparticles. *Int. J. Biol. Macromol.* **2017**, *104*, 1794–1806.
38. Sahu, S.K.; Maiti, S.; Maiti, T.K.; Ghosh, S.K.; Pramanik, P. Hydrophobically modified carboxymethyl chitosan nanoparticles targeted delivery of paclitaxel. *J. Drug Target.* **2010**, *19*, 104–113. [CrossRef] [PubMed]
39. Mohammadpour, D.N.; Eskandari, R.; Avadi, M.R.; Zolfagharian, H.; Mir Mohammad Sadeghi, A.; Rezayat, M. Preparation and in vitro characterization of chitosan nanoparticles containing Mesobuthus eupeus scorpion venom as an antigen delivery system. *J. Venom. Anim. Toxins Incl. Trop. Dis.* **2012**, *18*, 44–52.
40. Kafshgari, M.H.; Khorram, M.; Khodadoost, M.; Khavari, S. Reinforcement of Chitosan Nanoparticles Obtained by and Ionic Cross-Linking Process. *Iran. Polym. J.* **2011**, *20*, 445–456.
41. Gomathi, T.; Govindarajan, C.; Rose, H.R.M.H.; Sudha, P.N.; Imran, P.K.; Venkatesan, J.; Kim, S.K. Studies on drug-polymer interaction, in vitro release and cytotoxicity from chitosan particles excipient. *Int. J. Pharm.* **2014**, *468*, 214–222. [CrossRef] [PubMed]
42. Tan, J.M.; Karthivashan, G.; Gani, S.A.; Fakurazi, S.; Hussein, M.Z. In vitro drug release characteristic and cytotoxic activity of silibinin-loaded single walled carbon nanotubes functionalized with biocompatible polymers. *Chem. Cent. J.* **2016**, *10*, 81. [CrossRef] [PubMed]
43. Nagpal, K.; Singh, S.K.; Mishra, D.N. Chitosan Nanoparticles: A Promising System in Novel Drug Delivery. *Chem. Pharm. Bull.* **2010**, *58*, 1423–1430. [CrossRef] [PubMed]
44. Riss, T.L.; Moravec, R.A.; Niles, A.L.; Duellman, S.; Benink, H.A.; Worzella, T.J.; Minor, L. Cell Viability Assays. In *Assay Guidance Manual*; Eli Lilly & Company and the National Centre for Advancing Translational Sciences: Bethesda, MD, USA, 2013.
45. Masarudin, M.J. Chitosan Nanoparticles as a Delivery Vehicle for [^{14}C]-Doxorubicin and the Formaldehyde Releasing Prodrug AN-250. Ph.D. Thesis, La Trobe University, Bundoora, Australia, 2012.
46. Zhang, J.; Chen, X.G.; Li, Y.Y.; Liu, C.S. Self-assembled nanoparticles based on hydrophobically modified chitosan as carriers for doxorubicin. *Nanomed. Nanotechnol. Biol. Med.* **2007**, *3*, 258–265. [CrossRef] [PubMed]

47. Chiu, Y.L.; Ho, Y.C.; Chen, Y.M.; Peng, S.F.; Ke, C.J.; Chen, K.J.; Mi, F.L.; Sung, H.W. The characteristics, cellular uptake and intracellular trafficking of nanoparticles made of hydrophobically-modified chitosan. *J. Control. Release* **2010**, *146*, 152–159. [CrossRef] [PubMed]
48. Mateen, S.; Tyagi, A.; Agarwal, C.; Singh, R.P.; Agarwal, R. Silibinin inhibits human nonsmall cell lung cancer cell growth through cell-cycle arrest by modulating expression and function of key cell-cycle regulators. *Mol. Carcinog.* **2010**, *49*, 247–258. [CrossRef] [PubMed]
49. Wang, Y.; Li, P.; Truong-Dinh Tran, T.; Zhang, J.; Kong, L. Manufacturing Techniques and Surface Engineering of Polymer Based Nanoparticles for Targeted Drug Delivery to Cancer. *Nanomaterials* **2016**, *6*, 26. [CrossRef] [PubMed]

Permissions

All chapters in this book were first published by MDPI; hereby published with permission under the Creative Commons Attribution License or equivalent. Every chapter published in this book has been scrutinized by our experts. Their significance has been extensively debated. The topics covered herein carry significant findings which will fuel the growth of the discipline. They may even be implemented as practical applications or may be referred to as a beginning point for another development.

The contributors of this book come from diverse backgrounds, making this book a truly international effort. This book will bring forth new frontiers with its revolutionizing research information and detailed analysis of the nascent developments around the world.

We would like to thank all the contributing authors for lending their expertise to make the book truly unique. They have played a crucial role in the development of this book. Without their invaluable contributions this book wouldn't have been possible. They have made vital efforts to compile up to date information on the varied aspects of this subject to make this book a valuable addition to the collection of many professionals and students.

This book was conceptualized with the vision of imparting up-to-date information and advanced data in this field. To ensure the same, a matchless editorial board was set up. Every individual on the board went through rigorous rounds of assessment to prove their worth. After which they invested a large part of their time researching and compiling the most relevant data for our readers.

The editorial board has been involved in producing this book since its inception. They have spent rigorous hours researching and exploring the diverse topics which have resulted in the successful publishing of this book. They have passed on their knowledge of decades through this book. To expedite this challenging task, the publisher supported the team at every step. A small team of assistant editors was also appointed to further simplify the editing procedure and attain best results for the readers.

Apart from the editorial board, the designing team has also invested a significant amount of their time in understanding the subject and creating the most relevant covers. They scrutinized every image to scout for the most suitable representation of the subject and create an appropriate cover for the book.

The publishing team has been an ardent support to the editorial, designing and production team. Their endless efforts to recruit the best for this project, has resulted in the accomplishment of this book. They are a veteran in the field of academics and their pool of knowledge is as vast as their experience in printing. Their expertise and guidance has proved useful at every step. Their uncompromising quality standards have made this book an exceptional effort. Their encouragement from time to time has been an inspiration for everyone.

The publisher and the editorial board hope that this book will prove to be a valuable piece of knowledge for researchers, students, practitioners and scholars across the globe.

List of Contributors

Yana Zorkina and Anna Morozova
Department Basic and Applied Neurobiology, V.P. Serbsky Federal Medical Research Centre of Psychiatry and Narcology, 119034 Moscow, Russia
Healthcare Department, Mental-Health Clinic No. 1 Named after N.A. Alexeev of Moscow, 117152 Moscow, Russia

Olga Abramova, Eugene Zubkov, Marat Valikhov and Pavel Melnikov
Department Basic and Applied Neurobiology, V.P. Serbsky Federal Medical Research Centre of Psychiatry and Narcology, 119034 Moscow, Russia

Valeriya Ushakova
Department Basic and Applied Neurobiology, V.P. Serbsky Federal Medical Research Centre of Psychiatry and Narcology, 119034 Moscow, Russia
Department of Biology, Lomonosov Moscow State University, 119992 Moscow, Russia

Alexander Majouga
D. Mendeleev University of Chemical Technology of Russia, 125047 Moscow, Russia

Vladimir Chekhonin
Department Basic and Applied Neurobiology, V.P. Serbsky Federal Medical Research Centre of Psychiatry and Narcology, 119034 Moscow, Russia
Department of Medical Nanobiotechnology, Pirogov Russian National Research Medical University, 117997 Moscow, Russia

Reema Narayan and Usha Y. Nayak
Department of Pharmaceutics, Manipal College of Pharmaceutical Sciences, Manipal Academy of Higher Education, Manipal 576104, India

Ashok M. Raichur
Department of Materials Engineering, Indian Institute of Science, Bengaluru 560012, India

Sanjay Garg
School of Pharmacy and Medical Science, University of South Australia, Adelaide, SA 5000, Australia

Eline Teirlinck, Jing Liu, Juan C. Fraire, Ranhua Xiong, Katrien Forier and Stefaan C. De Smedt
Laboratory of General Biochemistry and Physical Pharmacy, University of Ghent, 9000 Ghent, Belgium
Centre for Nano- and Biophotonics, 9000 Ghent, Belgium

Alexandre Barras, Chengnan Li and Rabah Boukherroub
Univ. Lille, CNRS, Centrale Lille, ISEN, Univ. Valenciennes, UMR 8520—IEMN, 59000 Lille, France

Tatu Lajunen
Drug Research Program, Faculty of Pharmacy, University of Helsinki, Viikinkaari 5 E, 00790 Helsinki, Finland

Arto Urtti
Drug Research Program, Faculty of Pharmacy, University of Helsinki, Viikinkaari 5 E, 00790 Helsinki, Finland
School of Pharmacy, University of Eastern Finland, Yliopistonranta 1, 70211 Kuopio, Finland
Laboratory of Biohybrid Technologies, Institute of Chemistry, St. Petersburg State University, Universitetskii pr. 26, Peterhoff, St. 198504 Petersburg, Russia

Tom Coenye
Laboratory of Pharmaceutical Microbiology, University of Ghent, 9000 Ghent, Belgium

Kevin Braeckmans
Laboratory of General Biochemistry and Physical Pharmacy, University of Ghent, 9000 Ghent, Belgium
Centre for Nano- and Biophotonics, 9000 Ghent, Belgium
Univ. Lille, CNRS, Centrale Lille, ISEN, Univ. Valenciennes, UMR 8520—IEMN, 59000 Lille, France

Flavio Nucciarelli
Physics Department, Lancaster University, Lancaster LA1 4YB, UK
Grupo de Electrónica y Semiconductores, Departamento de Física Aplicada, Universidad Autónoma de Madrid, 28049 Madrid, Spain

Iria Bravo
Departamento de Química Analítica y Análisis Instrumental, Universidad Autónoma de Madrid, Cantoblanco, 28049 Madrid, Spain
Instituto Madrileño de Estudios Avanzados en Nanociencia (IMDEA-Nanociencia), Faraday, 9, Campus UAM, Cantoblanco, 28049 Madrid, Spain

Sergio Catalan-Gomez and Jose Luis Pau
Grupo de Electrónica y Semiconductores, Departamento de Física Aplicada, Universidad Autónoma de Madrid, 28049 Madrid, Spain

Luis Vázquez
Materials Science Factory, Instituto de Ciencia de Materiales de Madrid, CSIC, 28049 Madrid, Spain

Encarnación Lorenzo
Departamento de Química Analítica y Análisis Instrumental, Universidad Autónoma de Madrid, Cantoblanco, 28049 Madrid, Spain
Instituto Madrileño de Estudios Avanzados en Nanociencia (IMDEA-Nanociencia), Faraday, 9, Campus UAM, Cantoblanco, 28049 Madrid, Spain
Institute for Advanced Research in Chemical Sciences (IAdChem), Universidad Autónoma de Madrid, 28049 Madrid, Spain

Vieri Piazzini, Giulia Graverini, Anna Rita Bilia and Maria Camilla Bergonzi
Department of Chemistry, University of Florence, Via Ugo Schiff 6, Sesto Fiorentino, 50019 Florence, Italy

Elisa Landucci and Domenico E. Pellegrini-Giampietro
Department of Health Sciences, Section of Clinical Pharmacology and Oncology, University of Florence, Viale Pieraccini 6, 50139 Florence, Italy

Elita Montanari, Chiara Di Meo, Tommasina Coviello and Pietro Matricardi
Department of Drug Chemistry and Technologies, Sapienza University of Rome, P.le Aldo Moro 5, 00185 Rome, Italy

Virginie Gueguen and Graciela Pavon-Djavid
INSERM U1148, Laboratory for Vascular Translational Science, Cardiovascular Bioengineering, Paris 13 University, Sorbonne Paris Cite 99, Av. Jean-Baptiste Clément, 93430 Villetaneuse, France

Jieru Qiu
Department of Radiology, Shanghai Tenth People's Hospital, Tongji University School of Medicine, Shanghai 200072, China
College of Chemistry, Chemical Engineering and Biotechnology, Donghua University, Shanghai 201620, China

Lingdan Kong, Xueyan Cao, Aijun Li, Ping Wei and Lu Wang
Department of Radiology, Shanghai Tenth People's Hospital, Tongji University School of Medicine, Shanghai 200072, China

Serge Mignani
Université Paris Descartes, PRES Sorbonne Paris Cité, CNRS UMR 860, Laboratoire de Chimie et de Biochimie Pharmacologiques et Toxicologique, 45, rue des Saints Peres, 75006 Paris, France
CQM—Centro de Química da Madeira, MMRG, Universidade da Madeira, Campus da Penteada, 9020-105 Funchal, Portugal

Anne-Marie Caminade and Jean-Pierre Majora
Laboratoire de Chimie de Coordination du CNRS, 205 Route de Narbonne, BP 44099, 31077 Toulouse CEDEX 4, France
Université de Toulouse, UPS, INPT, 31077 Toulouse CEDEX 4, France

Xiangyang Shi
Department of Radiology, Shanghai Tenth People's Hospital, Tongji University School of Medicine, Shanghai 200072, China
College of Chemistry, Chemical Engineering and Biotechnology, Donghua University, Shanghai 201620, China
CQM—Centro de Química da Madeira, MMRG, Universidade da Madeira, Campus da Penteada, 9020-105 Funchal, Portugal

Agostina Grillone
Smart Bio-Interfaces, Istituto Italiano di Tecnologia, Viale Rinaldo Piaggio 34, 56025 Pontedera, Italy

Tianshu Li
Research Organization for Nano & Life innovation, Waseda University, 2-2 Wakamatsu-cho, Shinjuku-ku, Tokyo 162-8480, Japan

Matteo Battaglini
Smart Bio-Interfaces, Istituto Italiano di Tecnologia, Viale Rinaldo Piaggio 34, 56025 Pontedera, Italy
The Biorobotics Institute, Scuola Superiore Sant'Anna, Viale Rinaldo Piaggio 34, 56025 Pontedera, Italy

Alice Scarpellini
Electron Microscopy Facility, Istituto Italiano di Tecnologia, Via Morego 30, 16163 Genova, Italy

Mirko Prato
Materials Characterization Facility, Istituto Italiano di Tecnologia, Via Morego 30, 16163 Genova, Italy

Shinji Takeoka
Department of Life Science and Medical Bioscience, Graduate School of Advanced Science and Engineering (TWIns), Waseda University, 2-2 Wakamatsu-cho, Shinjuku-ku, Tokyo 162-8480, Japan

Gianni Ciofani
Smart Bio-Interfaces, Istituto Italiano di Tecnologia, Viale Rinaldo Piaggio 34, 56025 Pontedera, Italy
Department of Mechanical and Aerospace Engineering, Politecnico di Torino, Corso Duca degli Abruzzi 24, 10129 Torino, Italy

Roberto Pinna, Enrica Filigheddu and Giuliana Solinas
Department of Biomedical Sciences, University of Sassari, 07100 Sassari, Italy

Claudia Juliano and Giacomo Petretto
Department of Chemistry and Pharmacy, University of Sassari, 07100 Sassari, Italy

Alessandra Palmieri
Department of Medicine, Surgery and Experimental Science, University of Sassari, 07100 Sassari, Italy

Maria Manconi, Carla Caddeo and Maria Letizia Manca
Department of Life and Environmental Sciences, University of Cagliari, 09124 Cagliari, Italy

Guy D'hallewin
Institute of Science of Food Production UOS Sassari-CNR, 07040 Sassari, Italy

Margherita Maioli
Department of Biomedical Sciences, University of Sassari, 07100 Sassari, Italy
Laboratory of Molecular Biology and Stem Cell Engineering, National Institute of Biostructures and Biosystems, 40129 Bologna, Italy

Antonella Bortone
Dental Unite, Azienda Ospedaliero-Universitaria, 07100 Sassari, Italy

Vincenzo Campanella
Department of Clinical and Translational Medicine, Tor Vergata University of Rome, 00133 Rome, Italy

Egle Milia
Department of Medicine, Surgery and Experimental Science, University of Sassari, 07100 Sassari, Italy
Dental Unite, Azienda Ospedaliero-Universitaria, 07100 Sassari, Italy

Cha Yee Kuen and Mas Jaffri Masarudin
Department of Cell and Molecular Biology, Faculty of Biotechnology and Biomolecular Sciences, Universiti Putra Malaysia, 43400 Serdang, Selangor, Malaysia
Cancer Research Laboratory, Institute of Biosciences, Universiti Putra Malaysia, 43400 Serdang, Selangor, Malaysia

Sharida Fakurazi
Department of Human Anatomy, Faculty of Medicine and Health Sciences, Universiti Putra Malaysia, 43400 Serdang, Selangor, Malaysia

Siti Sarah Othman
Department of Cell and Molecular Biology, Faculty of Biotechnology and Biomolecular Sciences, Universiti Putra Malaysia, 43400 Serdang, Selangor, Malaysia

Index

www.ingramcontent.com/pod-product-compliance
Lightning Source LLC
LaVergne TN
LVHW082136200926
848484LV00008B/2062